Pocket Guide
to
Low Sodium
Foods

Bobbie Mostyn

Third Edition
Revised

InData Group, Inc.

Pocket Guide to Low-Sodium Foods. Copyright 2003, 2006, 2013 by Bobbie Mostyn. All rights reserved. This book, or parts thereof, may not be reproduced in any form without permission from the publisher, exceptions are made for brief excerpts used in published reviews. Published by InData Group, Inc., P.O. Box 256, Allyn, WA 98524.

Printed in the United States of America

Pocket Guide to Low-Sodium Foods website:

www.LowSaltFoods.com

The Library of Congress has cataloged the earlier edition as follows:

Mostyn, Bobbie
   Pocket guide to low sodium foods / Bobbie Mostyn. -- 2006 ed., completely rev.
      p.cm.
      Includes index.
      LCCN 2002117596
      ISBN 0-9673969-6-4

      1. Food--Sodium content--Tables. I. Title.
TX553.S65M67 2006   613.2'85

CONTENTS

CONTENTS

PART 2 - FAST FOOD AND CASUAL DINING RESTAURANTS

4

INTRODUCTION

First came cholesterol, then fats, and now sodium. The efforts of government and health organizations to raise consumer awareness about the foods we consume are now moving to salt.

It's about time! In the last eight years since the first edition of the *Pocket Guide to Low Sodium Foods* came out, the number of adults with high blood pressure (or hypertension) has increased. According to the Centers for Disease Control one in three adults are now hypertensive with a majority of those 65 and older having the malady.

GOVERNMENT CAMPAIGNS TO REDUCE SALT CONSUMPTION
Here is what has happened and what is on the horizon:

- The USDA 2010 Dietary Guidelines lowered the recommended daily amount of sodium intake from 2,400 milligrams (mg) to 2,300 mg. Additionally, individuals 51 and older, people who have or are at risk for high blood pressure, African Americans, and those with diabetes or chronic kidney disease should have no more than 1,500 mg per day.[1]

  The 1,500 mg recommendation applies to most adults and about half the general population. However, the American Heart Association is recommending all adults limit their daily sodium intake to less than 1,500 mg.

- In 2010 New York Mayor Michael Bloomberg, along with a coalition of cities and health organizations, began the National Salt Reduction Initiative (NSRI) to encourage restaurants and food companies to cut salt levels by 25% over 5 years. This initiative is modeled after a program in the UK, where food manufacturers have reduced salt levels in some products by 40% or more.

  Several other countries, including Canada, Australia, and France, have also launched campaigns to help reduce the sodium in food. As of this writing, 28 food manufacturers and fast food chains, including Campbells, Kraft, Starbucks, and Subway have pledged to lower the salt in many of their products.[2]

- The government is proposing that schools receiving subsidized meals serve healthier items, which includes cutting the amount of sodium in half.

---

[1] U.S. Dept of Agriculture, Center for Nutrition Policy and Promotion, Dietary Guidelines, **www.cnpp.usda.gov/dietaryguidelines.htm**

[2] NY City Dept of Health & Mental Hygiene, **www.nyc.gov/html/doh/html/cardio/cardio-salt-initiative.shtml**

- Food manufacturers have developed a voluntary front-of-package (FOP) nutrition labeling system that will provide calories, saturated fat, sodium, and sugar information on the front of food products. However, as of this writing, there is still some debate from medical and government agencies as to a simple way to identify a product's healthfulness.

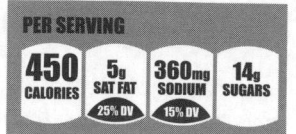

- While some food makers are cutting the salt, many are doing the opposite *(see Author's Note, pg 20)*. But there is good news... there are many more lower salt products on the market today than in previous years and the market will continue to grow, as consumer demand for lower sodium products increases.

USE LESS SALT

As the population ages and the risk for high blood pressure increases, most adults should consume less salt. Sodium, like a sponge, causes the body to hold fluid, forcing the heart to work harder, which raises blood pressure. Less salt means less fluid retention and better control of hypertension.

TIPS TO REDUCE SALT

Eliminate the saltshaker. Don't salt before you taste. Break the habit of automatically reaching for the saltshaker.

Choose lower sodium foods. Eat more fruits and vegetables and use less prepared foods (the less processing, the less sodium). Look for foods labeled *sodium free, low sodium, reduced sodium, unsalted* and *no salt added. (See page 13, for more information.)*

Read the label. Know how much sodium is in each serving. Be alert to "salty" terms, like *brine, cured, marinated, pickled,* and *smoked.* Notice serving sizes. What is listed may be smaller than what you will actually eat.

Use less salt in cooking. In most recipes salt can be reduced or, in many cases, omitted without compromising the flavor. Use more herbs and spices, particularly onion and garlic powder. Also, low-sodium bouillon can add extra flavor, as can wine, vinegar, lemon or lime juice.

Prepare low-salt recipes. Get a good low-sodium cookbook, such as our companion cookbook, *The Hasty Gourmet Low Salt Favorites.* Also, search the Internet where there is an abundance of low-salt recipes.

Order low-sodium foods at restaurants. Ask how foods are prepared and whenever possible request that no salt be added to your entree. Find restaurants that feature *heart-healthy* meals or will accommodate your dietary restrictions. NOTE: Heart-healthy usually indicates a menu item is low fat or low cholesterol and may not always be low sodium. *(See page 17 for more dining out tips.)*

Reducing one's intake of salt is not easy. Nearly everything we eat contains some natural sodium, even small amounts occur naturally in fruits and vegetables, but the vast majority comes off the grocery shelves and from restaurant meals. Surprisingly, less than 15% of the salt we consume comes from the saltshaker.

Thanks in part to our busy lifestyles, we have become accustomed to salty snacks and foods. Because we have less time to plan meals, we rely more on convenience and fast foods, which are loaded with sodium. Unfortunately, the more salt we consume, the more we crave. It's a vicious cycle, but it can be modified.

Although lifestyle changes may be difficult, particularly when it comes to eating, you can retrain your tastebuds to enjoy less salt in about 6-8 weeks. If you start gradually, using a little less salt each day, not only will your use of sodium decrease, but also your craving. In fact, many foods that previously tasted good will now taste salty.

BECOME SODIUM CONSCIOUS

Although experts have been warning us for years to cut back on salt, most consumers are not listening. The problem is most of us are unaware of how much sodium we actually take in. Many people mistakenly think the amount they are consuming is okay, because they do not use salt at the table or in their cooking. Although the saltshaker contributes little to the

---

FOODS HIGH IN SODIUM

Bakery items – bagels, breads, donuts, and muffins

Canned foods – soups, meats, fish, sauerkraut, beans, and vegetables

Convenience foods – frozen dinners, pizza, cereals, and packaged mixes , such as pancakes, food "helpers," stuffing, and rice dishes

Dairy products – cheese and cottage cheese

Deli items – bacon, luncheon meats, corned beef, smoked meats or fish, anchovies, and mayonnaise-based salads, like cole slaw and potato salad

Snack foods – crackers, chips, and dips

Condiments – mustard, ketchup, mayonnaise, salad dressings, pickles, olives, capers, salsas, and packaged seasoning mixes

Sauces – gravy, steak, pasta, teriyaki, soy, and most Asian sauces

Baking needs – self-rising flour, baking and biscuit mixes, bouillon cubes, batter and coating mixes, bread crumbs, cooking wines, meat tenderizers, monosodium glutamate (MSG), baking powder and baking soda

Beverages – tomato and vegetable juices, Bloody Mary and chocolate drink mixes

salt we consume, the majority comes from your pantry. The bottom line, if you don't know how much sodium is in a product, you cannot take control of your diet.

As you become more aware of the amount of sodium in grocery items, you will discover two things: (1) nearly every food has a low-salt alternative and (2) there is a large disparity among brands. For instance, some pasta sauces contain as much as 850 mg sodium per serving, others have around 200 mg, and no-salt-added sauces have less than 50 mg. Another example is teriyaki marinade, averaging 690 mg per tablespoon, and lite varieties averaging 320 mg sodium. As a substitute, try one of the many grilling sauces with less than 140mg. Use the *Pocket Guide to Low-Sodium Foods* to find low-salt substitutes for high-sodium products.

HIDDEN SOURCES OF SODIUM

Did you know that many over-the-counter health aids have hidden sources of sodium? For example, certain dentifrices, aspirin, and medications containing ibuprofen (such as *Advil* and *Nuprin*) have sodium, as do antacids, like *Rolaids* and *Alka-Seltzer* (some have as much as 761 mg). Check labels for low-sodium alternatives or ask your pharmacist or healthcare provider for suggestions.

Also, many households have water-softening systems that contain sodium chloride. To remedy this, there are some alternatives: (1) use potassium chloride (where potassium replaces the salt) in your softener, or (2) install a salt-free water softener (or descaler). Of course, if it is still a concern you can always drink bottled water.

NOTE TO THE HYPERTENSIVE

"High blood pressure is a time bomb in your blood vessels, just waiting to explode in a stroke or heart attack," says Pat Kendall, Ph.D., R.D., a nutrition specialist at Colorado State University Cooperative Extension. "It just keeps ticking away, speeding the artery-clogging process until the blood vessels finally burst."

THE DASH DIET

Scary stuff, but research has determined diet can have a positive effect on blood pressure. The Dietary Approaches to Stop Hypertension (DASH) clinical study, funded by the National Heart, Lung and Blood Institute (NHLBI), shows that the DASH diet not only lowers blood pressure, but also may help prevent and control hypertension.

According to the DASH study, sodium reduction lowers blood pressure regardless of race or sex and has the greatest effect on hypertensive individuals. Subsequent research indicates tho lower the salt intake, the better the results.

The DASH diet, based on 2,000 calories a day, is low in fats and cholesterol. It is also high in fiber and plentiful in fruits, vegetables, and low-fat dairy products. What's more, following the DASH diet may also reduce your risk of cancer, osteoporosis, and diabetes.

Diet is only one part of the prevention and treatment of hypertension. Other factors include exercise, maintaining a healthy weight, and quitting smoking. Before making any major changes in salt consumption or beginning an exercise program, talk with your healthcare provider.

SALT SUBSTITUTES

If you are taking certain diuretics and other prescription drugs, such as ace inhibitors, for the treatment of hypertension, be cautious of salt substitutes. Many contain potassium which may adversely affect your medication. Additionally, many foods that are low in sodium also have added potassium. Check with your healthcare provider before using salt substitutes or consuming potassium-enhanced foods.

OTHER CULPRITS THAT MAY RAISE BLOOD PRESSURE

Caffeine (including coffee, tea, soft drinks, chocolate, and some medications) – may temporarily increase blood pressure[1]

Licorice – consumed in large amounts[2]

Phenylalanine (used in sugar-free foods with aspartame, such as *Nutra-Sweet* and *Equal*) – may elevate blood pressure in sensitive individuals[3]

Alcohol – more than one or two drinks may cause a rise in blood pressure[4]

Cold and cough remedies – decongestants (such as, pseudoephedrine, phenylpropanolamine, dextromethorphan) found in many cough and cold medications may elevate blood pressure[5]

Appetite suppressants – ingredients (like diethylpropion) found in many weight reducing agents may raise blood pressure[6]

Cold weather – low temperatures narrow blood vessels, so more pressure is needed to force blood through your arterial system[7]

---

[1] Mayo Clinic, **mayoclinic.com/health/blood-pressure/AN00792**

[2] U.S. Nat'l Library of Medicine, **nlm.nih.gov/medlineplus/druginfo/natural/881.html**

[3] Southern Medical Journal, **journals.lww.com/smajournalonline/Fulltext/2008/09000/Resistant_Hypertension__Identifying_Causes_and.34.aspx**

[4] Mayo Clinic, **mayoclinic.com/health/blood-pressure/AN00318**

[5] American Heart Assn, **www.heart.org**, search for "decongestants and HBP"

[6] Nat'l Institute of Diabetes & Digestive & Kidney Diseases (NIDDK) , **win.niddk.nih.gov/publications/prescription.htm**

[7] Mayo Clinic, **www.mayoclinic.com/health/blood-pressure/AN01786**

FOOD LABELING GUIDELINES

The Food and Drug Administration (FDA) regulates food labeling to assure consumers that the information they receive is accurate and not misleading. Labels contain a lot of useful information to help you compare products and make healthy food choices.

WHAT THE LABEL TELLS YOU

Serving Size – Identified in familiar units (such as cups or tablespoons) followed by the metric equivalent (i.e. grams) and is determined by the amount typically eaten.

Amount per Serving – Nutritional information is based on one serving. In the example below, the serving size is 1 cup. If you eat 2 cups you need to double the calories, nutrients, and *% Daily Value*.

Calories from Fat – This is the amount of fat multiplied by 9 (number of calories per gram of fat). Dietary guidelines suggest no more than 30% of daily calories come from fat. To calculate percentage, divide *Calories from Fat* by *Calories* (in this example, $10 \div 170 = 6\%$).

Nutrition Facts

Serving Size 1 cup (55g)
Servings Per Container about 8

Amount Per Serving

Calories 170   Calories from Fat 10

	% Daily Value*
Total Fat 1 g	**2** %
Saturated Fat 0g	**0** %
Trans Fat 0g	
Cholesterol 0mg	**0** %
Sodium 85mg	**4** %
Total Carbohydrate 41g	**14** %
Dietary Fiber 7g	**28** %
Sugars 21g	
Protein 6g	

Vitamin A 0%	▪	Vitamin C 0%
Calcium 0%	▪	Iron 6%

*Percent Daily Values are based on a 2,000 calorie diet. Your daily values may be higher or lower depending on your calorie needs.

	Calories	2,000	2,500
Total Fat	Less than	65g	80g
Sat Fat	Less than	20g	25g
Cholesterol	Less than	300mg	300mg
Sodium	Less than	2,400mg	2,400mg
Total Carbohydrate		300m	375mg
Dietary Fiber		25g	30g

Nutrients – Values are listed in grams except for *Cholesterol* and *Sodium* which are in milligrams. Use these figures to compare fat, sodium, etc. between products. If a nutrient is not shown, there is no significant amount in the product.

% Daily Value – This shows how much of the *Recommended Daily Values* (RDVs) each nutrient provides and is another way to compare similar products. Calculations are based on 2,000 calories. In this example, the amount of sodium per serving (85mg) is divided by the total RDV for sodium (2,400mg), which means this serving equals 4% of your RDV for sodium.

Ingredients – Listed in order from most to least amount. Generally, if sodium is one of the first 3 ingredients, there is probably too much in this product for a low-salt diet.

NUTRITIONAL CONTENT CLAIMS

Label content claims describe the level of a nutrient or dietary substance in the product, using terms, such as *free*, *high*, and *low*. They can also compare the nutrient amount in a particular food to that of another food using terms, such as *more*, *reduced*, and *lite*. The following claims are used on nutritional labels and are based on one serving.

	FREE	LOW	REDUCED/ LESS	LIGHT/ LITE
Cal	< 5 calories	40 calories or less	25% less than normal	50% less than normal
Fat	< 0.5g fat	3g or less fat	25% less than normal	50% less than normal
Sat Fat	< 0.5g sat fat and < 0.5g trans fatty acids	1g or less saturated fat	25% less than normal	50% less than normal
Chol	< 2mg chol and 2g or less sat fat	< 20mg chol and 2g or less sat fat	25% less than normal	50% less than normal
Sug	< 0.5g sugar		25% less than normal	50% less than normal

	FREE	VERY LOW	LOW	UNSALTED/NSA
Sod	< 5mg /100g (approx 3.6 oz)	< 35mg /100g (approx 3.6 oz)	<140mg /100g (approx 3.6 oz)	No salt added to normally salted food

NOTE: *Low-fat* and *non-fat* do not mean low sodium or low sugar; manufacturers often replace the fat with added salt and sugar.

CALORIES AND NUTRIENTS

CALORIES

Calories measure the amount of energy contained in foods and are calculated based on the amount of carbohydrates, fat, and protein within the food. (Alcohol also provides calories.)

Once consumed and digested, food is converted to glucose which fuels everything the body does, like walking, talking, and breathing. The amount of calories needed is different for every individual. For example, the more active an individual, the greater the caloric need. However, when the body takes in more calories than it requires, the extra energy is stored as body fat.

CHOLESTEROL AND FATS

Cholesterol and fats are essential to the human body, however, too much of either can be detrimental to your health.

CHOLESTEROL

Cholesterol is a waxy, fat-like substance produced naturally in the body and is necessary for many bodily functions. The body manufactures all the cholesterol it needs and circulates it via the bloodstream, which separates it into "good" and "bad" lipoproteins.

The bad, or low-density lipoproteins (LDL), stick to the blood vessel walls contributing to clogged arteries and hypertension, and is the leading cause for heart disease. The good, or high-density lipoproteins (HDL), unstick LDLs and help move them through the bloodstream and out of the body. This is why the ratio of HDL to LDL is important.

Over time the LDL deposits (along with fat) build up, causing the arteries to clog. As the arteries narrow, the flow of blood decreases and blood pressure increases. This build-up of fatty deposits is also a major factor in coronary disease and strokes.

Research indicates that saturated fats and trans-fatty acids have a greater impact in raising cholesterol than from eating dietary cholesterol. It should be noted, that most foods high in cholesterol are also high in saturated fats, and vice versa.

Cholesterol is found mainly in animal foods (meat, poultry, fish, egg yolks, and dairy products), it is not found in plant foods. The daily recommendation for cholesterol is less than 300mg.

FAT

Not all fats are harmful and have been classified as either good or bad. Saturated fat is considered bad, as too much of it raises LDL cholesterol levels. Monounsaturated and polyunsaturated fats help lower cholesterol and are considered good.

TYPES OF FAT

Saturated – Usually solid at room temperature (comes mainly from animal products, such as butter, cheese, meat products, egg yolks, and whole milk dairy products).

Monounsaturated – Liquid at room temperature, but solidifies in the refrigerator (found in plant foods, such as olive oil, canola oil, avocados, and nuts).

Polyunsaturated – Liquid at room temperature and also in the refrigerator (examples are vegetable oils, including corn oil, safflower oil, and sunflower oil).

Trans fatty acids – Result of hydrogenation and used for shelf stability or solidifying a fat product (found in margarine, crackers, cookies, potato chips, and fast foods, such as french fries).

Trans fatty acids, considered saturated and classified as bad, not only raise LDLs, but also decrease HDLs. Many experts believe trans fats are as bad as, if not worse than, saturated fats.

If a product lists *hydrogenated* or *partially hydrogenated* in the ingredients, it has trans-fatty acids. Be aware that many low-fat, low-cholesterol products may have trans fats.

The American Heart Association (AHA) suggests no more than 30% of total calories come from fat and no more than 10% from saturated fat (7% if you have heart disease, diabetes, or high LDL cholesterol). As a general rule, any food that has 5% or less fat is considered low in fat; 20% or more, is high. Choose fats with 2g or less saturated fat per serving.

CARBOHYDRATES, FIBER AND SUGAR

Carbohydrates are the body's supplier of energy. Once consumed carbohydrates convert into two basic forms: simple carbohydrates (found in sugars) and complex carbohydrates (comprised of starches and fibers). Except for fiber, which is not digestible, all carbohydrates turn directly into sugar (glucose) in the bloodstream and affect blood glucose in different ways.

> ### CARBOHYDRATES
>
> **Simple carbohydrates** – Generally have no nutritive value and produce a rapid rise in blood glucose followed by a rapid fall.
> **Complex carbohydrates** – More nutritious and produce a slower, more sustained blood glucose response.

Foods high in complex carbohydrates are usually low in calories, saturated fat, and cholesterol. They are found primarily in plant foods, such as fruits, vegetables, whole grains, beans, and legumes. They also are present in dairy products.

Daily caloric intake of carbohydrates should be between 55-60% (or 25-35 grams) with an emphasis on complex carbohydrates.

FIBER

Fiber is the part of food that is not digested. The amount of fiber also affects blood glucose. The more fiber in a food, the slower the digestion and absorption of sugars. To help understand fiber's influence on blood glucose, the glycemic index (GI) was developed. Using glucose (the highest rated GI) as a standard, a food is ranked by how fast it is digested and how much it causes blood glucose to rise. We will not get into GI rankings in this book, but suffice to say, this new information is changing the way nutritionists and the medical society are looking at carbohydrates. There are two types of fiber – soluble and insoluble.

Soluble fiber – Dissolves in fluids of the large intestine. Soluble fiber is found in oats, barley, rye, nuts, fruits, vegetables, psyllium seeds (used in fiber laxatives), beans, and legumes. Consumed in large amounts, soluble fiber can decrease blood cholesterol, improve blood glucose levels, and appears to reduce hypertension. It also may help with weight loss by increasing the feeling of fullness.

Insoluble fiber – Instead of dissolving, it passes straight through the intestines and helps maintain regularity. It is found in whole grains, seeds, bran, fruit, and vegetable skins. It also is associated with reduced risk of colon cancer.

The recommended level of total soluble and insoluble fiber is 20-35 grams per day. Look for a minimum of 3 grams of fiber, but 5 grams or more is better.

SUGAR

Sugar consumption has been on the increase and experts believe diets high in sugar are contributing to many of today's health problems, including hypertension and heart disease.

Current research indicates long-term consumption of a diet high in refined (simple) carbohydrates produces higher insulin levels. As insulin levels elevate, adrenaline production is stimulated, which can cause blood vessel constriction and increased sodium retention. Additionally, high carbohydrate intake has been linked to increased LDL and decreased HDL cholesterol.

Even though the RDVs have no sugar guidelines, the US Department of Agriculture (USDA) advises limiting sugar to 10 teaspoons (47g) a day (based on a 2,000-calorie diet).

SODIUM

Sodium is essential to the body. About 500mg a day is needed to help regulate fluids and maintain normal functioning of nerves and muscles. If excess sodium is not used, fluid builds up (water retention) increasing the work of the heart and kidneys.

Select foods that contain less than 5 percent of the daily value for sodium (or about 100mg per serving). Experts suggest limiting any foods that have more than 480mg sodium per serving.

DINING OUT

The most difficult time to control salt consumption is when dining out. Making good nutritional choices can be difficult, especially when we do not know what has been added to the foods we order. For example, a healthy garden salad with lowfat dressing oftentimes has more sodium than a hamburger and french fries. Hard to believe, but depending on how it is prepared, what we think is healthy may not be low sodium.

Another fast food misconception is chicken or fish sandwiches being a better choice than beef. There may be less fat, but not salt. In most instances added seasonings, coatings, deep frying, and other preparations create a much higher sodium meal.

Follow the suggestions below in selecting healthier, low-sodium menu items.

WATCH THE SALT

Order low-sodium foods. Ask how foods are prepared; choose steamed, broiled, grilled, or roasted entrees without sauces.

Avoid fried foods. Most batters are salted, plus additional saturated or trans-fats are in the frying liquid.

Stay away from soups and creamed sauces. Most have way too much sodium to be included in a low-salt diet.

Go easy on the bread. One small piece may have several hundred milligrams of sodium, and that's before you add the margarine or butter.

Use oil and vinegar on salads. Watch out for the salad bar, many items are mayonnaise-based or pickled, which have too much salt.

Order the smallest portion. For larger portions, eat half or save the rest for the next day.

Request condiments and sauces served on the side. Then you control the amount you use.

Ask that salt not be added to your meal. Most restaurants can accommodate you, however, fast food eateries often premake many items and may not be able to handle special requests.

PLAN AHEAD

If you know you will be dining out, eat a low-salt breakfast and lunch. If you have too much salt at one meal, keep your sodium intake low for the next couple of meals. You can also place low-sodium condiments, like ketchup, mustard, mayonnaise and salad dressing, in small plastic containers and take them with you. The important thing is you do not have to deprive yourself. Just use moderation. Remember, low salt does not mean no salt.

USING THIS GUIDE

With our increasingly busy lifestyles, making healthy, low-sodium food choices at the supermarket and when dining out is challenging. Most of us do not have time to compare the labels of thousands of grocery items. We also have no idea of what's in the restaurant foods we are consuming.

This is where the *Pocket Guide to Low Sodium Foods* can help. It includes common products found in most grocery stores and menu items from more than 160 national restaurant chains. It's small enough to put in a purse or coat pocket and can be used as a quick reference when grocery shopping or eating out.

Only low-salt foods within acceptable low-sodium diet guidelines are listed. Calories, fat, saturated fat, cholesterol, carbohydrates, fiber, sugar, and sodium are shown for each food product. These are the most important nutrients to consider for healthy eating.

The book is broken down into two parts: *Grocery Products* and *Fast Food and Casual Dining Restaurants*.

GROCERY PRODUCTS
All foods are listed alphabetically within the following 15 categories and approximates the aisles of your supermarket.

Baking and Cooking Needs
Beverages
Bread and Flour Products
Breakfast Foods
Condiments and Sauces
Dairy and Non-Dairy Alternatives
Desserts and Sweets
Dinners, Light Meals and Entrees
Ethnic Foods
Fish and Seafood
Fruits and Vegetables
Meat, Poultry and Meatless Alternatives
Noodles, Pasta, Rice and Grains
Snack Foods
Soups and Chili

Generic nutrient analysis is shown for each food type and represents the average or typical values for that particular food. This is followed by brand named products listed in alphabetical order. Only low-salt foods are listed, generally items with 140mg sodium or less. Some products exceeding these guidelines may be shown if there are few low-sodium brands, such as, frozen dinners, pizza, soups, etc. In these cases, you'll see a subheading, *Reduced sodium (less than generic)*. This indicates the product exceeds 140mg, but has substantially less sodium than the generic average.

FAST FOOD AND CASUAL DINING RESTAURANTS

This section includes national fast food and casual dining restaurant chains listed in alphabetical order. Although fast foods are loaded with fat and sodium and are not necessarily the best choices for healthy, low-sodium diets, they are a fact of life. Use the *Pocket Guide to Low-Sodium Foods* to help you make the wisest selections.

Restaurant menu selections are broken down into categories, such as *Sandwiches, Salads, Side Dishes*, and *Desserts*. Also shown is the amount of sodium, ranging from the least to the highest amount, of all items in each category, for example: Burgers / Sandwiches... 780–2,160. Menu items with the least sodium are listed below each heading with the amount of sodium in brackets. If all choices within a category exceed sodium guidelines, the menu item with the least amount of salt may be listed as a reference.

Because restaurants are continually changing their menus, it is recommended that you view their menus online. Most restaurant chains have nutritional data available, so you can make your selections before venturing out.

DISCLAIMER

All information contained in the *Pocket Guide to Low-Sodium Foods* is based on nutritional data provided by the US Department of Agriculture, food manufacturers, restaurant chains, and author calculations.

Data is for informational purposes only and is subject to change. No endorsement is intended of companies and their products, nor is any adverse judgment implied for companies and products not mentioned.

Availability of products, menu items and variations in serving sizes or product ingredients may occur dependent upon geographical region, local suppliers, season of the year and production changes. Read manufacturer's product labels or contact individual restaurants for the most up-to-date analysis of food items. Data was collected during 2011-2012.

Consequently, read labels and continue to re-read them. You may be surprised to discover a favorite low-sodium food suddenly having more salt listed than the last time you used it.

AUTHOR'S NOTE

Although several organizations, including the American Public Health Association, are urging the food industry to reduce sodium, food manufacturers have been opposed to these changes. They contend that low-sodium products often do not fare well in the marketplace. Taste is the main reason people buy a particular product and when salt is removed, consumers react negatively to the loss of flavor.

Unfortunately, food manufacturers cannot be forced to produce low-salt items. It is much easier for them to stop manufacturing a product than it is to create a new item, particularly one that probably will not be embraced by consumers.

In the process of gathering data for this third edition of the *Pocket Guide to Low Sodium Foods*, it became evident that many food makers and quick-serve restaurants are not lowering the sodium in their products, instead they are adding more sodium! Has our appetite for salt continued to increase? Or are some food makers raising the amount of sodium in anticipation of more pressure to lower the salt?

While the number of low-sodium foods has increased in recent years, many smaller manufacturers that previously produced low-salt products are either out-of-business or no longer producing them. A sad state for those of us who are concerned about the salt in our diets. It's crucial that we continue to support products that are lower in sodium; food makers need to hear a loud and clear message... more low-salt foods!

ABBREVIATIONS AND SYMBOLS

all	all varieties/flavors	NSA	no salt added
approx	approximately	orig	original
avg	average	oz	ounce
cal	calories	pc	piece(s)
carb	carbohydrate	pkg	package
choc	chocolate	pkt	packet
chol	cholesterol	prep	prepared to product
cinn	cinnamon		directions
envl	envelop	refrg	refrigerated
FF	fat free	reg	regular
fl oz	fluid ounce	sat	saturated fat
g	gram	serv	serving
lb	pound	sl	slice
LF	low fat	sm	small
lrg	large	sod	sodium
mayo	mayonnaise	sq	square
med	medium-sized	tbsp	tablespoon
mg	milligram(s)	tsp	teaspoon
misc	miscellaneous	veg	vegetable
most	most varieties	w/	with
NF	nonfat	w/o	without

FOOD MEASUREMENTS AND EQUIVALENTS

1 1/2 tsp	=	1/2 tbsp	=	0.25 oz	=	7 grams
3 tsp	=	1 tbsp	=	0.5 oz	=	14 grams
2 tbsp	=	1/8 cup	=	1 oz	=	28 grams
4 tbsp	=	1/4 cup	=	2 oz	=	55 grams
8 tbsp	=	1/2 cup	=	4 oz	=	115 grams
16 tbsp	=	1 cup	=	8 oz	=	225 grams

LIQUID

1/2 fl oz	=	tbsp		2 cups	=	1 pint
1 fl oz	=	1/8 cup		2 pints	=	1 quart
2 fl oz	=	1/4 cup		4 quarts	=	1 gallon
4 fl oz	=	1/2 cup				
8 fl oz	=	1 cup				
16 fl oz	=	1 pint				

READING THE NUTRITIVE VALUES

GROCERY ITEMS

Food	Cal	Fat	Sat	Chol	Carb	Fib	Sug	Sod
FROSTING								
Vanilla, ready-to-spread, 2 tbsp	140	5	2	0	23	0	20	70
Cream cheese, ready-to-spread, 2 tbsp....	140	5	2	0	23	0	20	80
Chocolate, ready-to-spread, 2 tbsp..........	130	5	2	0	21	0	18	90

1 applies to the three rows above.

Brands . . . *(1/4 cup unless noted)*

READY-TO-SPREAD

Vanilla frosting – *Most brands within generic average (70mg).*

ABC Food Manufacturer

Food	Cal	Fat	Sat	Chol	Carb	Fib	Sug	Sod
Vanilla or Choc, 2 tbsp......................	93	3	1	0	8	0	1	27
Cream Cheese, 2 tbsp	140	5	2	20	18	0	6	80
Very Tasty Foods, all, prep, 2 tbsp	67	1	0	0	13	0	–	0

2 applies to the three rows above.

1 Generic foods are listed first. Generic values are an average of all brands of this food type.

2 Brand name products follow and are listed alphabetically. Items within each brand are listed from least to most sodium.

All nutrient values are rounded off to the nearest whole number. If the nutrient value on a food label is:

<5	(less than 5mg or 5g), the Pocket Guide uses:	5
<1	(less than 1mg or 1g), the Pocket Guide uses:	1
tr	(trace amount present*), the Pocket Guide uses:	0

*If the nutrient value is not listed, there is no significant amount present; the Pocket Guide uses 0. If no nutritional information is available, the Pocket Guide uses –.

All nutrient values listed are based on FDA food label guidelines:

Fat, saturated fat, carbohydrates, fiber and sugar are in grams. Cholesterol and sodium are in milligrams.

QUICK-SERVE AND CASUAL DINING

1 **BURGERS/SANDWICHES** **440–2,200**

HAMBURGERS: Original w/o mayo [440] • Original [510]

2 Turkey & Swiss on Wheat [576] • Grilled Chicken Sandwich [805]

HOT DRINKS **70–370**

Cappuccino, 12 oz/18 oz/20 oz [70–135]

1 The first line shows the food category and the sodium range for all menu items in that category. For example, in Burgers/Sandwiches, the burger or sandwich with the least sodium has 440mg, the item with the most has 2,200mg.

2 Items in that category with the least sodium are listed with the amount of sodium in brackets , i.e. [440]. Individual items are separated by •.

All sodium amounts shown are in milligrams (mg).

PART 1

GROCERY PRODUCTS

BAKING AND COOKING NEEDS

See RESOURCES, page 305, for a partial list of manufacturers and retailers
offering low-salt products online or visit **LowSaltFoods.com** for additional
sources.

BAKING AND COOKING NEEDS

BAKING CHOCOLATE AND MORSELS

	Cal	Fat	Sat	Chol	Carb	Fib	Sug	Sod
Baking chocolate:								
Semi-sweet, 1 oz	140	9	5	0	16	2	12	0
Sweet, 1 oz	120	8	5	0	16	2	14	0
Unsweetened, 1 oz	140	14	9	0	8	4	0	0
White, 1 oz	160	9	5	0	18	0	18	20
Morsels:								
Choc, semi-sweet, 1 oz	140	8	5	0	18	2	16	0
Carob, grain sweetened, 1 oz	70	4	3	0	10	1	5	0
Butterscotch, 1 oz	160	8	7	0	18	0	16	30
White, 1 oz	160	8	7	0	18	0	18	40
Peanut butter, 1 oz	160	8	8	0	14	0	12	70
Cocoa powder, unsweetened, 2 tbsp	25	1	1	0	6	4	0	2

Brands . . . *Most brands within generic average.*

BAKING MIX – ALL-PURPOSE

(also see Biscuits/Popovers, pg 47; Bread Mixes, pg 51; Muffins/Scones, pg 56; Brownies/Dessert Bars, pg 113; Cake, pg 114; Cheesecake, pg 118; Cookies, pg 119; Dessert Mixes, pg 122)

	Cal	Fat	Sat	Chol	Carb	Fib	Sug	Sod
All-purpose baking mix, 1/3 cup	160	6	2	0	35	0	1	490

Brands . . . *(1/3 cup mix unless noted)*

	Cal	Fat	Sat	Chol	Carb	Fib	Sug	Sod
Atkins Cuisine All Purpose Baking Mix	150	5	1	0	11	6	1	25
Bob's Red Mill Low Carb Baking Mix	100	2	0	0	11	5	0	115
Carbquik Biscuit & Baking Mix	50	4	0	0	9	7	0	110
Chébé All-Purpose Mix	70	0	0	0	17	0	0	103
Dixie's Gluten Free Bakesquick	49	0	0	0	12	2	0	122
Ener-G								
Rice Mix, 1/4 cup	130	0	0	0	28	1	0	85
Potato Mix, 1/4 cup	160	0	0	0	40	1	0	130
Gluten-Free Essentials All Purpose Mix	111	1	0	0	25	1	0	0
Hodgson Mill Multi-Purpose Mix	100	1	0	0	22	3	0	0

BAKING POWDER AND BAKING SODA

(see Leavening Agents, pg 27)

BREAD CRUMBS AND COATING MIXES

(also see Rubs/BBQ Seasonings, pg 32)

	Cal	Fat	Sat	Chol	Carb	Fib	Sug	Sod
Matzo meal, 1/4 cup	110	0	0	0	24	1	0	0
Cracker meal, 1/4 cup	100	0	0	0	21	1	0	10
Panko breading, unseasoned, 1/4 cup	50	0	0	0	9	0	1	45
Seasoned panko breading, 1/4 cup	120	4	1	0	19	1	1	300
Graham cracker crumbs, 1/4 cup	107	5	1	0	31	1	9	140
Corn flake crumbs, 1/4 cup	80	0	0	0	18	0	2	160
Bread crumbs, plain, 1/4 cup	120	2	0	0	21	2	2	270
Seasoned, 1/4 cup	120	2	0	0	21	2	2	450
Coating and Batter Mixes:								
Tempura batter mix, 1/4 cup	100	0	0	0	23	0	0	175
Seasoned coating mix, 2 tsp	60	1	0	0	10	1	0	390
Batter mix, 1/4 cup	100	0	0	0	22	1	0	690

Brands . . . *(1/4 cup unless noted)*

BAKING AND COOKING NEEDS
Coconut

	Cal	Fat	Sat	Chol	Carb	Fib	Sug	Sod
BREAD CRUMBS								
4C Seasoned Bread Crumbs, SF	110	1	0	0	23	2	2	5
Edward & Sons Lightly Salted, 1/3 cup	110	1	0	0	21	1	2	110
Ener-G Bread Crumbs	100	5	0	0	13	2	0	100
Gonnella French Style Bread Crumbs	60	0	0	0	13	0	0	135
Kikkoman Panko Bread Crumbs	55	0	0	0	12	1	1	20
Nu-World Foods Amaranth Bread Crumbs	122	2	0	0	22	3	0	2
Pereg Seasoned, all varieties, 3 tbsp	98	1	0	0	21	1	2	60
Schar Gluten-Free Bread Crumbs, 3 tbsp	120	4	2	10	19	2	1	120
Shabtai Gluten Free Bread Crumbs, 1 oz	120	5	0	30	15	0	0	30
OTHER CRUMBS AND BREADING								
Cracker meal – *Most brands within generic average (10mg).*								
Matzo meal – *Most brands within generic average (0mg).*								
Hol-Grain Brown Rice Crumbs, SF	40	0	0	0	9	0	0	0
OrgraN All-Purpose Rice Crumbs, 0.9 oz	84	0	0	0	20	0	0	3
Corn Crispy Crumbs, 0.9 oz	89	0	0	0	19	1	0	9
Southern Homestyle								
Tortilla Crumbs, 2 tbsp	40	0	0	0	9	0	1	50
Corn Flake Crumbs, 2 tbsp	40	0	0	0	9	0	1	50
COATING AND BATTER MIXES								
Andy's LS Fish Breading, 1 tbsp	40	0	0	0	7	0	0	75
Fry Krisp SF Seasoned Batter Mix	100	1	0	0	22	1	1	10
Coating Mix	110	1	0	0	23	1	0	10
Hime Tempura Batter Mix	100	0	0	0	23	1	0	45
Hooters Wing Breading, 1.5 tbsp	80	0	0	0	18	1	1	130
Louisiana Fish Fry								
Fish Fry, 2 tsp	20	0	0	0	5	0	0	5
Seasoned Fish Fry, 3 tsp	20	0	0	0	5	0	0	135
Tony Chachere's Fish Fry Creole	120	0	0	0	26	1	2	35
Zatarain's Wonderful Fish Fry, 1 tbsp	45	0	0	0	10	0	0	0
REDUCED SODIUM (LESS THAN GENERIC):								
McCormick *Golden Dipt* Tempura Batter	100	0	0	0	21	0	0	150
Shake 'N Bake Hot & Spicy, 1/8 pkt	40	1	0	0	7	0	0	170

CAKE FROSTING, ICING AND DECORATIONS

(see Cake Frosting/Icing/Decorations, pg 117)

COCONUT

	Cal	Fat	Sat	Chol	Carb	Fib	Sug	Sod
Raw coconut meat, 1 oz	99	9	8	0	4	3	2	2
Coconut, shredded, unsweetened, 2 tbsp	80	7	6	0	3	1	1	3
Flaked, sweetened, 2 tbsp	70	5	5	0	6	1	5	40
Coconut milk, 1/4 cup	138	14	13	0	3	1	2	9

Brands . . . *Most brands within generic average.*

CORNMEAL

(see Flour/Cornmeal, pg 27)

CORNSTARCH

	Cal	Fat	Sat	Chol	Carb	Fib	Sug	Sod
Cornstarch, 1 tbsp	29	0	0	0	7	0	0	0

Brands . . . *Most brands within generic average.*

EGGS – DRIED/POWDERED

	Cal	Fat	Sat	Chol	Carb	Fib	Sug	Sod
Egg whites, powdered, 1 tbsp	26	0	0	0	0	0	0	87

	Cal	Fat	Sat	Chol	Carb	Fib	Sug	Sod
Brands . . . *(1 tbsp unless noted)*								
Bob's Red Mill Egg Replacer	30	1	0	0	2	1	1	20
Deb El								
Just Whites, 2 tsp	12	0	0	0	0	0	0	51
Whole Eggs, 2 tsp	80	6	2	245	1	0	1	75
Ener-G Egg Replacer, 1 1/2 tsp	15	0	0	0	4	0	0	5
OrgraN No Egg, 1 tsp	9	0	0	0	2	0	0	0

FATS, OILS AND COOKING SPRAYS

	Cal	Fat	Sat	Chol	Carb	Fib	Sug	Sod
Cooking spray, 1 spray	0	0	0	0	0	0	0	0
Lard or shortening, 1 tbsp	110	12	3	0	0	0	0	0
Oil, all varieties, 1 tbsp (avg)	120	14	2	0	0	0	0	0

Brands . . . *Most brands within generic average.*

FLAVORINGS AND EXTRACTS

	Cal	Fat	Sat	Chol	Carb	Fib	Sug	Sod
Flavorings and extracts, 1 tsp (avg)	10	0	0	0	0	0	0	0

Brands . . . *Most brands within generic average.*

FLOUR AND CORNMEAL

	Cal	Fat	Sat	Chol	Carb	Fib	Sug	Sod
Flours:								
All-purpose flour, 1/4 cup	100	1	0	0	22	3	1	0
Self-rising, 1/4 cup	100	0	0	0	22	1	0	360
Whole wheat flour, 1/4 cup	110	1	0	0	23	4	1	0
Rye flour, light, 1/4 cup	100	1	0	0	21	1	1	0
Dark, 1/4 cup	110	1	0	0	21	7	1	0
Soy flour, 1/4 cup	120	6	1	0	8	3	2	0
Rice flour, white, 1/4 cup	150	1	0	0	32	1	0	0
Brown, 1/4 cup	140	1	0	0	31	2	0	5
Potato flour, 1/4 cup	160	1	0	0	36	3	0	13
Meals:								
Cake meal, 1/4 cup	140	0	0	0	31	1	0	0
Matzo meal, 1/4 cup	110	0	0	0	24	1	0	0
Cornmeal, blue, 1/4 cup	98	1	0	0	19	3	0	0
White or yellow, 1/4 cup	110	0	0	0	23	5	0	10
Self-rising, white or yellow, 1/4 cup	102	1	0	0	21	2	0	380

Brands . . . *Most brands within generic average.*

FROSTING, ICING AND DECORATIONS

(see Cake Frosting, Icing/Decorations, pg 117)

LEAVENING AGENTS

	Cal	Fat	Sat	Chol	Carb	Fib	Sug	Sod
Yeast, 1 tbsp	35	1	0	0	5	3	0	6
Baking powder, 1 tsp	0	0	0	0	1	0	0	480
Baking soda, 1 tsp	0	0	0	0	0	0	0	1231
Brands . . . *(1 tsp unless noted)*								
Ener-G SF Baking Powder or SF Baking Soda	0	0	0	0	0	0	0	0
Hain Featherweight Baking Powder, SF	0	0	0	0	0	0	0	0

MARSHMALLOWS

	Cal	Fat	Sat	Chol	Carb	Fib	Sug	Sod
Marshmallow creme, 2 tbsp	40	0	0	0	10	0	6	10
Marshmallows, 1 oz (2/3 c miniatures or 4 lrg)	89	0	0	0	23	0	16	22

Brands . . . *Most brands within generic average.*

BAKING AND COOKING NEEDS
Milk and Milk Substitutes–Canned/Powdered

	Cal	Fat	Sat	Chol	Carb	Fib	Sug	Sod
MILK AND MILK SUBSTITUTES – CANNED/POWDERED								
Coconut milk, canned, 1/2 cup	223	24	21	0	3	0	3	30
Goat milk, powdered, 1/2 cup prep.................	70	4	2	13	6	0	6	58
NF, powdered, 1/2 cup prep	40	0	0	3	6	0	6	65
Canned liquid, 1/2 cup............................	140	8	6	20	12	0	12	120
Buttermilk, powdered,1/2 cup prep.................	47	1	0	9	6	0	6	64
Evaporated milk, canned, 1/2 cup..................	169	10	6	37	13	0	13	134
Skim, canned, 1/2 cup.............................	100	0	0	5	15	0	15	147
Condensed milk, sweetened, canned, 1/2 cup ..	491	13	8	52	83	0	83	194

Brands . . . *(1/2 cup unless noted)*
Evaporated milk – *Most brands within generic average (134-147mg).*
Goat milk, powdered – *Most brands within generic average (58-65mg).*
Goat milk, canned liquid – *Most brands within generic average (120mg).*

	Cal	Fat	Sat	Chol	Carb	Fib	Sug	Sod
Bernard Ber-No-Lac, powdered, 1 cup prep	110	5	3	0	15	0	7	20
Meyenberg Condensed Milk........................	70	4	2	13	6	0	6	58
REDUCED SODIUM (LESS THAN GENERIC):								
Santini Sweetened Condensed	520	12	8	40	92	0	92	160

MOLASSES

(see Sweeteners, pg 32)

NUTS – BAKING

(see Nut/Seeds, pg 224)

PASTRY DOUGH

(see Pie Crusts/Shells, pg 30; Bread/Pastry Dough/Mixes, pg 51)

PASTRY AND PIE FILLINGS

(also see Pudding/Mousse, pg 131)

	Cal	Fat	Sat	Chol	Carb	Fib	Sug	Sod
Pastry Filling:								
Almond paste, 1 oz	180	11	1	0	19	1	17	0
Marzipan, 1 oz..	170	4	0	0	29	0	24	0
Fruit, most varieties, 1 oz...........................	70	0	0	0	18	0	12	10
Poppyseed, 1 oz......................................	120	4	0	0	20	1	15	20
Nut filling, 1 oz.......................................	120	5	1	0	19	1	14	35
Pie Filling (canned):								
Blueberry pie filling, 1/3 cup	156	0	0	0	38	2	33	10
Cherry pie filling, 1/3 cup...........................	89	0	0	0	22	1	18	14
Peach pie filling, 1/3 cup	80	0	0	0	19	1	17	20
Apple pie filling, 1/3 cup	77	0	0	0	20	1	11	36
Pumpkin pie mix, 1/3 cup...........................	90	1	0	0	20	3	17	120
Lemon cream pie filling, 1/3 cup	100	0	0	0	25	0	17	160
Mincemeat pie filling, 1/3 cup	200	2	0	0	48	1	35	270
Cheesecake filling, 1/3 cup........................	260	22	13	85	13	0	12	330
Pudding and Pie Filling (mix):								
Chocolate, regular, 1/4 pkg..........................	90	1	0	0	22	1	11	87
Instant, 1/4 pkg...................................	94	0	0	0	22	1	17	354
Lemon, regular, 1/4 pkg.............................	77	0	0	0	20	0	18	108
Instant, 1/4 pkg	94	0	0	0	24	0	22	330
Coconut cream, regular, 1/4 pkg	95	3	3	0	18	0	14	150
Instant, 1/4 pkg...................................	96	1	0	0	23	1	16	257
Banana cream, regular, 1/4 pkg	80	0	0	0	20	0	15	150
Instant, 1/4 pkg....................................	90	0	0	0	23	0	18	360

Cal Fat Sat Chol Carb Fib Sug Sod

Brands . . . *(1 serving unless noted)*
PASTRY FILLING – *Most brands within generic average (0-35mg).*
PIE FILLING

MIXES

	Cal	Fat	Sat	Chol	Carb	Fib	Sug	Sod
America's Choice Cook & Serve								
Pudding & Pie Filling, Choc	100	1	0	0	25	0	18	130
Calorie Control Cheesecake mixes, all	60	2	1	5	7	0	4	80
Concord Foods Banana Pudding & Pie	100	2	2	0	21	0	14	60
Dr. Oetker Lemon or Key Lime Pie & Dessert	100	0	0	0	26	0	18	80
Organics Pudding & Pie Filling:								
Mocha or Banana	90	0	0	0	23	0	17	100
Coconut, Butterscotch, or Vanilla (avg)	100	2	2	0	24	0	18	100
Chocolate	120	0	0	0	30	0	23	100
Durkee Lemon Pie Filling	50	0	0	0	11	0	7	70
Hannaford Choc Cook/Serve Pudding/Pie Filling	100	1	0	0	23	0	17	120
Vanilla Cook & Serve Pudding & Pie Filling	80	0	0	0	21	0	16	130
Hy-Vee Cooked Pudding & Pie, Choc or Vanilla	100	0	0	0	23	0	17	130
Jell-O Cook & Serve Pudding								
Lemon	50	0	0	0	12	0	6	70
Chocolate	90	0	0	0	22	1	15	110
Choc Sugar Free	30	0	0	0	7	1	0	110
Vanilla Sugar Free	20	0	0	0	5	0	0	115
Butterscotch	100	0	0	0	24	0	19	130
Vanilla	80	0	0	0	20	0	16	135
Lem Pie Filling & Pudding	40	0	0	0	10	0	4	25
Meijer Cook/Serve Pudding/Pie, Choc or Vanilla	100	0	0	0	23	0	17	130
*My*T*Fine* Pudding & Pie, Sugar Free Choc	50	0	0	0	12	1	0	85
Pudding & Pie Filling, Lemon	50	0	0	0	12	0	5	120
Pudding & Pie Filling, Vanilla	70	0	0	0	18	0	13	120
Pudding & Pie Filling, Chocolate Fudge	80	0	0	0	20	1	12	125
Pudding & Pie Filling, Chocolate	80	0	0	0	20	1	13	130
Royal Regular Pudding & Pie Filling, Lemon	120	0	0	0	30	0	23	40
Regular Pudding & Pie Filling, Chocolate	80	0	0	0	20	1	13	80
San Sucre Key Lime Pie Filling	50	3	2	0	8	0	0	25
Pumpkin Pie Filling	50	1	1	0	7	1	4	80

READY-TO-USE

Fruit fillings – *Most brands within generic average (10mg-36mg).*

	Cal	Fat	Sat	Chol	Carb	Fib	Sug	Sod
Bruce's Sweet Potato Filling, 1/3 cup	140	0	0	0	33	1	27	100
Comstock Quick & Easy Lemon	130	2	0	0	28	0	20	120
Lemon Creme	130	2	1	0	28	0	20	135
Farmers Market Pumpkin Pie Mix	100	0	0	0	25	2	20	0
Sweet Potato Puree	130	0	0	0	30	2	15	96
Lucky Leaf Banana Creme	110	0	0	0	28	0	20	75
Choc Creme	100	0	0	0	26	0	16	95
Coconut Creme	110	2	0	0	25	3	12	140
Musslemans Banana Creme	110	0	0	0	28	0	20	75
Choc Creme	100	0	0	0	26	0	16	95
Coconut Creme	110	2	0	0	25	3	12	140
Norfolk Manor Mincemeat	170	3	2	0	37	1	32	15
Steel's Blueberry, Cherry, or Peach, 1/3 cup	80	0	0	0	20	1	18	0
Apple Pie Filling, 1/3 cup	90	0	0	0	25	1	20	0
Tree of Life Organic Pumpkin Pie Mix	100	0	0	0	25	2	20	5
Wilderness Quick & Easy Lemon	130	2	0	0	28	0	20	120
Lemon Creme	130	2	1	0	28	0	20	135

PIE CRUSTS AND SHELLS

	Cal	Fat	Sat	Chol	Carb	Fib	Sug	Sod
Flour pie crust, frozen, 1/8	110	7	3	5	12	0	0	100
Cookie crumb shell, shelf-stable,1/8	140	5	2	0	14	0	6	110
Graham cracker shell, shelf-stable, 1/8	110	5	1	2	14	1	6	115
Mini shell, shelf-stable	110	5	1	0	15	1	6	125
Flour pie crust, refrigerated, unroll, 1/8	110	7	3	5	13	0	1	140
Mix, prep, 1/8	100	6	2	0	9	0	0	145

Brands . . . *(1/8 of 9" shell unless noted)*

FROZEN/REFRIGERATED

	Cal	Fat	Sat	Chol	Carb	Fib	Sug	Sod
Country's Delight	80	5	1	0	8	0	1	75
Food Club Regular	80	4	2	5	9	0	1	70
Jewel Ready-to-Bake	80	4	2	5	9	0	0	70
Lowes Ready-to-Bake	80	4	2	5	9	0	0	70
Our Family Regular	80	4	2	5	9	0	1	70
Deep Dish	90	5	2	5	11	0	1	85
Pillsbury Pet-Ritz Regular	80	4	2	0	9	0	1	70
Deep Dish or All Veg Deep Dish	90	5	1	0	11	0	1	85
Just Unroll!	120	7	3	5	13	0	1	110

MIXES

	Cal	Fat	Sat	Chol	Carb	Fib	Sug	Sod
Arrowhead Mills Graham Mix	100	5	3	0	14	1	6	65
Betty Crocker Pie Crust	110	7	0	0	9	0	0	135
Dixie Carb Counters Graham Cracker, 1/9	63	4	0	0	5	4	1	1
Gluten-Free Pantry Perfect Pie, 1/6	120	0	0	0	29	0	0	140
Jiffy Pie Crust Mix	80	5	2	5	8	0	0	120
Krusteaz Pie Crust Mix	100	6	2	0	10	1	1	90
ShopRite Pie Crust Mix	90	6	2	0	8	0	0	135

SHELF-STABLE (READY-TO-USE)

Most shelf-stable shells are within the generic average (115mg), the following have 100mg or less sodium per serving.

	Cal	Fat	Sat	Chol	Carb	Fib	Sug	Sod
America's Choice Graham Cracker	110	6	1	0	13	1	4	65
Arrowhead Mills Graham Cracker	100	5	2	0	12	0	6	55
Choc Cookie	110	6	3	0	14	1	7	95
Fifty50 Sugar Free Graham Cracker	110	6	2	0	13	0	0	65
Giant Graham Cracker	110	6	2	0	12	0	5	70
Heartland Granola	110	6	2	0	12	1	5	50
Honey Maid Graham Cracker	110	6	3	0	14	1	6	85
Keebler Ready Crust Graham, Reduced Fat	100	4	1	0	15	1	6	100
Kemach Graham Cracker	100	4	1	0	14	1	5	50
Meijer Graham Cracker	110	7	2	0	12	2	6	50
Midwest Country Fare Graham Cracker	100	5	1	0	14	1	4	90
Mother's Own Graham Cracker	110	5	1	0	14	1	4	90
Nabisco Nilla	140	8	2	5	18	0	10	85
Roland Fluted Dessert Shell, 3.6 oz	510	25	0	55	63	2	20	0
ShopRite Graham Cracker	110	7	2	0	12	2	6	50
Spartan Graham Cracker	100	5	1	0	14	1	4	90
Wholly Wholesome Graham Cracker	110	5	3	0	14	1	5	70
Choc Pie Crust	110	5	3	0	14	1	5	100

SEASONINGS – SALT AND SALT SUBSTITUTES

	Cal	Fat	Sat	Chol	Carb	Fib	Sug	Sod
Salt substitute, 1 tsp	2	0	0	0	0	0	0	0
Lite table salt, 1 tsp	0	0	0	0	0	0	0	1160
Seasoned salt, 1 tsp	0	0	0	0	0	0	0	1280
Garlic salt, 1 tsp	0	0	0	0	0	0	0	1480

	Cal	Fat	Sat	Chol	Carb	Fib	Sug	Sod
Table salt or sea salt, 1 tsp............................	0	0	0	0	0	0	0	2325

Brands . . . *(1 tsp unless noted)*

Salt substitutes – *Most brands within generic average (0mg).*

	Cal	Fat	Sat	Chol	Carb	Fib	Sug	Sod
Eden Gomasio (sesame salt), all varieties	15	2	0	0	1	0	0	80
J&D's Bacon Salt Jalapeno or Maple, 1/4 tsp..	5	0	0	5	1	0	0	100
Cheddar, 1/4 tsp..	5	0	0	5	0	0	0	105
Applewood, Mesquite or Peppered, 1/4 tsp	0	0	0	5	0	0	0	130
Original, Natural, or Hickory, 1/4 tsp.............	0	0	0	5	0	0	0	135

SEASONINGS – HERBS, SPICES AND OTHER SEASONINGS

	Cal	Fat	Sat	Chol	Carb	Fib	Sug	Sod
Chili powder, 1 tbsp......................................	24	1	0	0	4	3	1	76
MSG, 1 tbsp	0	0	0	0	0	0	0	150
Old Bay seasoning, 1/4 tsp.............................	0	0	0	0	0	0	0	160
30% less salt, 1/4 tsp..................................	0	0	0	0	0	0	0	95
Meat tenderizer, 1/4 tsp	0	0	0	0	0	0	0	380

Brands . . . *(1 tsp unless noted)*

HERBS, SPICES AND SEASONING BLENDS

Individual herbs and spices have little or no sodium, however herb and spice blends may contain added salt.

	Cal	Fat	Sat	Chol	Carb	Fib	Sug	Sod
Adolph's Marinade in Minutes SF, 3/4 tsp	5	0	0	0	2	0	1	0
Ball's Cajun SF Seasoning	0	0	0	0	0	0	0	0
Bell's SF Seasoning	0	0	0	0	0	0	0	0
Benson's Gourmet SF Seasonings, all	0	0	0	0	0	0	0	0
Bittersweet Herb Farm Seasonings, all	0	0	0	0	0	0	0	0
Blue Crab SF Seasonings, all........................	0	0	0	0	0	0	0	0
BBQ Shrimp, Seafood, or Voodoo	0	0	0	0	0	0	0	0
Chicken Fajita, Fajita, or Chorizo Mix.............	0	0	0	0	0	0	0	0
Creole Pot Roast or Jambalaya	0	0	0	0	0	0	0	0
Etouffe, Gumbo, or Spicy Cajun	0	0	0	0	0	0	0	0
Meatloaf or Mardi Gras Chopped...................	0	0	0	0	0	0	0	0
Red Beans & Rice Seasoning........................	0	0	0	0	0	0	0	0
New Orleans Style Chicken	0	0	0	0	0	0	0	0
Bolner's Fiesta Salt-Free Seasonings, all	0	0	0	0	0	0	0	0
Boscoli Foods Chicken Grande Seasoning, 1/4 jar	57	7	1	0	0	0	0	0
Shrimp Mosca Seasoning, 1/6 jar	57	7	1	0	0	0	0	0
Bragg Sprinkle 24 Herbs & Spices, 1/4 tsp	0	0	0	0	0	0	0	0
Chef Paul Prudhomme								
Magic SF Seasonings, all	0	0	0	0	0	0	0	0
Pizza & Pasta Magic	0	0	0	0	0	0	0	0
DiFiore Italian Seasoning	0	0	0	0	0	0	0	0
Eden Dulce Flakes	3	0	0	0	0	0	0	15
Eden Shake (Furikake), 1/2 tsp....................	5	0	0	0	1	1	0	25
Emeril's Italian Essence, 1/2 tsp	0	0	0	0	0	0	0	0
Fortner's SF Seasonings, all	0	0	0	0	0	0	0	0
Frontier SF Seasonings, all............................	0	0	0	0	0	0	0	0
Great American Spice Co.								
SF Seasonings	0	0	0	0	0	0	0	0
Bloody Mary Spice Mix	0	0	0	0	0	0	0	0
Beefeaters Roast Beef Seasoning	0	0	0	0	0	0	0	0
Cajun Marinade or Herbal Seasonings.............	0	0	0	0	0	0	0	0
Doctor's Choice or Jambalaya Seasonings......	0	0	0	0	0	0	0	0
SF North Bay Shrimp & Crab Boil..................	0	0	0	0	0	0	0	0
Southwest Chili Mix, No Salt	0	0	0	0	0	0	0	0
Lawry's SF 17	0	0	0	0	0	0	0	0

BAKING AND COOKING NEEDS
Sweeteners

	Cal	Fat	Sat	Chol	Carb	Fib	Sug	Sod
Maison Louisianne Creole Spices	0	0	0	0	0	0	0	0
McCormick Salt Free, all	5	0	0	0	0	0	0	0
Morton & Bassett SF Cajun Spice Blend	0	0	0	0	0	0	0	0
SF Mexican Spice Blend	0	0	0	0	0	0	0	0
Mrs. Dash SF, all	8	0	0	0	0	0	0	4
New Orleans Gourmet SF seasonings, all	0	0	0	0	0	0	0	0
Nutrifit Spice Blend, all	5	0	0	0	0	0	0	0
Omaha Steaks SF Steak Seasoning	0	0	0	0	0	0	0	0
Silver Cloud Estates SF Seasoning	0	0	0	0	0	0	0	0
Simply Organic Seasoning blends, all............	0	0	0	0	0	0	0	0
Southern Delight Garlic/Mustard Seasoning ...	0	0	0	0	0	0	0	5
The Spice Hunter SF blends & spices, all	0	0	0	0	0	0	0	0
Spice Island SF, all	0	0	0	0	1	0	0	0
Spike SF Magic! or 5 Herb Magic!	2	0	0	0	0	0	0	15
Sylvia's Secret Seasoning, SF	0	0	0	0	0	0	0	0
Tony Chachere SF Seasoning	0	0	0	0	0	0	0	0
Vanns Spices SF Blends, all	0	0	0	0	0	0	0	0
Wassi's Own SF Sausage Seasoning, all	0	0	0	0	0	0	0	0
Wayzata Bay Spice Co, most seasonings	0	0	0	0	0	0	0	
Zatarain's								
Shrimp/Crab Boil, 1 cap concentrate.............	0	0	0	0	0	0	0	0

RUBS AND BBQ SEASONINGS
Blazing Blends Chile Blends, all....................	0	0	0	0	0	0	0	0
Great Am Spice Co Dr. Larry's NS Rub..........	0	0	0	0	0	0	0	0
Longhorn Grill LS Mesquite, 1/4 tsp..............	0	0	0	0	0	0	0	5
Mickey & T's Gourmet Rubs & Spices, all	0	0	0	0	0	0	0	0
Morton & Bassett								
SF Tailgate or Tex-Mex Rub..........................	0	0	0	0	0	0	0	0
Nantucket Off-Shore Rubs								
Nantucket for Grilling Seafood, 2 tbsp...........	25	0	0	0	5	1	0	0
Rasta for Chicken & Pork, 2 tbsp	30	1	0	0	6	1	2	0
Prairie for Steaks & Burgers, 2 tbsp.............	40	2	0	0	4	1	0	0
Holiday Turkey or Renaissance, 2 tbsp	40	2	0	0	4	2	0	0
The Spice Hunter								
BBQ Spice Blend, 1/4 tsp	0	0	0	0	0	0	0	0
Vanns Spices								
Cancun SF or Caribbean SF Rub	0	0	0	0	0	0	0	0
Wayzata Bay Spice Co								
Tommy's Blend SF Grilling	0	0	0	0	0	0	0	0

SEASONING MIXES
(also see Asian Seasoning Mixes, pg 155; Hispanic/Latino Seasoning Mixes, pg 167; Dips, pg 220, 223; Chili Seasoning, pg 230)

Cedar Hill Seasonings Meat Loaf Mix............	90	2	0	0	15	4	5	15
Stir-Fry Mix..	140	8	0	0	11	3	1	25
Taco/Chili Mix	115	3	0	0	24	9	3	30
Turkey Loaf Mix	60	1	0	0	16	3	9	35
Kraft Parmesan Seasoning Blends								
Rosemary & Garlic..	35	3	2	5	1	0	0	125
Hearty Tuscan Herbs....................................	35	3	2	5	1	0	0	125
Cracked Black Pepper & Toasted Onion, 1/6 pkg	35	3	2	5	1	0	0	130

(SWEETENERS)

Sugar Substitutes:								
Fructose, 1 tsp	15	0	0	0	4	0	4	0

	Cal	Fat	Sat	Chol	Carb	Fib	Sug	Sod
Sweetener w/aspartame, 1 tsp	8	0	0	0	1	0	0	0
Sweetener w/saccharin, 1 tsp	4	0	0	0	1	0	0	0
Sucralose, 1 tsp	0	0	0	0	0	0	0	0
Agave, 1 tbsp	60	0	0	0	16	0	16	0
Sugar, powdered, 1/4 cup.............................	11	7	0	0	30	0	29	0
Granulated, 1/4 cup	194	0	0	0	50	0	50	0
Brown, packed, 1/4 cup	207	0	0	0	54	0	53	21
Honey, 1/4 cup	258	0	0	0	70	0	70	3
Rice syrup, brown, 1/4 cup...........................	170	0	0	0	42	0	19	5
Fruit sweetener, 1/4 cup..............................	120	0	0	0	30	2	28	10
Molasses, 1/4 cup	244	0	0	0	63	0	47	31
Corn syrup, light, 1/4 cup.............................	241	0	0	0	65	0	22	53
Dark, 1/4 cup...	235	0	0	0	64	0	22	127

Brands . . . *Most brands within generic average.*

(**WHEAT GERM**)

Wheat germ, 2 tbsp	50	1	0	0	6	2	1	0

Brands . . . *Most brands within generic average.*

(**YEAST**)

(see Leavening Agents, pg 27)

BEVERAGES

See RESOURCES, *page 305, for a partial list of manufacturers and retailers offering low-salt products online or visit* **LowSaltFoods.com** *for additional sources.*

34

BEVERAGES

ALCOHOLIC BEVERAGES

(also see Cooking Wine, pg 77)

	Cal	Fat	Sat	Chol	Carb	Fib	Sug	Sod
Beer and ale:								
Beer, regular, 12 fl oz	153	0	0	0	13	0	0	14
Non-alcoholic, 12 fl oz	70	0	0	0	15	0	3	10
Light, 12 fl oz	103	0	0	0	6	0	0	14
Liquor and spirits:								
Distilled, all (i.e. gin, rum, whiskey), 1 fl oz	64	0	0	0	0	0	0	0
Creme de menthe, 1 fl oz	125	0	0	0	14	0	14	2
Coffee liqueur w/cream, 1 fl oz	102	5	3	5	7	0	7	29
Ready-to-drink/prepared cocktails:								
Daiquiri, canned, 6.8 fl oz	259	0	0	0	32	0	31	83
Whiskey sour, mix, 1 pkt	130	0	0	0	30	0	29	90
Tequila sunrise, canned, 6.8 fl oz	232	0	0	0	24	0	22	120
Pina colada, canned, 6.8 fl oz	526	17	15	0	61	0	58	158
Wine and champagne:								
Sake, 3.5 fl oz	136	0	0	0	5	0	0	2
Red wine, 5 fl oz (avg)	125	0	0	0	4	0	1	6
White wine and champagne, 5 fl oz (avg)	121	0	0	0	4	0	1	7
Dessert wines, dry, 3.5 fl oz	157	0	0	0	12	0	1	9
Sweet, 3.5 fl oz	165	0	0	0	14	0	8	9

Brands . . .
Most beer, ale, liquor, spirits, wine, and champagne are within the generic average (0-29mg).

READY-TO-DRINK COCKTAILS

	Cal	Fat	Sat	Chol	Carb	Fib	Sug	Sod
Seagrams Escape Coolers, all, 12 fl oz	180	0	0	0	47	0	44	40

BREAKFAST DRINKS

(see Diet/Meal Replacement/Nutrition Drinks, pg 39)

COCKTAIL MIXERS

(also see Water/Tonic/Seltzer, pg 44)

	Cal	Fat	Sat	Chol	Carb	Fib	Sug	Sod
Daiquiri mix, 4 fl oz	70	0	0	0	18	0	17	0
Grenadine, 2 tbsp	90	0	0	0	22	0	21	10
Cosmopolitan mix, 1.5 fl oz	60	0	0	0	14	0	13	15
Manhattan mix, 4 fl oz	200	0	0	0	39	0	33	33
Cream of coconut, 1 fl oz	85	2	2	0	18	1	17	45
Whiskey sour mix, 4 fl oz	90	0	0	0	23	0	22	45
Sweet and sour mix, 4 fl oz	90	0	0	0	23	0	22	45
Margarita mix, 4 fl oz	50	0	0	0	13	0	12	50
Mojito mix, 4 fl oz	107	0	0	0	27	0	27	53
Pina colada mix, 4 fl oz	160	0	0	0	38	0	36	115
Collins mix, 4 fl oz	210	0	0	0	49	0	48	115
Bloody Mary mix, 4 fl oz	25	0	0	0	5	0	3	640
Reduced sodium Bloody Mary mix, 4 fl oz	35	0	0	0	7	0	5	460

Brands . . . *(4 fl oz unless noted)*

FROZEN/REFRIGERATED

	Cal	Fat	Sat	Chol	Carb	Fib	Sug	Sod
Bacardi Margarita Mix, 8 fl oz	90	0	0	0	25	0	23	0
Real Fruit Mixers Pina Colada	170	4	3	0	35	0	35	20
Trader Vic's Tom & Jerry Batter, 1 tbsp	60	1	0	15	13	0	13	20

BEVERAGES
Cocoa and Hot Cider Mixes

	Cal	Fat	Sat	Chol	Carb	Fib	Sug	Sod
Hot Butter Rum Batter, 2 tsp	70	3	2	5	11	0	11	20
MIXES								
Baja Bob's Mudslide Mix, 1 pkt	0	0	0	0	0	0	0	15
Bar-Tenders Cosmopolitan Mix, 1/6	130	0	0	0	33	0	24	0
Lemon Drop Cocktail Mix, 1/6	100	0	0	0	25	0	24	0
Fire Station 5 Margarita Mixes, all	30	0	0	0	8	0	8	0
Island Delites Low Carb Mixes, all	15	0	0	0	3	0	0	5
Roland Pina Colada Mix	120	6	0	0	17	0	16	30
The Spice Hunter Hot Butter Rum Mix	60	0	0	0	15	0	14	0
SEASONING MIXES								
The Aspen Mulling Co Cider Spices, 2 tsp	40	0	0	0	9	0	9	0
Sugar Free Mulling Spices, 1 tbsp	15	0	0	5	3	0	0	0
Mulling Spices, 2 tsp (avg)	40	0	0	0	9	2	2	0
Hot Butter Rum Mix, 3 tsp	80	0	0	0	10	0	10	0
Cook in the Kitchen Bloody Mary Mix	0	0	0	0	0	0	0	55
Papa Timmy's Bloody Mary Mix, 3/4 tsp	0	0	0	0	0	0	0	55
READY-TO-USE								
Coco Lopez Pina Colada Mix, 1/3 cup	130	4	3	0	25	1	24	10
Margarita Mix, 5 fl oz	100	0	0	0	25	0	20	25
Daily's Strawberry Margarita Fruit Mixer	180	0	0	0	47	0	44	25
Margarita Fruit Mixer, 3 fl oz	140	0	0	0	37	0	35	40
Finest Call Mai Tai Mix	90	0	0	0	23	0	21	0
Cosmopolitan Martini Mix	87	0	0	0	21	0	21	5
Tom Collins Mix or Sweet & Sour Mix (avg)	140	0	0	0	33	0	32	10
Pina Colada Mix	170	0	0	0	39	0	36	20
Holland House Manhattan Mix, 2 fl oz	60	0	0	0	15	0	14	10
Strawberry Daiquiri-Margarita	180	0	0	0	46	0	44	30
Pina Colada Mix	170	0	0	0	44	0	42	40
Major Peters Pina Colada Mix	200	2	0	0	50	0	47	31
Master of Mixes Margarita	140	0	0	0	44	0	43	25
Mr & Mrs T Manhattan Mix	150	0	0	0	29	0	25	25
Margarita Mix or Old Fashioned Mix (avg)	180	0	0	0	43	0	39	30
Strawberry-Daiquiri Margarita Mix	190	0	0	0	46	0	44	35
Pina Colada Mix	180	0	0	0	43	0	42	45
Mai Tai Mix	140	0	0	0	33	0	32	65
Stirrings Mojito Mixer, 2 fl oz	50	0	0	0	13	0	13	0
Pomegranate Martini Mixer, 3 fl oz	70	0	0	0	18	0	17	0
T.G.I. Friday's Strawberry Daiquiri Mixer	110	0	0	0	27	0	27	5
Vigo Pina Colada Mix, 3 fl oz	120	6	6	0	17	0	0	30
Wegmans Lemon Drop Martini, 3 fl oz	60	0	0	0	15	0	14	0
Chocolate Martini, 3 fl oz	60	0	0	0	16	0	16	0
Watermelon Margarita	60	0	0	0	17	0	16	5
Orange Pomegranate Martini, 3 fl oz	50	0	0	0	14	0	14	5
Mojito, 6 fl oz	110	0	0	0	29	0	26	5
Margarita	50	0	0	0	13	0	12	10
Cosmopolitan or Apple Martini, 3 fl oz (avg)	55	0	0	0	15	0	15	10

COCOA AND HOT CIDER MIXES

(also see Drink Mixes/Syrups for Milk, pg 39)

	Cal	Fat	Sat	Chol	Carb	Fib	Sug	Sod
Apple cider mix, 1 envl	80	0	0	0	20	0	20	30
Cocoa powder, sugar-free, 1 envl	68	0	0	0	10	1	11	124
Cocoa powder, 3 heaping tsp or 1 envl	111	1	0	0	11	1	18	141
Gourmet hot choc mix, 1 serv	160	0	0	0	28	0	22	240

Brands . . . *(1 serving unless noted)*

There are many low-sodium cocoa and hot cider mixes, the following have 100mg or less per serving.

	Cal	Fat	Sat	Chol	Carb	Fib	Sug	Sod
Ah!Laska Organic Cocoa Non-Dairy	110	1	0	0	25	2	24	5
Organic Cocoa Mix, Low Fat	100	1	0	0	24	1	22	25
The Aspen Mulling Co Spice Apple Cider Mix	110	0	0	0	28	0	26	0
Bellagio Sipping Choc Original	90	1	1	0	22	6	15	30
Big Train Low Carb Hot Choc Mix	50	3	3	0	10	1	2	55
Caffe D'Amore Sipping Choc	110	1	1	0	23	2	16	0
Bellagio White Hot Choc	150	4	3	0	28	0	17	40
Latin Blends Dulce de Leche	130	5	3	0	22	0	17	50
Latin Blends Mexican Spiced Cocoa	165	3	2	0	35	1	25	50
Bellagio Hot Choc, all other flavors	140	4	3	0	28	0	17	85
CarbSmart Sugar Free Hot Cocoa	35	2	0	0	3	0	0	60
Dixie Carb Counters Holy Cow Cocoa Mix	21	0	0	0	2	0	0	81
Droste Cocoa	15	1	1	0	2	1	1	35
Equal Exchange Drinking Choc	180	6	2	0	28	5	18	0
Spicy Hot Cocoa Mix	70	1	0	0	16	2	12	0
Hot Cocoa	70	0	0	0	13	1	11	60
Ghiradelli Hot Choc Mix, most (avg)	80	2	1	0	19	1	16	0
Double Choc	80	2	1	0	19	1	17	30
Ground Choc & Cocoa	140	2	1	0	34	2	30	60
Hershey's Dark Cocoa	10	1	0	0	3	2	0	60
Keurig White Hot Choc K-Cup	90	5	4	0	10	0	7	100
Cafe Escapes Dark Choc K-Cup	60	2	2	0	11	1	7	135
Rabbit Creek Gourmet Hot Choc, most	90	1	0	0	23	0	21	5
Winter or Peppermint Hot Choc Drink (avg)	105	1	0	0	28	0	22	10
Rich Classic Choc, Sugar Free	20	2	2	0	2	0	0	0
Classic Choc	60	1	0	0	14	0	12	0
The Spice Hunter Cioccolata	120	5	3	0	23	3	16	15
Stonewall Kitchen								
Peppermint Hot Choc	220	9	5	15	39	3	34	35
Hot Choc & Marshmallows	230	9	5	15	41	3	36	35
Gingerbread Hot Choc	170	4	3	15	32	1	29	55
Eggnog Hot Choc Mix	170	4	3	15	32	1	29	95
Twinings of London Choc Indulgence	80	4	3	0	10	3	6	0
Wegmans Hot Cocoa Blend	140	7	5	0	19	2	16	10
White Velvet								
White Choc	70	1	1	0	14	0	13	10
White Choc, Sugar Free	25	2	2	0	2	0	0	20

COFFEE AND COFFEE-FLAVORED DRINKS

	Cal	Fat	Sat	Chol	Carb	Fib	Sug	Sod
Coffee, brewed or instant, prep, 6 fl oz	2	0	0	0	0	0	0	4
Coffee, espresso, 6 fl oz	4	0	0	0	0	0	0	25
Mocha-flavor, instant, 1 serv	140	4	3	0	24	1	19	95
Coffee drink, ready-to-drink, 9.5 oz	190	3	2	12	39	0	30	110
Cappuccino-flavor, instant, 1 serv	140	3	3	0	25	0	20	120

Brands . . . *(8 fl oz unless noted)*
Most brands are low in sodium, the following have 90mg or less per serving.

COFFEE AND ESPRESSO – *Most brands within generic average (4mg-25mg).*

COFFEE-FLAVORED DRINK MIXES

	Cal	Fat	Sat	Chol	Carb	Fib	Sug	Sod
Bellagio Mocha, most	110	3	2	0	23	1	14	15
Big Train Caramel Latte, Low Carb Blended	30	2	1	0	10	4	1	65
Vanilla Latte, Low Carb Blended Ice Coffee	30	2	0	0	10	4	1	75

BEVERAGES
Coffee Creamers and Flavorings

	Cal	Fat	Sat	Chol	Carb	Fib	Sug	Sod
Caramel Latte Blended Ice Coffee	190	7	7	0	29	0	19	75
Caffe D'Amore Frappe Freeze, Mocha	110	3	2	0	22	0	14	35
Frappe Freeze, Coffee Toffee	120	2	2	0	23	1	15	45
Caffe D'Vita								
Cappuccino Mint Mocha or Pumpkin Spice	60	2	2	0	10	0	8	20
Cappuccino White Choc	60	2	1	0	12	0	7	25
Cappuccino Caramel, Irish Cr, or Hazelnut	60	3	3	0	10	0	7	30
Cappuccino Mocha or French Vanilla (avg)	65	2	2	0	11	1	5	30
Cappuccino Orange Mocha	60	1	1	0	12	0	5	40
Blended Ice Coffee Coffee Latte	220	8	7	0	38	0	31	50
Blended Ice Coffee Double Mocha Latte	220	8	7	0	38	1	31	55
Cappuccino English Toffee	60	2	2	0	12	0	7	60
Cappuccino Sugar Free, Fr Vanilla or Mocha	35	2	2	0	3	0	0	60
Blended Ice Coffee Caramel or Vanilla Latte	230	8	7	0	40	0	32	85
Hills Bros *Cappuccino* Sugar Free Fr Vanilla	50	2	2	0	8	0	0	50
Maxwell House Int'l								
Suisse Mocha Sugar Free or Decaf	30	2	2	0	2	0	0	30
Suisse Mocha	60	2	2	0	10	0	8	40
French Vanilla Cafe Sugar Free or Decaf	30	3	2	0	2	0	0	50
Vanilla Nut	60	2	2	0	11	0	9	50
Hazelnut or French Vanilla (avg)	65	3	2	0	11	0	9	55
Vienna Cafe Sugar Free	30	2	2	0	2	0	0	60
Cappuccino Cinnamon Dulce	70	2	2	0	14	0	11	65
Cappuccino Toasted Hazelnut	70	3	2	0	12	0	9	70
Cafe Francais	60	3	3	0	8	0	5	90

READY-TO-DRINK COFFEE DRINKS
	Cal	Fat	Sat	Chol	Carb	Fib	Sug	Sod
Mr. Bond Iced Coffee Original, 8.3 fl oz	133	2	1	7	19	0	15	49
Starbucks DoubleShot Light	90	5	3	20	7	0	6	60
Frappuccino Mocha	85	3	2	10	10	0	9	80
Frappuccino Coffee, Caramel, or Vanilla (avg)	170	3	2	10	31	0	26	85
DoubleShot Energy Mocha	110	2	1	10	18	0	14	85
DoubleShot Energy, Coffee or Cinn Dulce	110	2	1	10	19	0	14	90

COFFEE CREAMERS AND FLAVORINGS
	Cal	Fat	Sat	Chol	Carb	Fib	Sug	Sod
Soy creamer, liquid, 1 tbsp	20	2	0	0	2	0	1	0
Cream, liquid, 1 tbsp	29	3	2	10	1	0	0	6
Syrup flavoring, all, 1 fl oz	85	0	0	0	21	0	20	8
Non-dairy creamer, powder, 1 tbsp	33	3	3	0	3	0	3	12
Liquid, 1 tbsp	20	2	0	0	2	0	2	12
Flavored creamer, powder, 1 tbsp	59	3	2	0	8	0	7	24
Liquid, 1 tbsp	35	2	0	0	5	0	5	25

Brands . . . *(1 tbsp unless noted)*
COFFEE CREAMERS – *Most brands within generic average (0mg-12mg).*
FLAVORED CREAMERS – LIQUID
Most brands are low sodium, the following have 15mg or less per serving.

	Cal	Fat	Sat	Chol	Carb	Fib	Sug	Sod
Nestle Coffee-Mate Coconut Creme	35	2	0	0	5	0	5	0
FF Cinnamon Vanilla Creme or FF Hazelnut	25	0	0	0	5	0	4	0
Gingerbread, Pumpkin Spice	35	2	0	0	5	0	5	5
Peppermint Mocha	35	2	0	0	5	0	5	5
Amaretto, Creme Brulee, or French Vanilla	35	2	0	0	5	0	5	10
Hazelnut or Cinnamon Vanilla Creme	35	2	0	0	5	0	5	10
Irish Creme	35	2	0	0	5	0	5	10
Toffee Nut, Vanilla Nut or Vanilla Caramel	35	2	0	0	5	0	5	10

	Cal	Fat	Sat	Chol	Carb	Fib	Sug	Sod
Choc Raspberry	33	2	0	0	5	0	5	15
FF French Vanilla..	50	0	0	0	11	0	6	15

FLAVORED CREAMERS – POWDERED

	Cal	Fat	Sat	Chol	Carb	Fib	Sug	Sod
Nestle Coffee-Mate FF French Vanilla	50	0	0	0	11	0	6	15
French Vanilla, Hazelnut or Hazelnut Biscotti	60	3	2	0	9	0	7	15
Italian Sweet Creme or Vanilla Caramel.........	60	3	3	0	9	0	7	15
Sugar Free, French Vanilla or Hazelnut	30	3	2	0	2	0	0	15
Sugar Free, Vanilla Caramel.........................	30	3	2	0	2	0	0	15
Gingerbread or Peppermint Mocha...............	60	3	3	0	8	0	7	15

COFFEE SUBSTITUTES

	Cal	Fat	Sat	Chol	Carb	Fib	Sug	Sod
Cereal grain, prep w/water, 6 fl oz	11	0	0	0	2	1	0	9
Cereal grain, prep w/milk, 6 fl oz...................	120	6	4	24	10	0	8	91

Brands . . . *Most brands within generic average.*

DIET, MEAL REPLACEMENT AND NUTRITION DRINKS

(also see Energy/Sports/Enhanced Drinks, pg 40)

	Cal	Fat	Sat	Chol	Carb	Fib	Sug	Sod
Meal replacement, powder, choc, 1 envl	132	1	0	4	24	0	24	142
Ready-to-drink, vanilla, 11 fl oz	250	5	2	10	34	0	31	180
Ready-to-drink, choc, 11 fl oz.......................	260	5	2	10	41	1	39	230
Nutritional, ready-to-drink, choc, 8 fl oz	250	6	1	5	40	1	22	190
Ready-to-drink, vanilla, 8 fl oz	250	6	1	5	40	0	23	200

Brands . . . *(8 fl oz unless noted)*

MIXES

	Cal	Fat	Sat	Chol	Carb	Fib	Sug	Sod
Alba Dairy Shakes (avg)	70	0	0	5	12	2	7	140
Carnation Instant Breakfast Essentials								
No Sugar Added, Rich Milk Choc....................	60	1	0	5	12	4	7	60
No Sugar Added, Classic French Vanilla...........	60	0	0	0	12	3	8	70
Rich Milk Choc or Dark Choc (avg)...............	130	1	0	5	27	1	19	90
Classic French Vanilla	130	0	0	0	27	0	18	120
Classic Choc Malt	130	1	1	5	27	1	20	140

READY-TO-DRINK

	Cal	Fat	Sat	Chol	Carb	Fib	Sug	Sod
Ensure Clear Nutritional Drink, 10 fl oz..........	180	0	0	5	35	0	18	50

DRINK MIXES – POWDERED

(also see Cocoa/Hot Cider Mixes, pg. 36; Coffee/Coffee-Flavored Drinks, pg 37; Tea/Chai, pg 43)

	Cal	Fat	Sat	Chol	Carb	Fib	Sug	Sod
Fruit-flavored drink mix, 8 fl oz prep	60	0	0	0	16	0	16	0
Sugar free fruit-flavored mix, 8 fl oz prep......	0	0	0	0	0	0	0	0

Brands . . . *Most brands within generic average.*

DRINK MIXES AND SYRUPS FOR MILK

	Cal	Fat	Sat	Chol	Carb	Fib	Sug	Sod
Syrups:								
Strawberry syrup, 2 tbsp............................	100	0	0	0	28	0	26	5
Choc syrup, 2 tbsp	109	0	0	0	25	1	19	28
Prepared w/whole milk, 8 fl oz..................	254	8	5	25	36	1	32	133
Mixes:								
Strawberry, powder, 1 serv	86	0	0	0	22	0	21	8
Carob flavor, powder, 1 tbsp	82	0	0	0	21	2	18	23
Choc, powder, 1 serv	89	1	0	0	20	1	18	46
Prepared w/whole milk, 8 fl oz..................	226	9	5	24	32	1	31	154
Malted milk, natural, powder, 1 tbsp	80	0	0	0	18	0	14	55
Malted milk, choc, powder, 1 tbsp.................	80	0	0	0	18	1	15	115

BEVERAGES
Energy, Sports and Enhanced Drinks

Brands . . . *(8 fl oz unless noted)*
SYRUPS – *Most brands within generic average (5mg-28mg).*

DRINK MIXES

	Cal	Fat	Sat	Chol	Carb	Fib	Sug	Sod
Concord Foods Smoothies								
Mango	70	0	0	0	17	0	14	0
Banana	50	0	0	0	13	0	11	10
Choc Banana	40	0	0	0	8	1	2	15
Strawberry	70	0	0	0	18	0	15	15
Orange	70	0	0	0	18	0	15	65
Pineapple	70	0	0	0	18	0	15	70
Green & Blacks Organic Hot Choc Drink	80	2	1	0	15	2	12	0
Nestle Abuelita Mexican Choc Drink	100	4	2	0	18	0	17	0
Nesquik Strawberry, 25% Less Sugar	60	0	0	0	15	0	15	0
Nesquik Chocolate, No Sugar Added	35	1	1	0	7	1	3	70
Sunkist Orange Ice Smoothie	45	0	0	0	13	0	9	0
Smart Smoothie Mix Banana or Strawberry	55	0	0	0	14	3	10	20
Lemon Ice Smoothie	100	1	0	0	21	0	20	55

EGG NOG

(see Egg Nog, pg 106)

ENERGY, SPORTS AND ENHANCED DRINKS

	Cal	Fat	Sat	Chol	Carb	Fib	Sug	Sod
Sports drink, fruit flavored, 8 fl oz	50	0	0	0	14	0	14	100
Energy drink, 8 fl oz	115	0	0	0	28	0	26	200

Brands . . . *(8 fl oz unless noted)*
There are many low-sodium brands, the following have 75mg or less.

MIXES

	Cal	Fat	Sat	Chol	Carb	Fib	Sug	Sod
Apex Max Whey Drink, Choc, 1 scoop	90	2	1	30	5	1	2	30
Max Whey Drink, Vanilla, 1 scoop	90	2	1	30	4	0	2	40
Chocolite Protein French Vanilla	130	3	1	4	15	12	0	20
Peanut Butter	135	4	1	4	13	9	0	20
Choc Supreme	135	4	1	4	13	9	0	30
Nutiva Hemp Shake Amazon Acai	100	3	0	0	15	8	3	5
Berry Pomegranate	90	2	0	0	20	8	11	5
Chocolate	80	2	1	0	19	12	7	5
Proformix 90% Whey Protein	100	0	0	0	1	0	0	40

READY-TO-DRINK

	Cal	Fat	Sat	Chol	Carb	Fib	Sug	Sod
Amp								
Energy Shot, 2 fl oz	40	0	0	0	9	0	9	20
Energy	110	0	0	0	29	0	29	65
Energy Traction or Energy Overdrive	110	0	0	0	29	0	29	70
Energy Lightning or Energy Elevate	110	0	0	0	29	0	29	70
Energy w/Green Tea	100	0	0	0	25	0	25	70
Energy w/Black Tea	100	0	0	0	25	0	25	75
Energy Sugar Free	5	0	0	0	1	0	0	75
Bawls Exxtra, 16 fl oz	0	0	0	0	0	0	0	35
Guarana, all, 10 fl oz (avg)	180	0	0	0	32	0	32	35
Big Water Joe w/Natural Caffeine	0	0	0	0	0	0	0	0
Elements Energy Drinks (avg)	120	0	0	0	29	0	27	10
Ginseng Up most (avg)	160	0	0	0	41	0	41	10
Apple, Ginger, or Ginger Beer (avg)	160	0	0	0	41	0	41	30
Glaceau Vitamin/Energy, all flavors	100	0	0	0	25	0	25	0
Grainaissance Amazake most (avg)	180	2	0	0	35	4	30	20
Gimme Green Rice Shake	190	3	1	0	37	4	29	35

	Cal	Fat	Sat	Chol	Carb	Fib	Sug	Sod
Amazing Mango	170	2	0	0	35	4	30	40
Rice Nog	190	2	0	0	39	4	34	65
Hansens *Rumba* Energy Juice	130	0	0	0	32	0	32	15
Hi-Ball *Energy* No Sugar, all flavors	10	0	0	0	0	0	0	0
Energy Low Sugar, all flavors	70	0	0	0	17	0	16	10
Monster *Mixxd* Energy Juice	110	0	0	0	27	0	27	10
Khaos Energy Juice	70	0	0	0	17	0	17	15
M-80 Energy Juice	90	0	0	0	23	0	23	15
Hitman Energy Shot, 2.5 fl oz	30	0	0	0	7	0	6	45
Ocean Spray *Cranergy*, 12 fl oz	50	0	0	0	12	0	12	75
Odwalla								
B Monster	140	0	0	0	34	0	23	10
Superfood, Original	130	1	0	0	30	0	25	10
Superfood, Berries GoMega	160	2	0	0	34	3	24	15
Superfood, Pink Poetry Smoothie	140	0	0	0	32	0	26	15
Superfood, Red Rhapsody Smoothie	110	0	0	0	26	0	22	15
Serious Focus, Mental Energy	170	0	0	0	40	0	37	15
C Monster or Mo'Beta	150	0	0	0	36	0	27	15
Serious Energy	160	0	0	0	39	0	30	20
Super Protein, Vanilla Al'Mondo	190	6	1	0	25	3	19	80
Phat Phruit *Energy*, all (avg)	40	0	0	0	10	0	8	30
Red Bull								
Energy Shot, 2 fl oz	25	0	0	0	6	0	6	40
Energy Shot, Sugar Free, 2 fl oz	2	0	0	0	0	0	0	40
Simply Cola	90	0	0	0	22	0	22	10
Rockstar								
Juiced Pomegranate	100	0	0	0	24	0	23	25
Juiced Guava	90	0	0	0	21	0	20	30
Energy Shots, all flavors, 2.5 fl oz	0	0	0	0	0	0	0	35
Juiced Mango	100	0	0	0	23	0	22	40
Punched Citrus	130	0	0	0	32	0	31	40
Energy Drink (original)	140	0	0	0	31	0	31	40
RW Knudsen								
Simply Nutritious:								
Lemon Ginger Echinacea	100	0	0	0	25	0	24	10
Plum Boost or Vita Pomegranate (avg)	120	0	0	0	33	0	27	10
Vita Blueberry or Vita Cranberry (avg)	125	0	0	0	30	0	27	10
Mega C	140	0	0	0	34	0	30	15
Mega Antioxidant	120	0	0	0	29	0	29	20
Morning Blend	130	0	0	0	30	0	28	25
Recharge, all	70	0	0	0	18	0	17	25
Simply Nutritious Mega Green	130	0	0	0	31	0	25	35
Simply Nutritious Vita Juice	120	0	0	0	31	0	27	40
SoBe								
Orange Carrot	90	0	0	0	23	0	23	10
Citrus Energy	110	0	0	0	27	0	27	15
Mango Melon	120	0	0	0	29	0	29	15
Cranberry Grapefruit	100	0	0	0	26	0	26	20
Black & Blue Berry Brew or Lizard Fuel (avg)	120	0	0	0	31	0	30	25
Power Fruit Punch	100	0	0	0	27	0	27	25
Orange Cream Tsunami	100	0	0	0	25	0	24	25
Fuji Apple Cranberry or Raspberry Lemonade	5	0	0	0	9	0	1	25
Lifewater, all flavors	0	0	0	0	6	0	0	25
Strawberry Banana Lizard Fuel	120	0	0	0	29	0	29	30

BEVERAGES
Fruit and Fruit-Blended Juices/Drinks

	Cal	Fat	Sat	Chol	Carb	Fib	Sug	Sod
Strawberry Daquiri Lizard Lava	120	0	0	0	31	0	30	30
Black & Blue Berry Brew	120	0	0	0	30	0	30	30
Pina Colada Liz Blizz	130	0	0	0	32	0	31	50
Vault Energy	119	0	0	0	32	0	32	30
Zero	4	0	0	0	0	0	0	30

FRUIT AND FRUIT-BLENDED JUICES/DRINKS

	Cal	Fat	Sat	Chol	Carb	Fib	Sug	Sod
Fruit juice, all citrus, 8 fl oz	112	0	0	0	27	0	21	2
Cranberry juice cocktail, 8 fl oz	137	0	0	0	34	0	30	5
Lemonade, frozen, prep, 8 fl oz	131	0	0	0	34	0	33	7
Mix, prep, 8 fl oz	60	0	0	0	16	0	16	25
Apricot nectar, 8 fl oz	141	0	0	0	36	2	31	8
Fruit punch, frozen, prep, 8 fl oz	114	0	0	0	29	0	29	10
Ready-to-drink, 8 fl oz	119	0	0	0	32	0	28	25
Apple juice, 8 fl oz	110	0	0	0	29	0	23	15
Grape drink, canned, 8 fl oz	153	0	0	0	40	0	33	40
Fruit and vegetable drink, 8 fl oz	110	0	0	0	29	0	26	80

NOTE: Some fruit blends with less than 25% juice may contain as much as 80mg sodium per serving.

Brands . . . *Most brands within generic average.*

MEAL REPLACEMENT/NUTRITION DRINKS

(see Diet/Meal Replacement/Nutrition Drinks, pg 39)

MILK DRINKS

(see Milk Products, pg 107)

RICE, SOY AND OTHER NON-DAIRY DRINKS

(see Non-Dairy Milk Alternatives, pg. 108)

SODAS AND SOFT DRINKS

(also see Energy/Sports/Enhanced Drinks, pg 40)

	Cal	Fat	Sat	Chol	Carb	Fib	Sug	Sod
Cream soda, 12 fl oz	180	0	0	0	46	0	46	45
Cream soda, diet, 12 fl oz	0	0	0	0	0	0	0	70
Orange, 12 fl oz	190	0	0	0	52	0	52	45
Orange, diet, 12 fl oz	0	0	0	0	0	0	0	130
Cola, 12 fl oz	140	0	0	0	39	0	29	50
Cola, diet, 12 fl oz	0	0	0	0	0	0	0	40
Ginger ale, 12 fl oz	140	0	0	0	36	0	35	50
Ginger ale, diet, 12 fl oz	0	0	0	0	0	0	0	120
Grape, 12 fl oz	190	0	0	0	51	0	51	55
Pepper-type, 12 fl oz	150	0	0	0	40	0	40	55
Pepper-type, diet, 12 fl oz	0	0	0	0	0	0	0	55
Root beer, 12 fl oz	180	0	0	0	46	0	46	60
Root beer, diet, 12 fl oz	0	0	0	0	0	0	0	100
Lemon-lime, 12 fl oz	140	0	0	0	39	0	39	75
Lemon-lime, diet, 12 fl oz	0	0	0	0	0	0	0	45
Lemonade, 12 fl oz	150	0	0	0	42	0	40	120

Brands . . . *(12 fl oz unless noted)*
Most soda and soft drinks are within the generic average, the following have 35mg or less per 12-oz serving.

	Cal	Fat	Sat	Chol	Carb	Fib	Sug	Sod
Canfield's Diet, all	0	0	0	0	0	0	0	0

	Cal	Fat	Sat	Chol	Carb	Fib	Sug	Sod
Diet Riet, all....................	0	0	0	0	0	0	0	0
Green River (avg)...........................	180	0	0	0	45	0	45	15
Minute Maid Light Orangeaid.......................	0	0	0	0	2	0	1	35
Polar, all (avg)............................	0	0	0	0	0	0	0	0
Specher Root Beer	110	0	0	0	27	0	27	20

ALTERNATIVE, ORGANIC AND NATURAL SODAS

	Cal	Fat	Sat	Chol	Carb	Fib	Sug	Sod
Blue Sky Natural, all (avg)	170	0	0	0	43	0	43	0
Lite, Natural, all....................	50	0	0	0	13	0	13	10
Organic or Premium Ginseng, all (avg)..........	160	0	0	0	40	0	40	10
GuS Grown-up Sodas (avg)	95	0	0	0	23	0	23	10
Hansen's Natural Cane Sodas, all (avg)	140	0	0	0	37	0	37	0
Honest Ade, all	100	0	0	0	12	0	12	5
Jones Pure Cane Soda, all (avg)	190	0	0	0	47	0	47	30
Izze Sparkling Juices.............................	100	0	0	0	23	0	22	10
Orangina	120	0	0	0	28	0	26	0
Reeds Ginger Brew	145	0	0	0	37	0	37	5
Santa Cruz Organic (avg)........................	150	0	0	0	35	0	31	0
Virgil's Root Beer	160	0	0	0	42	0	42	0

SOY, RICE AND OTHER NON-DAIRY DRINKS

(see Non-Dairy Milk Alternatives, pg. 108)

SPORTS DRINKS

(see Energy/Sports/Enhanced Drinks, pg 40; Water, Tonic, Seltzer, pg 44)

TEA AND CHAI

	Cal	Fat	Sat	Chol	Carb	Fib	Sug	Sod
Tea, instant, lemon-flavored, prep, 8 fl oz	39	0	0	0	9	0	1	6
Tea, regular, prep, 8 fl oz................................	2	0	0	0	1	0	0	7
Tea, ready-to-drink, flavored, 8 fl oz	100	0	0	0	25	0	23	10
Chai, prep mix or ready-to-drink, 8 fl oz	120	2	0	0	21	0	19	135

Brands . . . *(8 fl oz unless noted)*

TEA – *Most brands within generic average (6mg-10mg).*

CHAI

MIXES

	Cal	Fat	Sat	Chol	Carb	Fib	Sug	Sod
Big Train Spiced Low Carb Chai	60	3	1	0	11	0	2	90
Caffe D'Amore Chai Amore Tea Latte, all	150	4	3	0	29	0	17	25
Caffe D'Vita Enchanted Chai								
Raspberry or Vanilla Tea Latte....................	120	43	1	5	21	0	18	40
Chocolate Tea Latte...................................	118	3	1	4	21	0	18	57
Spiced Tea Latte	120	4	1	0	21	0	18	100
Carb Smart Sugar Free Chai Tea	33	3	0	0	3	0	0	40
Oregon Chai mix, all, 1/2 pkt	0	0	0	0	1	0	0	0
Concentrate:								
Sugar-Free Original, 4 oz.........................	0	0	0	0	1	0	0	0
Slightly Sweet Original, 4 oz....................	30	0	0	0	8	0	7	10
Vanilla, 4 oz...	80	0	0	0	21	0	19	30
Original or Peppermint Original, 4 oz	90	0	0	0	22	0	19	30
Vegan Original, 4 oz...............................	90	0	0	0	22	0	19	35
Vanilla Mix	100	2	1	5	24	0	20	25
Original Mix or Spiced Original Mix	80	1	1	5	19	0	16	30
Pacific Chai Latte, all	90	2	2	0	16	0	14	20

READY-TO-DRINK – REFRIGERATED

	Cal	Fat	Sat	Chol	Carb	Fib	Sug	Sod
Adina Iced Chai Latte, Indian......................	110	2	0	10	19	0	19	45

	Cal	Fat	Sat	Chol	Carb	Fib	Sug	Sod
Bolthouse Perfectly Protein Vanilla Chai	160	3	1	0	25	0	21	60
General Foods Int'l Chai Latte	70	2	2	0	12	0	10	60

VEGETABLE JUICE

	Cal	Fat	Sat	Chol	Carb	Fib	Sug	Sod
Mixed vegetable and fruit juice, 8 fl oz	72	0	0	0	18	0	5	52
Carrot juice, 8 fl oz	94	0	0	0	22	2	9	68
Tomato juice, 8 fl oz	41	0	0	0	10	1	9	653
Vegetable juice cocktail, 8 fl oz	46	0	0	0	11	2	8	655
Clam/tomato juice, 8 fl oz	116	0	0	0	26	1	8	875
Brands . . . *(8 fl oz unless noted)*								
After The Fall 24 Karrot Orange	120	0	0	0	28	0	25	55
Campbell's Tomato Juice, Low Sodium	50	0	0	0	10	2	7	140
Kagome Autumn Reds	120	0	0	0	29	0	24	20
Purple Roots & Fruits	130	0	0	0	30	1	26	55
Sweet Summer Tomato	50	0	0	0	11	1	9	100
Carrot Ginger Zest	100	0	0	0	21	0	19	115
Red Gold NSA Tomato Juice	45	0	0	0	10	2	7	25
RW Knudsen Very Veggie, LS	50	1	0	0	11	2	6	35
Very Veggie Organic, LS	70	0	0	0	14	2	8	35
Very Veggie Untomato	70	0	0	0	16	2	12	130
V8								
Fusion Vegetable & Fruit Juice:								
Light Peach Mango	50	0	0	0	13	0	10	40
Light Strawberry Banana	50	0	0	0	13	0	10	40
Light Pomegranate Blueberry	50	0	0	0	13	0	10	60
Pomegranate Blueberry	100	0	0	0	25	0	23	60
Acai Mixed Berry or Peach Mango	105	0	0	0	27	0	26	70
Passion Fruit Tangerine or Goji Raspberry	100	0	0	0	27	0	24	70
Tropical Orange or Strawberry Banana	120	0	0	0	28	0	25	80
Vegetable, LS	50	0	0	0	10	2	8	140

WATER, TONIC AND SELTZER

(also see Energy/Sports/Enhanced Drinks, pg 40)

	Cal	Fat	Sat	Chol	Carb	Fib	Sug	Sod
*Water, flavored, 8 fl oz	0	0	0	0	0	0	0	0
Water, bottled, 8 fl oz	0	0	0	0	0	0	0	5
Seltzer, includes fruit-flavored, 8 fl oz	0	0	0	0	0	0	0	10
Tonic, 8 fl oz	83	0	0	0	21	0	21	29
Diet tonic, 8 fl oz	0	0	0	0	0	0	0	35
Club soda, 8 fl oz	0	0	0	0	0	0	0	50
Low sodium club soda, 8 fl oz	0	0	0	0	0	0	0	35
Water, enhanced, 8 fl oz	30	0	0	0	8	0	1	70

Some flavored waters have as much as 70mg sodium.

Brands . . . *(8 fl oz unless noted)*

CLUB SODA – *Most brands within generic average (35mg-50mg).*

SELTZER/TONIC – *Most brands within generic average (10mg-35mg).*

WATER – BOTTLED/FLAVORED – *Most brands within generic average (0mg-5mg).*

WATER – ENHANCED

There is a wide variety of low-sodium enhanced waters, the following have 35mg or less per 8-oz serving.

	Cal	Fat	Sat	Chol	Carb	Fib	Sug	Sod
Eating Right Vitamin Enhanced Water								
Dragon Fruit or Fruit Punch	50	0	0	0	13	0	13	35
Zero Calorie, all flavors	0	0	0	0	0	0	0	35
Elations Glucosamine Drinks, all (avg)	30	0	0	0	8	0	1	0

	Cal	Fat	Sat	Chol	Carb	Fib	Sug	Sod
Glaceau Smartwater	0	0	0	0	0	0	0	0
Vitaminwater 10, all flavors (avg)	10	0	0	0	4	0	3	0
Vitaminwater, all flavors (avg)	50	0	0	0	13	0	13	0
SoBe Life Water, all (avg)	40	0	0	0	17	0	10	20

YOGURT DRINKS

(see Yogurt/Non-Dairy Drinks, pg 111)

BREAD AND FLOUR PRODUCTS

See RESOURCES, page 305, for a partial list of manufacturers and retailers offering low-salt products online or visit **LowSaltFoods.com** *for additional sources.*

BREAD AND FLOUR PRODUCTS

BAGELS

	Cal	Fat	Sat	Chol	Carb	Fib	Sug	Sod
Cinnamon raisin bagel, med, 3 oz	229	1	0	0	46	2	5	270
Plain bagel, medium, med, 3 oz	216	1	0	0	42	2	45	376
Mini, 1.5 oz	120	1	0	0	25	4	4	210
Large, 4 oz	288	2	1	0	57	3	6	502
Brands . . . *(3 oz unless noted)*								
Chatila's Bakery all varieties, 2.5 oz	90	1	0	0	10	6	0	50
David's Deli French Toast Bagel, 2.9 oz	230	2	1	5	48	1	12	85
Franz Mini 100% Whole Wheat, 1.5 oz	90	1	0	0	18	3	2	135
Mini Brown Sugar & Cinnamon, 1.5 oz	100	1	0	0	20	1	3	135
Just Bagels Energy, 1/2 of 4 oz bagel	160	2	0	0	31	2	4	110
Multigrain, 1/2 of 4 oz bagel	150	2	0	0	30	2	2	115
Sara Lee Soft & Smooth Mini Cinnamon, 1.3 oz.	100	1	0	0	21	2	4	130
Soft & Smooth Mini Plain or Blueberry, 1.3 oz	100	1	0	0	20	1	4	140
REDUCED SODIUM (LESS THAN GENERIC):								
Franz Bagelean Wheat, 1.5 oz	90	1	0	0	21	5	2	160
Bagelean Original, 1.5 oz	90	1	0	0	20	3	1	170
Kim's Light Bagels Blueberry, 2 oz	110	1	0	0	23	4	0	180
Plain, Wheat, Onion, or Cinnamon, 2 oz (avg)	110	1	0	0	23	4	0	190
Everything, 2 oz	110	1	0	0	23	4	0	200
Kraft Bagel-fuls Strawberry or Cinnamon, 2.5 oz	200	4	2	10	34	2	7	190
Bagel-fuls Original or Chive, 2.5 oz	200	5	3	15	31	2	4	200
Bagel-fuls Whole Grain, 2.5 oz	180	6	4	15	26	3	4	200
Otis Spunkmeyer Blueberry	210	1	0	0	44	1	5	220
Pepperidge Farms Mini Brown Sugar Cinn	120	1	0	0	24	2	6	150
Mini Cinnamon Raisin, 1.4 oz	110	1	0	0	23	1	6	180
Mini 100% Whole Wheat, 1.4 oz	100	1	0	0	20	3	3	180
Silver Hills Squirrelly or Flax (avg)	205	4	1	0	32	8	3	170
Thomas' Bagel Thins Cinnamon Raisin, 1.6 oz	110	1	0	0	25	5	6	160
Mini 100% Whole Wheat, 1.5 oz	110	1	0	0	22	3	3	180
Bagel Thins 100% Whole Wheat or Everything	110	1	0	0	24	5	3	190
Mini Blueberry, 1.5 oz	120	1	0	0	25	1	5	200

BISCUITS AND POPOVERS

(also see Baking Mix–All Purpose, pg 25)

	Cal	Fat	Sat	Chol	Carb	Fib	Sug	Sod
Crescent rolls, butter, refrig, 1 oz roll	110	6	2	0	11	0	2	210
Popovers, mix, 1 oz	105	1	0	0	20	0	-	257
Biscuit, plain or buttermilk, refrig, 2 1/2" (1.2 oz)	109	5	1	0	15	0	3	340
Plain/buttermilk, LF, refrg, 2 1/2" (1.2 oz)	87	2	0	0	16	1	2	424
Biscuit, ready-to-eat, 2 1/2" (1.2 oz)	128	6	1	0	17	1	1	368
Biscuit, mix, 1/3 cup	171	6	2	1	25	1	5	510
Brands . . . *(1 biscuit or roll unless noted)*								
MIXES								
Bernard LS Biscuit Mix	170	4	2	0	30	0	0	10
Barefoot Contessa Foolproof Popovers	100	0	0	0	20	1	2	130
Carbquik Biscuit & Baking Mix	50	4	0	0	9	7	0	110
King Arthur Flour Popover Mix	70	0	0	0	15	1	2	120
REDUCED SODIUM (LESS THAN GENERIC):								
Dixie Carb Counters Vegan Biscuit	51	0	0	0	10	1	0	167
Iveta Gourmet Biscuit Mixes, all	100	0	0	0	20	1	2	170

BREAD AND FLOUR PRODUCTS
Bread

	Cal	Fat	Sat	Chol	Carb	Fib	Sug	Sod

SHELF-STABLE (READY-TO-EAT)

	Cal	Fat	Sat	Chol	Carb	Fib	Sug	Sod
Cantanzaro's Red or White Wine Biscuits, 2	120	5	1	0	18	0	7	65

BREAD

(also see Bread/Pastry Dough/Mixes, pg 51; Buns/Sandwich Rolls, pg 53; English Muffins, pg 55; Cornbread, pg 58)

	Cal	Fat	Sat	Chol	Carb	Fib	Sug	Sod
Oat bran bread, 1.1 oz slice	76	1	0	0	13	1	2	130
Rice bran bread, 1.1 oz slice	78	1	0	0	14	2	1	141
Wheat bread, 1.1 oz slice	85	1	0	0	15	1	2	167
Oatmeal bread, 1.1 oz slice	86	1	0	0	16	1	3	192
French or sourdough bread, 1.1 oz slice	92	1	0	0	18	1	1	208
Rye bread, 1.1 oz slice	83	1	0	0	15	2	1	211
Pumpernickel bread, 1.1 oz slice	80	1	0	0	15	2	0	215
White bread, 1.1 oz slice	85	1	0	0	16	1	1	218
Boston brown, canned, 1.6 oz slice	88	1	0	0	19	2	1	284
Focaccia bread, 1 oz slice	78	1	0	0	15	1	1	308
Chibatta, 2 oz slice	140	0	0	0	29	0	1	310
French baguette, 2 oz slice	140	0	0	0	29	1	1	330

Brands . . . *(1 slice unless noted)*
There are many low-sodium breads, the following have 110mg or less per slice. Since there are fewer low-sodium selections for sourdough, rye, and pumpernickel, those listed have 125mg or less.

FROZEN/REFRIGERATED

	Cal	Fat	Sat	Chol	Carb	Fib	Sug	Sod
Better Bread Co French Baguettes, 1.5 oz	110	3	0	0	31	1	3	95
Food for Life Ezekiel, Low Sodium	80	1	0	0	15	3	0	0
Rice Pecan or Rice Almond (avg)	125	3	0	0	23	2	3	5
Genesis Sprouted Grain/Seed	80	2	0	0	14	3	0	65
Ezekiel Sprouted 7 Grain	80	1	0	0	15	3	1	75
Ezekiel Sesame or Sprouted 7 Grain	80	1	0	0	14	3	0	80
Shabtai Round Challah	100	5	2	35	12	0	0	95

SHELF-STABLE

	Cal	Fat	Sat	Chol	Carb	Fib	Sug	Sod
Alvarado St. Bakery Multi-Grain, SF	90	1	0	0	15	2	2	10
Sprouted Wheat Sourdough	80	1	0	0	15	2	2	125
Aunt Millies Healthy Goodness Light Whole Grain	35	1	0	0	9	3	1	83
Healthy Goodness Light Five Grain	40	1	0	0	9	3	1	90
Healthy Goodness 100% Whole Wheat	55	1	0	0	10	2	2	90
Healthy Goodness White	48	1	0	0	12	3	2	90
Healthy Goodness Light Potato	35	0	0	0	9	3	1	100
Beefsteak Dixie Rye	45	1	0	0	8	1	1	120
Bunny 100% Whole Wheat	55	1	0	0	11	2	2	110
Sliced French	65	1	0	0	13	1	2	120
Butternut Sandwich	55	1	0	0	11	0	2	110
Country Hearth English Muffin Toasting	70	1	0	0	13	0	1	85
Ener-G Rice Starch	90	2	0	0	20	5	4	0
Brown Rice	100	3	0	0	16	1	2	25
Light White Rice	50	2	0	0	8	1	1	40
Corn Loaf	40	2	0	0	8	3	2	50
Light Tapioca or Light White Rice Flax (avg)	45	2	0	0	7	1	1	60
Papas	70	3	0	0	11	2	0	65
Light Brown Rice	50	2	0	0	7	1	1	75
Seattle Brown	80	2	0	0	16	4	2	90
Tapioca, Thin Sliced	80	3	0	0	11	2	1	95
Four Flour	80	3	0	0	17	3	1	100
White Rice Flax	100	5	0	0	14	2	2	110

	Cal	Fat	Sat	Chol	Carb	Fib	Sug	Sod
Franz Net 4 Reduced Carbs	55	1	0	0	11	6	1	85
45 Calories Multigrain	45	1	0	0	9	3	1	85
45 Calories Whole Wheat	40	1	0	0	9	3	1	95
French Meadow Sprouted 16 Grain & Seed	110	3	0	0	17	4	2	80
Sprouted Grain	100	1	0	0	18	4	2	85
Gillian's Foods Sandwich Loaf (Gluten Free)	80	3	0	0	11	0	1	105
Gold Medal NSA White or NS Wheat	90	2	0	0	20	5	4	0
Healthy Life *40 Calories*, Flaxseed	40	1	0	0	9	3	1	80
35 Calories Whole Grain, White, or Italian	35	0	0	0	8	3	1	80
40 Calories Sugar Free, Whole Grain	40	1	0	0	8	1	0	85
Soft Style 100% Whole Grain	55	1	0	0	11	2	2	105
Jacobsen's *Snack Toast* Honey Maple	40	0	0	0	8	0	3	50
Snack Toast Original	40	1	0	0	8	1	3	65
Manna Organics *Manna Bread* Sun Seed, 2 oz	160	2	0	0	29	7	11	3
Manna Bread Millet Rice or Multigrain, 2 oz (avg)	130	0	0	0	27	4	8	10
Manna Bread Rye, 2 oz.	150	0	0	0	32	5	7	10
Milton's Healthy Gourmet White	110	1	0	0	23	1	5	110
Monks' Bread Wheat	80	1	0	0	10	2	2	110
Montana Mills Sunflower Millet	70	1	0	0	14	2	3	65
Woodstock	70	1	0	0	14	1	3	70
Honey Whole Wheat	70	0	0	0	14	2	2	80
Bavarian Rye	65	0	0	0	13	1	0	85
Sesame Garlic Cheddar	70	2	0	50	12	1	1	90
Spinach Feta	60	1	0	0	12	1	1	100
Mrs Baird's Honey Wheat	70	1	0	0	13	1	2	100
Whole Grain Wheat, 1 slice	75	1	0	0	14	2	2	105
100% Whole Wheat (avg)	60	1	0	0	12	2	1	110
Extra Thin White or Honey 7 Grain (avg)	72	1	0	0	13	0	1	110
Split Top Wheat	70	1	0	0	13	1	2	105
Natural Ovens *Weight Sense* Right Wheat	50	1	0	0	9	3	1	65
Sunny Millet	100	2	0	0	15	4	1	100
Whole Grain Grain Oat Nut Crunch	100	3	0	0	15	4	2	110
Nature's Pride 100% Whole Wheat (soft)	70	1	0	0	13	2	2	100
Honey Wheat (soft)	70	1	0	0	13	1	3	100
Nickles Bakery Swiss Maid LS	60	1	0	0	14	1	0	20
Light 35 Wheat	35	0	0	0	8	2	-	95
Light 35 White	35	0	0	0	8	2	-	100
Wheat Pullman or Whole Grain White (avg)	58	1	0	0	12	1	-	110
Rye Pullman	60	1	0	0	12	1	-	115
Light Deli Rye or Dark Deli Rye	60	1	0	0	12	1	-	120
Oroweat *Light* 100% Whole Wheat	40	0	0	0	9	4	2	110
Pepperidge Farm 100% Whole Wheat	70	1	0	0	12	2	1	65
Whole Grain Small Slice Whole Wheat	70	1	0	0	13	3	2	70
Whole Grain Small Slice 15 Grain	70	1	0	0	13	3	2	75
Original White	70	1	0	0	13	1	2	75
Very Thin 100% Whole Wheat, 1 slice	37	1	0	0	7	1	1	77
Light Style Extra Fiber, 1 slice	40	0	0	0	8	2	1	83
Very Thin White, 1 slice	40	0	0	0	8	0	1	83
Oatmeal	70	1	0	0	12	1	1	85
Light Style Oatmeal, 1 slice	47	0	0	0	9	1	1	87
Light Style Seven Grain, 1 slice	43	0	0	0	9	1	1	90
Light Style Soft Wheat, 1 slice	43	0	0	0	8	1	1	90
Whole Grain White	55	1	0	0	11	2	2	100
Rubschlager Cocktail Bread, all, 2 sl (avg)	53	1	0	0	9	1	1	120
Rudolph's SF Rye	124	1	0	0	26	4	0	2

BREAD AND FLOUR PRODUCTS
Bread

	Cal	Fat	Sat	Chol	Carb	Fib	Sug	Sod
Sami's Bakery Flax for Life	70	1	0	0	15	2	2	70
Slimmer You	50	1	0	0	10	2	2	70
Millet & Flax or Plain Millet	76	1	0	0	25	2	0	90
Sara Lee *45 Calories Delightful* Multi-Grain	45	1	0	0	9	3	1	80
Soft & Smooth Whole Grain White	75	1	0	0	14	2	2	95
Soft & Smooth Plus Whole Grain White	75	1	0	0	14	1	2	95
White or Classic 100% Whole Wheat	75	1	0	0	14	2	3	105
Soft & Smooth 100% Whole Wheat	75	2	1	0	13	2	3	105
45 Calories Delightful Wheat	45	1	0	0	10	3	1	110
Hearty & Delicious Jewish or Russian Rye (avg)	70	1	0	0	12	1	1	120
Schwebel's *Lite* Wheat	70	0	0	0	16	6	2	75
Lite White	80	1	0	0	18	5	2	85
ShaSha Co Ezekiel or Spelt	75	1	0	0	15	2	2	90
Silver Hills Steady Eddie Sprouted Wheat	100	1	0	0	18	5	1	105
Sunbeam Sandwich White	60	1	0	0	12	1	1	110
Village Hearth Light 12 Grain	40	1	0	0	8	2	1	110
Wegman's *Food You Feel Good About Lite* Wheat	40	0	0	0	10	2	1	105
Weight Watcher's Multi-Grain	50	1	0	0	9	2	0	85
Whole Wheat	45	1	0	0	8	2	1	90
Wonder *Smart White* or Whole Grain White (avg)	60	1	0	0	12	3	2	100
Soft 100% Whole Wheat	55	1	0	0	10	2	2	110

SANDWICH THINS
REDUCED SODIUM (LESS THAN GENERIC):

	Cal	Fat	Sat	Chol	Carb	Fib	Sug	Sod
Arnold Seedless Rye, 1.5 oz	100	1	0	0	22	5	2	210
Thomas Breakfast Thins, 1.5 oz (avg)	100	1	0	0	22	5	2	170

SWEET/DESSERT BREADS
The following sweet/dessert breads have 115mg or less sodium per serving.

	Cal	Fat	Sat	Chol	Carb	Fib	Sug	Sod
Arnold Bakery Raisin Cinnamon	80	2	0	0	15	1	7	95
Country Hearth Cinnamon Burst	80	1	1	0	15	1	4	110
Ener-G Raisin	100	3	0	0	16	1	7	85
Fiber One Cinnamon Raisin	75	1	0	0	18	4	6	85
Food for Life Cinnamon Raisin	80	0	0	0	18	2	5	65
French Meadow Bakery Sprouted Cinn Raisin.	100	1	0	0	19	3	4	90
Jacobsen's *Snack Toast*								
Blueberry or Raspberry (avg)	40	0	0	0	8	1	3	45
Manna Organics *Manna Bread*								
Banana Walnut Hemp, 2 oz	140	4	0	0	27	2	12	5
Carrot Raisin or Fruit & Nut, 2 oz (avg)	135	1	0	0	27	5	13	7
Fig Fennel, 2 oz	120	2	0	0	26	5	8	10
Cinnamon Date, 2 oz	150	0	0	0	29	5	6	15
Montana Mills Raspberry Cheese Danish	60	1	0	5	12	1	2	70
Cranberry Orange or Cinn Raisin Walnut (avg)	70	1	0	0	15	2	2	70
Apple Raisin Challah	70	0	0	10	14	2	1	75
Blueberry Cheese Danish	60	1	0	5	12	1	3	75
German Fruit/Nut Stollen or Sticky Bun	70	1	0	5	15	1	3	75
Maple Raisin Walnut or Blueberry Pancake	70	1	0	0	15	1	4	75
Red, White & Blue or Blueberry Cobbler	80	1	0	0	16	1	5	75
King's Cake	60	0	0	5	14	1	5	75
Almond Bear Claw or Cheese Danish	80	2	0	7	14	1	3	85
Hot Cross or Linzer Nut Tart (avg)	75	2	0	6	14	1	3	85
Cherry Choc, Choc Bobka, or Raspberry Apricot	70	1	0	0	14	1	2	85
Apple Raisin Cinnamon Swirl or Apricot Almond	70	0	0	0	14	1	3	90
Cherry Apple Strudel	70	1	0	5	10	1	3	90
Cherry Cheesecake	70	1	0	0	14	1	4	90

	Cal	Fat	Sat	Chol	Carb	Fib	Sug	Sod
Blueberry Cheesecake or Blueberry White Choc...	70	1	0	0	14	1	4	95
Cranberry Pecan Cornbread	80	2	0	0	14	1	4	95
Holiday Fruit..	60	0	0	0	14	1	2	95
Peaches 'n Creme or Stars 'n Stripes (avg)	75	1	0	5	15	1	4	95
Cinnamon Swirl or Cinnamon Crunch (avg)....	75	1	0	0	15	1	4	100
Pecan Pie or Pumpkin Nut Swirl (avg)	85	3	0	8	15	1	3	105
Caramel Apple	80	1	0	0	16	1	5	115
Traditional Fruit Challah	80	2	0	25	15	1	2	115
Pepperidge Farm *Swirl* Raisin Cinnamon........	80	2	0	0	15	1	5	100
Sara Lee Cinnamon w/Raisins	95	2	1	0	16	2	8	80
Brown Sugar Cinnamon	100	3	2	0	15	2	7	95
Blueberry Crumble Breakfast Bread	90	2	1	0	17	2	5	105
Schwebel's Raisin	80	1	0	0	17	1	6	95
Sun-Maid Raisin Cinnamon Swirl	80	2	1	0	16	1	7	100
Wholly Wholesome Banana Nut, 1.9 oz	210	11	1	25	26	1	13	75
Blueberry Crumb Bread, 1.9 oz	210	10	2	35	27	0	11	80
Cranberry Orange Bread, 1.9 oz..................	210	9	2	35	28	1	12	80
Wonder Cinnamon Raisin	80	2	0	0	14	0	2	100

BREAD/PASTRY DOUGH AND MIXES

(also see Dinner Rolls/Croissants, pg 55; Cornbread, pg 58)

(also see Dinner Rolls/Croissants, pg 55; Cornbread, pg 58)

	Cal	Fat	Sat	Chol	Carb	Fib	Sug	Sod
Bread dough, frozen/refrigerated:								
Whole wheat, ready-to-bake, 1.9-oz slice......	130	2	0	0	24	3	4	220
White, ready-to-bake, 1.9-oz slice...............	140	2	0	0	24	2	2	280
Bread mixes:								
Whole wheat, mix, 1 slice...........................	130	1	0	0	20	3	4	240
Rye, mix, 1 slice	130	1	0	0	27	3	1	240
Wheat or white, bread machine, 1.5 oz slice......	150	2	0	0	28	1	5	280
Sweet/dessert breads:								
Raisin bread, 1.1 oz slice...........................	88	1	0	0	17	1	2	115
Quick/sweet bread mix, banana, 1/12...........	130	3	1	0	25	01	12	190
Pastry dough:								
Fillo (phyllo) dough, 2.5 sheets (2 oz)..........	180	2	0	0	37	1	0	230
Puff pastry, 1/6 sheet (1.5 oz)	170	11	6	0	14	1	0	270
Puff pastry mini shell, 4 shells (1.6 oz)..........	180	9	6	0	15	1	1	290
Puff pastry shell, 1 shell (1.7 oz).................	190	13	7	0	16	1	0	300

Brands . . . *(1 slice unless noted)*

BREAD DOUGH – FROZEN/REFRIGERATED

	Cal	Fat	Sat	Chol	Carb	Fib	Sug	Sod
Upper Crust Banana Bread, 2 oz..................	177	7	3	22	26	1	17	113
REDUCED SODIUM (LESS THAN GENERIC):								
Fetting's Family Breads White..................	140	2	0	0	26	1	2	160
Upper Crust Pumpkin Bread, 2 oz..............	180	7	3	25	21	1	19	150

BREAD MIXES

Some mixes require additional ingredients which may raise sodium content.

	Cal	Fat	Sat	Chol	Carb	Fib	Sug	Sod
Bob's Red Mill Low-Carb Bread....................	90	2	0	0	9	4	0	92
Chébé Cheese Bread..................................	70	0	0	0	17	0	0	103
Gluten Free Pantry								
French Bread & Pizza	110	0	0	0	25	0	0	120
King Arthur								
Garlic Grilling Bread & Pizza........................	130	0	0	0	27	1	1	75
Little Chef Fry Bread	100	0	0	0	21	1	3	105
McCann's Irish Brown.................................	90	1	0	0	17	2	0	100

BREAD AND FLOUR PRODUCTS
Bread/Pastry Dough and Mixes

	Cal	Fat	Sat	Chol	Carb	Fib	Sug	Sod
Schar Gluten-Free Classic White	100	1	0	0	23	2	2	120
Sylvan Border Farm								
Wheat-Free Dark or White	140	4	1	35	24	1	6	120
Toro *Celiac-Safe* White or Whole Meal Bread	70	1	0	0	16	0	1	90
SWEET/DESSERT BREAD MIXES								
Chébé Cinnamon Roll-ups, 0.8 oz	73	0	0	0	18	0	0	100
Chiquita Banana Bread Mix, 1/12	130	2	0	0	26	0	13	130
Concord Foods Fresh Cranberry, 1/12	130	2	0	0	27	1	13	125
Dixie Carb Counters								
Banana Nut	32	1	0	0	5	2	1	124
Cranberry Orange	23	0	0	0	5	2	1	129
Cinnamon Swirl	25	0	0	0	7	4	1	133
Gluten Free Essentials								
Lemon Poppy Seed Bread & Muffins, 1/24	76	1	0	0	17	1	4	70
Holiday Gingerbread, 1/18	77	1	0	0	17	1	4	120
Harborside Bakery Lemon Poppy Seed, 1/15	120	1	0	0	27	1	12	75
King Arthur Almond Filled Sweet	180	3	0	0	34	1	15	50
Cinnamon Caramel Monkey Bread	140	0	0	0	32	1	16	55
Pillsbury Blueberry	120	2	1	0	24	1	14	100
Apple Cinnamon, Cranberry, or Date (avg)	125	2	1	0	26	1	14	115
Lemon Poppyseed	130	3	1	0	25	1	13	120
Nut	120	3	1	0	23	1	12	135
Pecan Swirl, Cinn Swirl, or Choc Chip Swirl (avg)	150	5	2	0	27	0	17	140
Rabbit Creek Gourmet *Flower Pot Breads*								
Cinnamon Swirl or Cranberry Orange (avg)	87	0	0	0	22	1	16	88
Cinnamon Raisin w/Glaze	120	0	0	0	30	1	21	88
Caramel Pecan or Funky Monkey Banana (avg)	90	2	0	0	19	1	14	90
Apple Spice Pecan	100	2	0	0	20	1	16	90
Cinnamon Oatmeal	100	1	0	0	23	1	13	90
Cranberry Nut Streusel	110	2	0	0	25	1	18	90
Maple Pecan w/Streusel	120	2	0	0	25	1	17	90
Raspberry Cream Cheese Swirl	101	0	0	0	24	0	18	93
Sweet Seasons Strawberry Bread	130	0	0	0	30	1	17	130
Caramel Apple	120	0	0	0	29	1	16	135
Lemon Bread	120	0	0	0	28	1	14	140
PASTRY DOUGH – FROZEN/REFRIGERATED (2 oz unless noted)								
Alessi Hand Rolled Mini Cannoli Shells, 1 shell	50	1	0	5	9	0	1	60
Hand Rolled Cannoli Shells, 1 shell	90	2	0	10	16	2	1	100
Apollo or **Athens** Mini Fillo Shells, 2 shells	35	2	0	0	4	0	0	25
Shredded Fillo Dough (Kataifi)	120	2	0	0	22	1	0	11
Bellino Cannoli Shells, 1 shell	45	0	0	5	8	0	1	50
Fillo Factory								
Mini Fillo Shells, 3 shells	45	2	0	0	7	0	0	30
Large Fillo Shells, 1 shell	80	2	0	0	13	0	0	55
Kataifi	180	2	0	0	35	4	1	140
Kineret Puff Pastry	200	12	5	0	22	0	0	110
Robert Rothschild Farm								
Mini Fillo Shells, 3	45	2	0	0	7	0	0	30
REDUCED SODIUM (LESS THAN GENERIC):								
Fillo Factory Organic Fillo Dough, 1.6 oz	130	1	0	0	28	1	0	160

(**BREAD CRUMBS**)

(see Bread Crumbs, pg 25)

	Cal	Fat	Sat	Chol	Carb	Fib	Sug	Sod

BREADSTICKS

	Cal	Fat	Sat	Chol	Carb	Fib	Sug	Sod
Plain, shelf-stable, 0.5 oz	60	2	0	0	11	1	0	150
Plain, ready-to-bake, 1 oz	63	1	0	0	10	0	0	167

Brands . . . *(0.5 oz unless noted)*

MIXES

	Cal	Fat	Sat	Chol	Carb	Fib	Sug	Sod
Chébé Breadsticks Onion & Garlic, 1/10	70	0	0	0	17	0	0	103

SHELF-STABLE

Aladdin Bakers *Old Little Italy* Breadsticks

	Cal	Fat	Sat	Chol	Carb	Fib	Sug	Sod
Onion	80	3	0	0	11	1	0	105
Wheat or Sesame	80	1	0	0	11	1	0	110
Garlic	60	1	0	0	12	1	0	120
Angonoa's *Deli-Style* Garlic Sesame	60	2	0	0	10	0	1	80
Sesame	70	3	0	0	10	1	0	110
Deli-Style Whole Wheat	60	2	0	0	9	2	1	120
Deli-Style or *Mini* Sesame	60	2	0	0	10	1	0	120
Cheese	60	1	0	0	11	1	1	120
Colavita Slim Breadsticks, 8	60	1	0	0	12	0	0	130
Dixie Carb Counters Plain	53	3	0	22	3	1	0	107
Garlic Parmesan	55	2	1	22	3	1	0	129
Fattorie & Pandea Grissini, Garlic	70	1	0	0	12	1	1	115
Whole Wheat	60	1	0	0	11	2	1	120
Sesame or Traditional (avg)	70	2	0	0	13	1	1	125
Glutino Sesame	60	2	1	0	13	0	0	100
Pizza Flavored	60	1	1	0	13	0	0	105
Granforno *Grissini* Sesame, 3	60	1	0	0	13	1	0	126
Onion, 3	66	1	0	0	14	1	0	132
Garlic or Rosemary, 3	72	1	0	0	14	1	0	138
Safeway Select Grissini, Toasted or Parmesan, 2	45	2	1	2	7	1	0	87
Sea Salt Grissini, 2	45	2	1	2	7	1	0	140
Seattle Int'l Italian or Sesame	60	1	0	0	12	1	0	120
Stella D'oro SF, 0.4 oz	45	1	0	0	7	0	1	0
Original, 0.4 oz	40	1	0	0	7	0	0	40
Sesame, 0.4 oz	50	2	0	0	7	0	0	45
Mini, Original, 0.6 oz	70	2	0	0	12	1	1	65
Mini, Sesame, 0.6 oz	80	4	1	0	11	1	1	75
Toufayan Sesame or Whole Wheat	45	1	0	0	9	1	1	80
Onion	55	1	0	0	11	1	1	90
Garlic, 2	55	1	0	0	11	1	1	95

BUNS AND SANDWICH ROLLS

(also see Dinner Rolls/Croissants, pg 55)

	Cal	Fat	Sat	Chol	Carb	Fib	Sug	Sod
Sandwich thins, 1.5 oz roll	100	1	0	0	21	6	2	230
Hot dog or hamburger bun, 1.5 oz	114	2	1	0	22	3	4	230
Kaiser roll, 2 oz	167	2	0	0	30	1	1	310
Hoagie/submarine, med, 3.4 oz	250	4	1	0	48	7	8	449

Brands . . . *(1 bun or roll unless noted)*

MIXES

REDUCED SODIUM (LESS THAN GENERIC):

	Cal	Fat	Sat	Chol	Carb	Fib	Sug	Sod
Dixie Carb Counters Bun & Roll Mix	23	0	0	0	4	3	0	197

SHELF-STABLE

	Cal	Fat	Sat	Chol	Carb	Fib	Sug	Sod
Barowsky's Organic Hamburger or Hot Dog	150	2	0	0	29	1	6	115
Cobblestone Mill Mini Sandwich	70	1	0	0	14	0	2	130

BREAD AND FLOUR PRODUCTS
Buns and Sandwich Rolls

	Cal	Fat	Sat	Chol	Carb	Fib	Sug	Sod
Get Healthy America! Gluten Free Hot Dog	120	3	1	30	20	1	3	120
Irenes Bakery Low-Carb Hot Dog or Hamburger..	40	0	0	0	5	0	0	60
Martin's Potato Rolls, Sliced, 1.3 oz	90	1	0	0	16	2	4	130
Potato Rolls, Whole Wheat, 1.3 oz	80	1	0	0	15	4	4	135
Natural Ovens Better Wheat Buns	170	3	0	0	30	3	5	140
Nature's Own Butter Sandwich Buns.............	120	2	2	5	23	1	2	115
S Rosen's Slammer Buns, 3" bun	140	1	0	0	19	1	2	105
Sami's Bakery Millet/Flax Hamburger or Hot Dog.	76	1	0	0	15	2	0	90
Sara Lee *Soft & Smooth* Mini Buns White........	90	1	0	0	18	1	3	110
REDUCED SODIUM (LESS THAN GENERIC):								
Arnold/Brownberry Potato Hot Dog...........	130	2	0	0	24	1	4	200
Aunt Millie's *Hearth* Organic Multigrain Hot Dog..	110	2	0	0	20	1	2	190
Hearth Deluxe Whole Grain Hot Dog	100	2	0	0	19	2	2	200
Better Bread Co Sandwich Rolls	170	6	2	10	34	3	4	200
Bread du Juor Italian Rolls	90	1	0	0	16	0	2	190
Cobblestone Mill Hot Dog	120	3	1	0	22	1	4	200
Country Hearth *Kids' Choice* Hot Dog/Burger	110	2	1	0	21	3	4	180
Country Kitchen Lite Wheat Hot Dog	80	2	0	0	17	4	1	160
EarthGrains *Thin Buns* 100% Multi-Grain.....	100	2	0	0	21	4	3	150
Thin Buns 100% Whole Wheat....................	100	2	0	0	22	4	3	160
Ener-G Tapioca Hamburger or Hot Dog..........	100	3	0	0	18	4	2	150
Seattle Brown Hamburger or Hot Dog...........	160	5	0	0	34	8	4	190
Food for Life *Ezekiel* Hamburger or Hot Dog ..	170	2	0	0	34	6	0	170
Ezekiel Sesame Hamburger	170	2	0	0	32	6	0	180
Franz Hot Dog, Potato or Whole Grain..........	110	2	0	0	22	3	3	200
Great Value Whole Wheat Hot Dog	110	2	0	0	21	3	2	170
Whole Wheat Hamburger	130	2	1	0	24	3	2	200
Healthy Life Wheat, Hot Dog or Sandwich....	80	1	0	0	19	5	3	200
Heiner's Hamburger.................................	100	2	0	0	18	1	3	190
King's Hawaiian Sweet Snacker Rolls	220	6	3	34	36	2	14	194
Martin's Potato Rolls, Party	130	2	0	0	26	3	6	190
Potato Rolls, Long or Sandwich (avg)..........	130	2	0	0	26	4	7	200
Mrs. Baird's Hot Dog..............................	110	2	0	0	20	1	3	170
100% Whole Wheat Hot Dog	110	2	0	0	19	3	3	180
Nature Bake Surviva Sandwich or Hot Dog...	160	3	0	0	28	4	5	190
Nature's Own Double Fiber Wheat Sandwich...	80	2	0	0	15	5	2	160
Whitewheat Hog Dog..............................	80	2	0	0	18	4	2	190
Nickles Bakery Sesame Hamburger.............	130	2	0	0	23	2	0	180
Small Beef Buns	90	1	0	0	19	1	0	190
Pepperidge Farm *Classic* Wheat Sliders........	100	2	0	0	17	1	3	150
Classic White Sliders...............................	100	2	0	0	18	1	3	160
Classic Hamburger	120	2	1	0	22	1	3	180
Classic 100% Whole Wheat Hamburger	120	2	0	0	18	2	3	190
Classic Whole Grain Hamburger	100	1	0	0	18	2	2	190
Classic Hot Dog....................................	140	3	1	0	26	1	4	190
Roman Meal Multi-Grain Burger or Hot Dog..	110	2	0	0	20	2	4	200
Sara Lee *80 Calorie & Delightful* Wheat Hot Dog..	80	1	0	0	15	6	4	160
80 Calorie & Delightful Wheat Hamburger ...	80	1	0	0	15	6	4	160
Soft & Smooth Whole Grain White Hot Dog....	120	2	0	0	22	2	3	190
Soft & Smooth Whole Grain White Hamburger..	120	2	0	0	22	2	3	190
Soft & Smooth Wheat Hot Dog or Hamburger..	120	2	0	0	22	2	3	190
Schwebel's *Lite* Hot Dog or *Lite* Sandwich	70	0	0	0	19	5	2	170
S Rosen's Mini Hot Dog	80	2	0	0	15	1	2	160
Mary Ann Hamburger	140	2	0	0	26	1	4	180
Thomas *Breakfast Thins*, 1.5 oz (avg)..........	100	1	0	0	22	5	2	170

	Cal	Fat	Sat	Chol	Carb	Fib	Sug	Sod
Village Hearth								
Light Italian or Wheat Hot Dog or Hamburger..	80	1	0	0	20	7	2	190
Slender Rounds Multigrain..........................	90	1	0	0	22	7	2	200
Wegmans Potato, Hot Dog or Hamburger.....	120	2	0	0	23	1	3	180
Food You Feel Good About Lite Hot Dog								
or *Lite* Hamburger	90	1	0	0	21	4	2	190

CORNBREAD

(see Cornbread, pg 58)

CREPES

(see Blintzes/Crepes, pg 138)

CROUTONS

(see Salad Toppings, pg 87)

DINNER ROLLS AND CROISSANTS

	Cal	Fat	Sat	Chol	Carb	Fib	Sug	Sod
Dinner roll, brown and serve, 1 oz	87	2	0	0	15	1	2	150
Dough, refrig, 1 oz.....................................	110	2	1	0	19	1	3	250
Croissant, butter, 1 oz................................	150	6	4	19	13	1	3	212
Crescent roll dough, refrig, 1 oz	110	6	2	0	11	0	2	220

Brands . . . *(1 roll unless noted)*
FROZEN/REFRIGERATED

	Cal	Fat	Sat	Chol	Carb	Fib	Sug	Sod
Rhodes White Dinner	95	2	0	0	17	0	2	140

SHELF-STABLE

	Cal	Fat	Sat	Chol	Carb	Fib	Sug	Sod
Butternut Brown N Serve...........................	70	1	0	0	13	1	1	135
Cobblestone Mill Pistolettes.......................	90	1	0	0	19	1	0	115
Ener-G Tapioca Dinner	100	3	0	0	18	4	2	125
Franz Brown 'n Serve................................	80	2	0	0	13	2	2	120
Gold Medal Finger Rolls	80	2	0	0	13	1	2	140
Heiner's Split Top Brown & Serve	70	2	0	0	14	1	1	130
King's Hawaiian Sweet Rolls.......................	100	3	2	15	16	1	6	80
Honey Wheat Rolls	90	2	1	15	14	1	4	95
Savory Butter Rolls	90	3	2	20	14	1	3	115
Marshall's Yeast Rolls, Parker House	90	4	1	5	13	0	-	115
Martin's Potato Rolls.................................	90	1	0	0	17	2	4	130
Mrs Baird's Dinner Rolls.............................	80	2	0	0	13	1	2	110
Nature's Own Honey Wheat Dinner..............	50	0	0	0	10	1	1	80
Nickles Bakery Finger Rolls........................	80	1	0	0	14	0	0	130
Pepperidge Farms Parkerhouse Dinner	80	2	1	0	14	1	2	95
Schwebel's Country Potato Minis	65	1	0	0	12	1	2	120
Sunbeam Heat 'n Serve Rolls......................	80	2	0	0	14	1	1	140
Wegmans *Food You Feel Good About*								
Dinner Rolls..	80	1	0	0	15	0	2	130

DONUTS

(see Donuts, pg 68)

ENGLISH MUFFINS

	Cal	Fat	Sat	Chol	Carb	Fib	Sug	Sod
Cinnamon-raisin english muffin, 2.3 oz	137	2	0	0	27	2	8	189
Plain or sourdough english muffin, 2.3 oz	134	1	0	0	26	2	2	264
Mixed-grain or granola english muffin, 2.3 oz	155	2	1	0	31	2	1	275
Whole wheat english muffin, 2.3 oz	134	1	0	0	27	4	5	312

BREAD AND FLOUR PRODUCTS
Matzo Balls and Dumplings

	Cal	Fat	Sat	Chol	Carb	Fib	Sug	Sod
Brands . . . *(1 muffin unless noted)*								
Food for Life Genesis 1:29	180	4	0	0	30	6	0	140
Gold Medal Premium	130	2	0	0	26	1	6	110
Healthy Life 100% Whole Wheat	100	1	0	0	18	2	2	60
Mediterranean Sweet Muffins......................	120	4	1	10	17	1	3	125
Thomas Triple Health	100	1	0	0	25	6	1	130
REDUCED SODIUM (LESS THAN GENERIC):								
Aunt Millie's Cinn Raisin English Muffin........	110	1	0	0	23	3	5	190
Whole Wheat..	100	1	0	0	21	3	2	200
David's Deli French Toast English Muffin ...	120	1	0	0	24	1	4	190
Fiber One Light Wheat..............................	100	1	0	0	24	8	2	150
Light Multigrain..	100	1	0	0	24	8	2	160
Food for Life Ezekiel 4:9	160	1	0	0	30	6	0	160
Ezekiel Cinnamon-Raisin	160	0	0	0	36	4	10	170
Franz 100 Calorie Multigrain	100	1	0	0	26	7	1	170
Old Fashioned Raisin	150	1	0	0	30	3	7	170
Hawaiian English Muffins............................	130	1	0	0	27	1	8	190
Gold Medal Multi-Wheat	130	2	0	0	25	1	3	180
Honey Wheat	120	1	0	0	23	1	3	190
Healthy Life Light Multi-Grain....................	80	1	0	0	17	4	0	150
Light English Muffins	90	0	0	0	21	6	1	200
Pepperidge Farm Original	130	2	1	0	25	1	1	170
Sun-Maid Raisin	170	1	0	0	36	2	13	180
Thomas Multi-Grain..................................	150	3	0	0	27	2	3	160
Cinnamon Raisin..	140	1	0	0	29	1	8	170
Light Multi-Grain..	100	1	0	5	26	8	1	180
Honey Wheat	130	1	0	0	26	1	3	180
Original Plain...	120	1	0	0	25	1	1	200
Health-Full 10 Grain	130	1	0	0	29	6	2	200
Vermont Bread Organic Cinnamon Raisin Spelt ..	140	1	0	0	30	4	7	180
Organic Honey Wheat................................	140	1	0	0	30	2	6	200
Wegman's 100% Whole Wheat....................	120	1	0	0	22	3	2	190
Lite Split...	90	0	0	0	21	6	1	200
Western Bagel Original or Sourdough	140	1	0	0	27	1	1	190

MATZO BALLS AND DUMPLINGS

	Cal	Fat	Sat	Chol	Carb	Fib	Sug	Sod
(also see Soups, pg 231)								
Matzo ball mix, 2 tbsp....................................	50	0	0	0	1	1	0	700
Brands . . . *(2 tbsp unless noted)*								
FROZEN/REFRIGERATED								
Mary B's Open Kettle Dumplings, 6 oz............	160	4	2	0	28	1	0	40
Meal Mart Matzoh Balls, 3.3 oz	130	5	1	95	16	1	1	30
MIXES								
REDUCED SODIUM (LESS THAN GENERIC):								
Croyden House Dumpling/Matzo Ball Mix.....	50	0	0	0	12	1	0	190
Goodman's Reduced Sodium Matzo Ball Mix ..	50	0	0	0	11	0	0	150
Haddar Shmura Matzo Ball Mix	75	0	0	0	17	1	0	200
Streit's Whole Wheat Matzo Ball Mix	50	0	0	0	12	0	0	170
Yehuda Matzos Matzo Ball Mix, 4 balls	65	0	0	0	13	0	0	210

MUFFINS AND SCONES

	Cal	Fat	Sat	Chol	Carb	Fib	Sug	Sod
Banana nut muffin, mix, 1/4 cup	150	5	1	5	23	0	11	205
Blueberry muffin, ready-to-eat, small, 2.4 oz ...	259	13	0	26	33	1	18	208
Mix, 1/12 pkg...	140	2	1	0	30	1	14	250

56

	Cal	Fat	Sat	Chol	Carb	Fib	Sug	Sod
Ready-to-eat, medium, 4 oz	444	22	0	45	56	2	31	356
Ready-to-eat, extra large, 6 oz	660	32	0	67	83	3	45	529
Oat bran muffin, ready-to-eat, small, 2.4 oz	178	5	1	0	32	3	5	259
Apple cinnamon muffin, mix, 1/4 cup	170	5	3	0	28	1	13	300
Corn muffin, small, 2.4 oz	201	6	1	17	34	2	5	344
Mix, 1/6 pkg	160	5	2	5	27	1	7	340
Scone mix, 1/12 pkg	170	9	2	0	20	1	4	410

Brands . . . *(1 muffin or scone unless noted)*

MUFFINS

FROZEN/REFRIGERATED
Isabella's Healthy Bakery

	Cal	Fat	Sat	Chol	Carb	Fib	Sug	Sod
FF Choc, 3.9 oz	220	0	0	0	48	4	26	110
FF Mt Blueberry or FF Blueberry, 3.9 oz	220	0	0	0	48	2	26	120
No Sugar Added Mountain Berry, 3.9 oz	300	10	2	50	52	2	2	120
No Sugar Added Raisin Bran, 3.9 oz	340	12	2	40	62	4	8	130
FF Cinnamon Apple, 3.9 oz	240	0	0	0	50	2	28	130
No Sugar Added Apple Explosion, 3.9 oz	300	10	2	40	58	2	2	130
No Sugar Added Banana Nut, 3.9 oz	320	12	2	50	54	2	4	130
No Sugar Added Cinnamon Streusel, 3.9 oz ..	340	12	3	40	60	2	2	130
No Sugar Added Blueberry Burst, 3.9 oz	300	10	2	50	56	2	2	140

REDUCED SODIUM (LESS THAN GENERIC):
Isabella's Healthy Bakery

	Cal	Fat	Sat	Chol	Carb	Fib	Sug	Sod
Sugar Free Lemon Poppy, 3.9 oz	340	12	2	50	60	2	24	160

MIXES

	Cal	Fat	Sat	Chol	Carb	Fib	Sug	Sod
Barefoot Contessa Foolproof Popover Mix ...	100	0	0	0	20	1	2	130
Cravings Place								
Dbl Choc Chunk Cookie/Muffin	70	2	1	0	11	1	4	30
Gluten Free Essentials Spice Cake/Muffin....	77	1	0	0	17	1	4	120
Iveta Gourmet								
Lemon Poppy Seed	90	0	0	0	19	1	8	95
Apricot White Choc or Blueberry (avg)	120	1	1	0	26	1	11	125
Double Dutch Choc	130	3	2	0	25	1	14	130
Cranberry Spice	120	0	0	0	26	1	13	135
King Arthur Flour								
Cinn Chip Muffin/Bread	160	1	0	0	35	1	17	115
Martha White								
LF Blueberry or Apple Cinnamon	130	2	1	0	27	1	16	135
LF Strawberry	130	2	1	0	27	1	16	140
Pantry Shelf Cinnamon Fudge	140	0	0	0	33	1	21	60
Golden Pumpkin	130	0	0	0	31	1	17	75
Blueberries 'N' Cream	130	2	0	0	26	0	15	120
Pelican Bay Apple Bread Muffin	140	0	0	0	33	1	19	85

REDUCED SODIUM (LESS THAN GENERIC):

	Cal	Fat	Sat	Chol	Carb	Fib	Sug	Sod
Authenic Foods Choc Chip	150	5	3	0	29	3	17	150
Bernard Hi-Pro Bran or Blueberry..............	155	4	2	0	27	3	15	160
Bob's Red Mill								
Oat Bran & Date Nut	120	2	0	0	22	2	1	160
Raisin Bran or Date Nut Bran (avg)	65	1	0	0	13	2	2	160
King Arthur Flour								
Cinnamon Struesel	290	1	0	0	66	2	37	150
Double Dutch Choc Muffin & Bread	170	3	2	0	38	2	22	150
Martha White								
Cranberry Orange	140	4	2	5	25	0	13	150
Apple Cinnamon or Cinnamon Sugar	140	4	2	5	24	0	13	150

BREAD AND FLOUR PRODUCTS
Muffins and Scones

	Cal	Fat	Sat	Chol	Carb	Fib	Sug	Sod
Whole Grains Apple Cinn or Blueberry	140	4	2	5	24	1	13	150
Strawberry, Raspberry, Blueberry or WildBerry	140	4	2	5	24	0	13	150
Lemon Poppy Seed or Pound Cake (avg)	150	4	2	7	27	1	14	160
Choc Choc or Choc Choc Chip	140	5	3	5	25	1	13	160
New Hope Mills Orange Cranberry Muffin/Bread	60	1	0	0	6	4	0	150
Pillsbury Lemon Poppy Seed	150	4	1	5	27	1	13	160
Stickey Fingers Morning Glory	220	7	3	20	35	1	13	160

MUFFINS – SHELF-STABLE

	Cal	Fat	Sat	Chol	Carb	Fib	Sug	Sod
Aunt Millie's Brownie Muffin 1.9 oz	220	9	2	15	35	2	24	130
Awrey's Apple, 1.5 oz	160	7	1	25	20	0	9	140
Blueberry or Cranberry, 1.5 oz	160	7	0	30	19	0	8	140
Petite Lemon Poppy Seed, 1.7 oz	190	11	2	30	20	0	10	140
Toaster Rounds Cranberry Orange, 1.5 oz	160	7	1	20	19	0	9	140
Toaster Rounds Blueberry, 1.5 oz	160	7	1	20	19	0	8	140
Breadsmith Apple Cinnamon Walnut, 5 oz	480	23	2	70	63	2	35	140
Chatila's Bakery Blueberry Muffin, 2.9 oz	130	3	0	10	28	4	1	140
Entemann's Little Bites 100 Calorie Choc Chip	100	5	1	10	13	0	9	65
100 Calorie Blueberry, 0.8 oz	100	4	1	10	12	0	7	90
Banana Choc Chip, 1.7 oz	180	8	2	20	20	1	17	125
Choc Chip, 1.7 oz	190	9	3	20	26	1	17	135
Golden Star Bakery Apple Cinnamon, 2 oz	134	0	0	0	30	2	7	25
Raisin Bran Muffins, 2 oz	108	0	0	0	24	4	9	25
Blueberry Muffin, 2 oz	158	0	0	0	30	2	7	25
Hill & Valley Sugar Free Blueberry Mini, 1 oz	80	3	1	15	11	0	1	130
Sugar Free Apple Walnut Mini, 1 oz	80	4	1	15	11	0	0	135
Sugar Free Lemon Poppy Mini, 1 oz	80	4	1	20	12	0	0	140
Hostess 100 Calorie Banana, 1.1 oz (3)	100	4	1	10	19	4	7	120
Isabella's Activate Probiotic Raisin Bran, 3 oz	210	8	2	30	34	7	14	85
Little Debbie Lemon	200	8	2	10	28	0	17	130
Double Choc	200	8	2	10	28	1	17	140
VitaMuffin VitaTops Banana Nut, 2 oz	100	2	0	0	19	5	3	120
Banana Nut, Sugar Free, 2 oz	90	3	0	0	21	5	0	125
Apple-Berry Bran, 2 oz	100	0	0	0	23	6	8	140
Multi-Bran or Cran-Bran, 2 oz	100	0	0	0	22	5	11	140
VitaTops CranBran or MultiBran, 2 oz	100	1	0	0	22	5	11	140
Blue-Bran, 2 oz	100	0	0	0	20	5	9	140
VitaTops BlueBran or Deep Choc, 2 oz (avg)	100	2	0	0	21	5	9	140
Chocolate, Sugar Free, 2 oz	80	2	1	0	23	6	0	140
VitaTops Apple Berry, 2 oz	100	1	0	0	23	6	8	140
VitaTops Dark Choc Pomegranate, 2 oz	100	2	0	0	21	6	11	140
VitaTops Velvety Choc, Sugar Free, 2 oz	80	2	1	0	23	6	0	140

REDUCED SODIUM (LESS THAN GENERIC):

	Cal	Fat	Sat	Chol	Carb	Fib	Sug	Sod
Aunt Millie's Blueberry, 1.9 oz	165	8	2	35	23	3	12	150
Coffee Cake or Choc Chip, 1.9 oz (avg)	190	9	3	35	25	3	16	150
Awrey's Banana, 1.5 oz	180	8	2	30	21	0	10	160
Petitie Blueberry or Banana Nut, 1.7 oz (avg)	175	9	2	30	20	0	10	160
Otis Spunkmeyer Reduced Fat Choc Chip	170	6	2	30	28	1	15	160
Reduced Fat Apple Cinnamon, 1.8 oz	170	5	1	30	27	1	15	160

CORNBREAD
FROZEN/REFRIGERATED
REDUCED SODIUM (LESS THAN GENERIC):

	Cal	Fat	Sat	Chol	Carb	Fib	Sug	Sod
Isabella's Sugar Free Native Corn	340	12	2	50	60	2	24	150
Upper Crust Corn Bread, 2 oz	180	5	2	25	33	1	16	170

	Cal	Fat	Sat	Chol	Carb	Fib	Sug	Sod
MIXES								
Bernard Cornbread & Muffin Mix	150	2	1	0	31	1	0	20
Chi-Chi's Fiest Sweet Corn Cakes Mix	100	0	0	0	23	0	11	130
Dixie Carb Counters Cornbread	32	1	0	0	5	2	1	124
El Torito Sweet Corn Cakes	100	1	0	0	22	0	11	120
Ener-G Corn Mix	110	1	0	0	24	1	0	135
Firenza Traditional Sweet Corn Bread...........	100	0	0	0	23	1	9	100
Sylvia's Golden Cornbread & Muffin	170	5	1	0	29	1	12	135
VitaMuffin Golden Corn Mix........................	90	1	0	0	25	6	9	135
REDUCED SODIUM (LESS THAN GENERIC)								
Dixie Carb Counters Cornbread	51	0	0	0	8	4	0	156
SHELF-STABLE								
VitaMuffin Golden Corn Muffins......................	100	1	0	0	25	6	9	135
REDUCED SODIUM (LESS THAN GENERIC):								
Awrey's Cornbread, 1.5 oz......................	180	9	2	30	22	0	11	160
Cornbread Toaster Rounds, 1.5 oz...........	180	9	2	30	22	0	11	160
SCONES								
MIXES								
Bette's Diner Raisin Scone Mix	229	0	0	0	30	1	9	129
Garvey's Organic Scone Mix	110	1	0	0	23	1	2	140
Gluten-Free Pantry Muffin & Scone	100	0	0	0	24	0	7	120
King Arthur Flour								
Choc Chunk Scone Mix	240	4	2	0	49	2	19	115
Cinnamon Filled Cream Scone Mix	240	1	0	0	54	1	26	120
Strawberries & Cream Scone Mix	210	1	0	0	48	2	21	135
Cranberry-Orange Scone Mix	200	1	0	0	45	1	16	135
Cherry Almond Scone Mix	230	2	0	0	49	2	20	135
Peaches & Cream Scone Mix......................	210	1	0	0	47	1	20	135
Vermont Maple-Oat Scone Mix	170	0	0	0	38	1	12	135
Lemon-Ginger Scone Mix	230	2	1	0	49	1	19	140
Rabbit Creek Gourmet								
Maple Pecan..	80	2	1	0	16	1	8	140
Cherry Almond, Key Lime, or Lemon Blueberry .	65	2	1	0	13	1	5	140
Lemon Blueberry or Peaches & Cream (avg)	67	2	1	0	13	1	5	140
Lemon Poppy or Raspberry Lemon Sparkler ..	80	2	0	0	15	1	7	140
Sarah's Choc Chip Raspberry	69	2	1	0	12	1	5	140
Snowball..	85	3	1	0	15	1	5	140
Grandpa Joe's Spicy Cranberry-Apple..........	80	2	1	0	17	1	8	140
Cinnamony Oatmeal w/Sprinkles................	80	2	1	0	16	1	5	140
Berry! Berry! Quite Contrary.....................	70	2	1	0	14	1	7	140
REDUCED SODIUM (LESS THAN GENERIC):								
Iveta Gourmet								
Ginger..	100	0	0	0	28	1	4	150
Vanilla, Maple, or Lemon (avg)	100	0	0	0	25	1	6	160
Sugar-Free Vanilla	100	0	0	0	23	1	0	160
Blueberry, Strawberry, or Raspberry (avg)...	130	0	0	0	29	1	10	160
Apple Spice, Golden Raisin, or Currant	130	0	0	0	29	1	10	160
Apricot...	130	0	0	0	23	1	5	160
Orange, Cranberry, or Cranberry Orange (avg) .	130	0	0	0	28	1	8	160
Lemon Ginger or Lemon Currant..............	130	0	0	0	28	1	8	160
Choc Chip or Cinnamon Chip	160	3	2	0	29	2	10	160
King Arthur Flour Cream Tea Scone Mix ...	200	1	0	0	43	1	11	150
Harvest Pumpkin Whole Wheat Scone Mix ...	200	1	0	0	45	5	22	150
Almond Filled Cream Scone Mix	260	3	0	0	53	1	24	150

BREAD AND FLOUR PRODUCTS
Pita and Pocket Breads

	Cal	Fat	Sat	Chol	Carb	Fib	Sug	Sod
Rabbit Creek Gourmet								
White Choc Raspberry	87	3	1	0	16	1	5	141
Aunt Catherine's Cranberry Orange	63	2	0	0	12	0	4	144
Aunt Hannah's Cinnamon Raisin..............	65	2	0	0	13	0	4	144
Uncle Edgar's Cinnamon Apple.................	65	2	0	0	13	0	5	144
Peanut Butter w/Sugar Sprinkles	90	3	2	0	16	1	6	150

PITA AND POCKET BREADS

	Cal	Fat	Sat	Chol	Carb	Fib	Sug	Sod
Whole Wheat pita, small 4" diam, 1	74	1	0	0	15	2	1	149
Large, 6.5" diam, 1	170	2	0	0	35	5	1	340
White pita, small 4" diam, 1...........................	77	0	0	0	16	1	0	150
Large, 6.5" diam, 1	165	1	0	0	33	1	1	322
Brands . . . *(1 pita unless noted)*								
Aladdin's Mini Plain Pocket Pita	70	0	0	0	15	1	1	140
Atie's Bakery Pocket Pita								
Sesame or Onion (avg).............................	95	0	0	0	20	2	1	60
White, or Whole Wheat (avg)......................	95	0	0	0	20	2	1	60
Damascus Bakeries								
Plain Pita, Salt Free	150	0	0	0	32	2	0	0
Mini Pita, Whole Wheat or Plain...................	65	0	0	0	14	2	0	75
Joseph's Soy Protein Pita, 1/2	120	0	0	0	18	1	2	130
Sandwich Size	80	0	0	0	15	1	1	130
Kangaroo								
Sandwich Pockets, Whole Grain	80	1	0	0	16	4	1	100
Salad Pockets, Wheat or White (avg)	85	0	0	0	17	2	1	140
King of Pita Gyro Pita................................	234	2	0	0	45	5	1	110
Toufayan Pita Bread, Whole Wheat...............	140	0	0	0	31	3	1	130
Yasmeen Bakery Pita Bread	138	1	0	0	29	5	2	80
REDUCED SODIUM (LESS THAN GENERIC):								
Joseph's Party Pita, 1.5 oz (6 pcs)	120	1	0	0	23	1	1	180
Whole Wheat..	120	1	0	0	23	4	1	180
Paramount Whole Wheat Pita....................	180	0	0	0	24	2	2	180
Toufayan White Pita Bread........................	160	0	0	0	33	1	2	160

ROLLS AND SANDWICH BUNS

(see Buns/Sandwich Rolls, pg 53; Dinner Rolls/Croissants, pg 55)

STUFFING/DRESSING

	Cal	Fat	Sat	Chol	Carb	Fib	Sug	Sod
Cornbread stuffing, dry mix, 1 oz	110	1	0	0	22	4	1	365
Prepared, 1 cup	179	9	2	0	22	3	4	455
Bread stuffing, dry mix, 1 oz...........................	109	1	0	0	22	1	2	451
Prepared, 1 cup	177	9	2	0	22	3	2	543
Brands . . . *(1 oz or 1 cup unless noted)*								
Franz Seasoned Stuffing...............................	110	2	0	0	20	2	2	120
Gillian's Foods Gluten Free Stuffing	15	1	0	0	2	0	0	20
Martin's Potatobread Stuffing soft cube..........	80	1	0	0	15	2	4	120
REDUCED SODIUM (LESS THAN GENERIC):								
Arrowhead Mills Savory Herb Stuffing, 1/2 c...	120	3	0	0	20	1	0	240
Classic Herb Cornbread, 1/3 cup	130	4	1	0	21	1	0	250
Canterbury Organics Herbes De Province Mix ..	140	5	1	0	19	1	1	160
Rosemary Sage Cornbread Mix, 1.3 oz........	150	34	1	0	30	1	16	210
Stove Top Chicken, lower sodium.................	110	1	0	0	22	1	2	250

WRAPS, FLATBREAD AND OTHER ROLL-UP BREADS

(also see Pizza Crust/Dough, pg 149; Tortillas/Taco Shells, pg 167)

	Cal	Fat	Sat	Chol	Carb	Fib	Sug	Sod
Lavash, plain, 2 oz	220	0	0	0	42	2	2	210
Flatbread, plain, 2 oz	260	2	1	0	38	2	2	320
Flour tortilla, 10"	218	5	1	0	36	2	1	445

Brands . . . *(1 wrap or flatbread unless noted)*

MIXES

	Cal	Fat	Sat	Chol	Carb	Fib	Sug	Sod
Little Chief Fry Bread	100	0	0	0	21	1	3	105

SHELF-STABLE

	Cal	Fat	Sat	Chol	Carb	Fib	Sug	Sod
Best Pita Whole Wheat	90	0	0	0	18	3	1	62
White	90	0	0	0	18	1	1	65
Boghosian *Valley Bread* White Lavash	130	3	0	0	23	1	2	125
Flatout Mini, Healthy Grain Flatbread	70	1	0	0	13	3	2	140
Garden City Foods Lavash, White	110	2	0	0	23	1	0	20
Whole Wheat	110	2	0	0	23	4	0	30
Indianlife Carb Life Roti	90	5	1	0	15	3	2	15
Indian Homestyle Roti	120	4	0	0	20	1	0	75
New Soft Roti or New Soft Chapati	130	4	0	0	20	3	0	95
Joseph's Lavash Roll-Ups	140	0	0	0	28	1	1	140
Nu-World Foods Amaranth Flatbread								
Sorghum, Buckwheat, or Garbanzo (avg)	161	4	1	0	30	5	0	12
Santa Fe Flatbread Co Garlic Onion	120	4	1	0	18	1	0	75
Tomato Oregano	120	4	1	0	19	1	0	80
Tumaro's *Soy-full Heart* Flatbread								
8 Grain 'N Soy	100	3	0	0	14	4	1	60
Apple Cinnamon or Wheat, Soy & Flax	90	3	0	0	14	4	1	65

REDUCED SODIUM (LESS THAN GENERIC):

	Cal	Fat	Sat	Chol	Carb	Fib	Sug	Sod
Damascus Bakeries								
Plain or Wheat Wrap, 1/2	130	0	0	0	29	1	1	150
Flatout Mini, Mediterranean Herb Flatbread	70	1	0	0	12	1	1	160
Kidz, Cinnamon Burst Flatbread	60	1	0	0	11	4	3	160
Mini, Southwest Chipotle Flatbread	70	1	0	0	13	1	1	170
Kidz, Original Flatbread	60	1	0	0	12	4	2	170
Mini, Whole Wheat Flatbread	70	1	0	0	14	2	2	180
Mini, Harvest Wheat Flatbread	70	1	0	0	13	3	2	190
Mini, French Toast Flatbread	70	1	0	0	14	1	3	190
JJ's Flats Breadflats, Flavorall	60	3	1	0	9	1	1	150
Pita Gourmet Flatbread, Whole Wheat	130	3	1	0	21	2	0	180
Flatbread, White	120	3	0	0	21	1	0	190
Sami's Bakery Slim Trim Lavash	65	1	0	0	11	11	0	160
Whole Wheat Lavash	84	0	0	0	17	12	0	160
Light Lavash	56	1	0	0	12	8	0	200
Santa Fe Flatbread Co Garlic Onion	110	3	1	0	19	1	1	150
Tumaro's *Wraps*								
Chipotle Chili & Peppers or Honey Wheat	170	2	0	0	34	2	1	200
Garden Spinach & Veg or Jalapeno & Cilantro	170	3	0	0	34	2	1	210
Tomato & Basil	170	2	0	0	34	2	2	210
Yasmeen Bakery Saj Bread	161	1	0	0	39	1	1	168

BREAKFAST FOODS

See RESOURCES, *page 305, for a partial list of manufacturers and retailers offering low-salt products online or visit* **LowSaltFoods.com** *for additional sources.*

BREAKFAST FOODS

BAGELS
(see Bagels, pg 47)

BREAKFAST BARS
(see Granola/Cereal/Breakfast Bars, pg 69)

BREAKFAST, MEAL REPLACEMENT AND NUTRITION DRINKS
(see Diet/Meal Replacement/Nutritional Drinks, pg 39)

BREAKFAST MEALS – FROZEN
(also see Pancakes/Waffles/French Toast, pg 70; Blintzes/Crepes, pg 138)

	Cal	Fat	Sat	Chol	Carb	Fib	Sug	Sod
Cinnamon french toast & sausage, 5.6 oz	415	23	7	98	38	2	0	502
Eggs, sausage & hash browns, 6.3 oz	361	27	7	283	17	1	0	772
Breakfast burrito, sausage, egg & cheese, 4.8 oz	350	21	8	139	28	1	2	810
Sausage, egg & cheese croissant, 4.5 oz	440	30	10	135	30	1	5	870
Sausage biscuit sandwich, 3.4 oz	385	22	7	32	23	1	0	881
Sausage biscuits & gravy, 6.7 oz	340	18	6	15	35	1	3	1070

Brands . . . *(4.5 oz serving unless noted)*

REDUCED SODIUM (LESS THAN GENERIC):

	Cal	Fat	Sat	Chol	Carb	Fib	Sug	Sod
Amy's Breakfast Scramble Wrap, 5.5 oz	380	19	5	10	30	4	1	490
Bob Evans Pigs in Blanket Sausage w/Cheese.	160	9	2	10	23	1	5	380
Brunch Bowls French Toast w/Berries, 10 oz	450	16	9	140	72	2	42	480
Sausage Sandwiches, 2	310	16	-	30	22	0	-	490
Oatmeal Bowl Hearty Blueberry	240	4	1	0	50	5	14	490
Oatmeal Bowl Cinnamon Raisin	270	4	1	0	57	5	21	490
Oatmeal Bowl Apple Cinnamon	280	4	1	0	58	5	22	490
Oatmeal Bowl Cranberry Pecan	290	7	2	0	53	5	17	490
El Monterey Brkfast Wrap Egg/Sausage/Cheese	280	16	7	150	21	0	2	450
Glutenfreeda Breakfast Burrito, 4 oz	199	8	3	27	23	2	1	150
Great Day Foods *Sausage Rolls* Cheddar, 2 oz	170	9	3	20	18	1	3	410
Sausage Rolls Jalapeno, 2 oz (1)	190	9	4	20	18	1	4	450
Piggies 'n Pancakes on a Stick, 2.5 oz	240	16	5	20	18	2	6	480
Mini Piggies 'n Pancakes, 2.6 oz (3)	260	25	4	35	19	1	5	480
Jimmy Dean Blueberry Pancakes/Sausage Stick	230	13	4	20	23	0	10	340
Original Pancakes & Sausage Stick	220	13	4	20	21	0	8	350
Minis Pancakes & Sausage, Blueberry	260	18	6	30	19	0	8	470
Kellogg's *Eggo Real Fruit Pizza*								
Mixed Berry Granola, 5.4 oz	390	13	6	15	62	4	17	390
Strawberry Granola, 5.4 oz	400	12	6	10	66	4	18	390
Lean Pockets Sausage, Egg & Cheese, 1	280	8	4	55	40	2	11	430
Ham, Egg & Cheese, 1	270	7	4	60	40	1	12	460
Applewood, Bacon, Egg & Cheese, 1	290	8	4	65	40	2	12	480
Las Campanas Breakfast Wraps, 1	190	8	2	55	25	1	0	350
Market Day Mini Cheese Omelets, 2 oz	60	2	2	5	2	0	0	170
Purnell's Country Sausage & Biscuits, 2	280	16	5	30	30	1	2	250
Country Sausage & Buttermilk Biscuits, 2	278	16	6	26	24	2	0	432
Tennessee Pride Turkey Sausage Biscuits, 2.	200	5	2	25	29	2	6	470
Sausage & Maple Pancakes, 2	240	14	5	30	21	0	8	470

BREAKFAST MEATS
(see Breakfast Meats, pg 191)

	Cal	Fat	Sat	Chol	Carb	Fib	Sug	Sod

CEREAL – COLD

	Cal	Fat	Sat	Chol	Carb	Fib	Sug	Sod
Puffed rice, 1 cup	56	0	0	0	13	0	0	0
Puffed wheat, 1 cup	44	0	0	0	10	1	0	0
Shredded wheat, 2 biscuits	155	1	0	0	36	6	0	3
Granola w/honey, nuts & raisins, 1/2 cup	210	6	4	0	38	5	15	35
Frosted corn flakes, 1 cup	152	0	0	0	37	1	16	198
Corn flakes, 1 cup	101	0	0	0	24	1	2	200
Crispy rice, 1 cup	108	0	0	0	24	0	3	266
Bran flakes with raisins, 1 cup	190	1	0	0	46	8	19	300
Wheat & barley, 1/2 cup	208	1	0	0	47	5	7	354

Brands . . . *(1 cup unless noted)*
There are many low-sodium cereals, the following have 100mg or less per serving.

	Cal	Fat	Sat	Chol	Carb	Fib	Sug	Sod
Alpen Original, 1.9 oz	200	3	0	0	44	4	11	30
No Sugar Added, 1.9 oz	200	3	0	0	40	4	7	30
Arrowhead Mills Amaranth Flakes	140	2	0	0	26	3	4	0
Puffed Cereal, all varieties (avg)	60	0	0	0	11	2	0	0
Shredded Wheat, all varieties (avg)	190	1	0	0	40	6	7	5
Corn or Kamut Flakes (avg)	120	0	0	0	26	2	2	70
Oat Bran Flakes	140	3	0	0	24	4	3	80
Kamut & Cranberries	170	1	0	0	36	3	7	90
Spelt Flakes	120	1	0	0	24	3	3	100
Back to Nature Cinnamon Crunch	200	2	0	0	43	4	15	15
Treasured Grains with Ginger	200	1	0	0	43	4	14	15
Barbara's Bakery Shredded Wheat, 2	140	1	0	0	31	5	0	0
Puffins Multigrain, 3/4 cup	110	0	0	0	25	3	6	80
Organic *Wild Puffs*, all, 3/4 cup	120	1	0	0	25	3	7	80
Organic Honey Nut O's, 3/4 cup	120	2	0	0	24	2	11	80
Organic Apple Cinnamon O's, 3/4 cup	120	2	0	0	24	2	11	85
Dixie Carb Counters Nutlettes, 1/2 cup	140	2	1	0	15	9	4	5
Smaps, 1/2 cup	71	2	0	0	9	7	1	33
Ener-G Pure Rice Bran, 1/2 cup	220	14	3	0	34	19	3	5
Envirokids Koala Crisp, 3/4 cup	110	1	0	0	25	2	11	100
Erewhon Crispy Brown Rice, NSA	110	0	0	0	25	1	1	10
Rice Twice	120	0	0	0	26	0	8	60
Aztec Crunchy Corn/Amaranth	110	0	0	0	26	1	1	70
Kamut Flakes, 2/3 cup	110	0	0	0	25	4	1	75
Corn Flakes, 1 1/4 cups	210	3	0	0	45	3	1	100
Raisin Bran	170	1	0	0	40	6	10	100
Crispy Brown Rice w/Mixed Berries	120	1	0	0	27	1	6	100
Fiber One Shredded Wheat	200	1	0	0	50	9	12	0
Food Club Frosted Shredded Wheat, Bite size	190	1	0	0	45	6	11	10
Full Circle Organic Raisin Bran	190	0	0	0	47	6	13	90
Organic Multigrain Flakes	100	0	0	0	24	4	5	90
Grainfields LS cereals (avg)	110	0	0	0	26	0	1	20
Great Value Frosted Shredded Wheat	200	1	0	0	42	5	11	0
Honey Crunch	100	0	0	0	24	1	15	50
Health Valley Organic Blue Corn Flakes	100	0	0	0	24	3	5	10
Cranberry Crunch, 3/4 cup	200	3	0	0	41	4	11	50
Golden Flax	190	4	1	0	37	6	9	65
Choc Blast'Ems, 3/4 cup	120	2	0	0	25	3	8	90
Amaranth Flakes	100	1	0	0	23	3	5	90
Cherry Lemon Orange Blast'Ems, 3/4 cup	120	1	0	0	25	2	7	95
Cranberry Crunch, 3/4 cup	190	4	0	0	38	3	13	100
Fiber 7	160	1	0	0	37	7	10	100

	Cal	Fat	Sat	Chol	Carb	Fib	Sug	Sod
Kashi Autumn Wheat	190	1	0	0	45	6	7	0
Cinnamon Harvest or Island Vanilla (avg)	185	1	0	0	44	5	9	0
7 Whole Grain Honey Puffs	120	1	0	0	25	2	6	0
7 Whole Grain Puffs	70	1	0	0	15	1	0	0
Heart to Heart Warm Cinnamon, 3/4 cup	110	2	0	0	24	5	5	80
Go Lean	140	1	0	0	30	10	6	85
Heart to Heart Honey Toasted Oat, 3/4 cup	110	2	0	0	25	5	5	90
Go Lean Crunch	190	3	0	0	36	8	13	95
Vive, 1 1/4 cup	170	3	1	0	43	12	10	100
Kellogg's Mini-Wheats (avg)	180	1	0	0	44	5	12	5
Honey Smacks	100	1	0	0	24	1	15	50
Malt-O-Meal Frosted Mini Spooners, all	190	1	0	0	45	6	11	10
Golden Puffs, 3/4 cup	110	0	0	0	24	0	15	65
Mom's Best Naturals Toasted Wheat-fulls	200	1	0	0	44	7	0	10
Sweetened or Blue Pom Wheat-fuls	210	1	0	0	45	6	11	10
Honey Wheat-fulls	110	0	0	0	24	0	15	65
Nature's Path Synergy 8 Grain, 3/4 cup	100	1	0	0	24	5	4	0
New Morning Oatios Apple Cinnamon	120	1	0	0	18	2	9	60
Fruit-e-O's	120	2	0	0	25	2	7	85
Cocoa Crispy Rice, 3/4 cup	120	1	0	0	26	1	10	100
Northern Gold								
Old Fashioned Oats, 1/2 cup	150	3	1	0	27	4	1	0
Nu-World Foods Cereal Snaps, all (avg)	183	3	0	0	25	5	4	2
Amaranth O's, Peach, 3/4 cup	65	2	0	0	15	9	3	26
Amaranth O's, Original, 3/4 cup	58	1	0	0	16	0	3	28
Post Shredded Wheat or Spoon-size (avg)	165	1	0	0	40	6	0	0
Spoon-size Frosted Shredded Wheat	180	1	0	0	43	5	12	0
Spoon-size Wheat'n Bran Shredded Wheat	200	1	0	0	49	8	1	0
Golden Crisp	110	0	0	0	24	1	14	25
Shredded Wheat Spoon-size Honey Nut	190	2	0	0	44	5	12	70
Quaker Puffed Rice or Puffed Wheat (avg)	45	0	0	0	10	0	0	0
Quisp	110	2	1	0	23	1	12	0
Shredded Wheat, 3 biscuits	220	2	1	0	50	7	1	0
Skinner's Raisin Bran	170	1	0	0	41	7	13	85
Spencer's Fruity O's, 3/4 cup	120	1	0	0	27	0	13	35
Frosted Honey Hives	100	1	0	0	23	1	10	90
Wegmans Fruit Hoops	120	1	0	0	26	0	9	60
Sweetened Wheat Puffs, 3/4 cup	110	0	0	0	24	0	15	65
Foods You Feel Good About Fall Harvest	230	5	1	0	43	3	12	90

GRANOLA AND MUSELI *(1/2 cup unless noted)*
Most granola/museli are low sodium, the following have 35mg or less per serving.

	Cal	Fat	Sat	Chol	Carb	Fib	Sug	Sod
Alpen (Museli) Original, 2/3 cup	200	3	0	0	41	4	11	30
Sugar Free, 2/3 cup	200	3	0	0	40	4	7	30
Alvarado St Bakery Classic Granola	220	6	1	0	37	6	6	0
Classic Granola w/Raisins	220	5	1	0	38	6	9	0
Back to Nature Choc Delight Granola	210	6	2	0	37	4	14	0
Classic Granola	200	3	1	0	39	4	12	0
Apple Blueberry or Organic Cherry Vanilla (avg)	200	3	0	0	39	4	13	10
Cranberry Pecan Granola	200	5	1	0	35	4	13	15
Granola to Go:								
Ginger Roasted Almonds	190	7	1	0	29	4	10	20
Honey Almond w/Flax Seed	190	7	1	0	29	4	10	20
Wild Blueberry Walnut w/Flax Seed	190	6	1	0	30	4	11	20
The Baker Pecan Granola	130	8	0	0	11	2	-	0

BREAKFAST FOODS
Cereal–Cold

	Cal	Fat	Sat	Chol	Carb	Fib	Sug	Sod
Honey Oat w/Almonds Granola	120	7	0	0	14	3	-	0
Cinnamon Raisin w/Flax Granola	120	6	0	0	16	3	-	0
Honey Crunch or Fruit & Nut Muesli (avg)	250	9	0	0	37	6	-	0
Forest Berry Muesli	200	3	0	0	40	6	-	15
Bakery on Main Granola, all but Fiber Power (avg)	245	12	1	0	29	4	10	20
Bear Naked Fruit & Nut Granola, 1/4 cup	140	7	2	0	18	2	6	0
Banana Nut Granola, 1/4 cup	140	7	2	0	18	2	5	5
Apple Cinnamon Granola, 1/4 cup	140	5	1	0	21	3	7	10
Fit, Vanilla Almond Crunch Granola, 1/4 cup	120	3	0	0	22	2	4	10
Fit, Triple Berry Crunch Granola, 1/4 cup	120	2	0	0	23	3	4	15
Mango Agave Almond Granola, 1/4 cup	130	5	1	0	19	2	6	25
Natural Blueberry Walnut Granola, 1/4 cup	140	6	1	0	17	2	6	25
Peak Protein 1/4 cup	140	6	1	0	17	2	6	25
Bob's Red Mill Museli, 1/4 cup	110	3	0	0	21	4	5	0
Honey Almond Granola	230	7	1	0	38	4	7	0
Crunchy Coconut Granola	260	10	4	0	36	6	8	0
Apple Blueberry or Natural	180	3	0	0	35	4	8	10
Apple Strawberry or Apple Cinnamon	180	3	0	0	35	4	8	10
Breadshop (Arrowhead Mills) Granola								
Crunchy Oat Bran w/Almonds & Raisins	210	8	1	0	33	4	9	0
Strawberry 'n Cream or Raspberry 'n Cream	220	8	1	0	34	4	9	0
Blueberry 'n Cream	210	6	1	0	36	4	9	0
Honey Gone Nuts	240	10	1	0	33	4	7	0
Super Natural w/Almonds & Raisins	220	8	1	0	34	3	10	5
Chappaqua Crunch Simply Granola, 1/3 cup	120	2	1	0	22	3	4	0
Original Granola, 1/3 cup	115	2	1	0	20	3	4	0
Granola w/Cranberries or Blueberries, 1/3 cup	120	2	1	0	22	2	6	0
Granola w/Raspberries, 1/3 cup	110	2	1	0	21	3	4	0
Granola w/Raisins, 1/3 cup	120	2	1	0	22	3	6	15
Dan-D-Pak Fruit & Nut Muesli	130	2	0	0	24	4	0	0
Fruity Berry Muesli	160	3	0	0	27	6	1	0
Deluxe Fruit & Nuts Muesli	150	4	1	0	23	4	5	5
Honey Raisin or Blueberry Apple Granola (avg)	130	5	1	0	20	3	5	25
Honey Nut Granola	260	9	1	0	36	5	8	25
Cranberry Coconut Granola	190	7	1	0	26	4	7	35
Enjoy Life Very Berry Crunch Granola	170	6	2	0	35	2	11	10
Cinnamon Crunch Granola	170	2	0	0	35	2	11	10
Cranapple Crunch Granola	170	3	0	0	34	2	10	20
Familia Swiss Museli, Original	220	3	1	0	41	4	14	0
Swiss Museli, No Sugar Added	210	3	1	0	41	4	7	0
Food Club 100% Natural Granola								
Oats, Honey & Almonds, 1/4 cup	230	9	2	0	31	5	10	15
Oats, Honey, Raisins & Almonds, 1/4 cup	220	8	2	0	33	4	13	15
Galaxy Granola, all varieties, 1/4 cup (avg)	115	1	0	0	22	4	5	0
Gluten Free Sensations								
French Vanilla Almond Granola, 1/3 cup	130	6	2	0	18	2	5	15
Cherry Vanilla Almond Granola, 1/3 cup	140	6	3	0	20	2	6	20
Glutenfreeda Raisin Almond Honey Granola	150	11	1	0	11	2	8	15
Cranberry Cashew Honey, 1/4 cup	120	5	1	0	17	2	6	25
Hodgson Mill Apple & More Museli, 1/4 cup	150	3	0	0	21	4	5	0
King Arthur Flour Mt Museli	220	6	1	0	38	5	9	20
Michaelene's Honey Crunch, all varieties (avg)	103	3	0	0	17	2	5	2
Gourmet Granola, most varieties (avg), 1/3 cup	106	3	1	0	17	3	5	12
Sweetnola for Life Granola, 1/3 cup	131	6	1	0	16	2	3	12
S'more Sweetnola Granola, 1/3 cup	119	5	1	0	16	2	4	23

	Cal	Fat	Sat	Chol	Carb	Fib	Sug	Sod
Mother's Oat & Honey Granola	210	0	4	0	55	5	12	20
Natural Ovens Great Granola	250	9	2	0	36	5	9	5
Nature's Hand Original Granola	220	9	2	0	29	4	8	0
Cinnamon Apple or Wild Blueberry Granola	140	6	1	0	20	4	5	0
Coconut Cashew or Raisin Hazelnut Granola (avg)	215	9	2	0	29	3	9	5
Cranberry Apricot Granola	200	7	1	0	28	3	8	20
Nature's Path Love Crunch Granola, 3/4 cup	260	9	2	0	38	4	10	25
HempPlus Granola, 3/4 cup	260	10	2	0	36	5	10	35
New England Naturals Natural Banana Walnut	190	3	1	0	35	4	6	10
All Natural Honey Nuts Granola	280	13	3	0	37	4	12	20
Organic Antioxidant Granola	200	6	1	0	32	4	6	32
Northern Gold Honey Almond Granola	250	9	2	0	36	5	8	0
Cashews & Raisins Granola	240	8	2	0	38	5	11	5
Quaker Natural Granola, Oats & Honey	210	6	4	0	35	3	12	25
Natural Granola, Honey & Raisins	210	6	4	0	38	3	15	25
Seitenbacher #21, Cashews & Almonds Musli	177	7	1	0	27	3	10	1
#22, Raspberries & Almonds Musli	174	6	1	0	29	3	10	1
#1, Natural Body Power Musli	180	5	1	0	23	6	9	3
#2, Berries Temptation Musli, 2/3 cup	160	3	0	0	26	4	9	5
#6, Gluten Free Musli	210	11	2	0	16	6	11	5
#23, Cherries & Almonds Musli	170	5	1	0	24	4	7	5
#9, Strawberry Delight Musli	160	2	0	0	29	4	12	9
#8, Cinnamon Magic Musli	180	4	1	0	29	6	12	13
#11, Apple Cinnamon Musli	190	7	2	0	30	3	10	17
#4, Men's Formula Musli, 3/4 cup	170	5	1	0	23	4	11	18
#5, Choco Max Musli, 2/3 cup	190	4	2	2	33	4	23	21
Udi's Granola, all, 1/4 cup (avg)	130	4	0	0	19	3	5	0
Wegmans Natural Granola	230	9	2	0	31	5	10	15
Natural Granola w/Raisins	220	8	2	0	33	4	13	15
Woodstock Farms Granola, most, 1/4 cup	120	5	1	0	18	3	7	0

CEREAL – HOT

	Cal	Fat	Sat	Chol	Carb	Fib	Sug	Sod
Regular or quick-cooking cereals:								
Wheat cereal, regular, cooked, 1 cup	150	1	0	0	3	4	0	0
Oat cereal, regular or quick cooked, 1 cup	147	2	0	0	25	4	1	2
Farina, cooked, 1 cup	112	0	0	0	24	1	0	5
Grits, regular or quick, cooked, 1 cup	143	0	0	0	31	1	0	5
Instant cereals:								
Oat cereal, instant, flavored, 1 pkt	172	2	0	0	35	3	15	243

There is a difference between "instant" and "quick cooking" cereals. Instant averages more than 200mg sodium per serving; quick-cooking has 2mg.

Brands . . . *(1 package/serving unless noted)*

REGULAR/QUICK-COOKING CEREAL – *Most brands within generic average (0–5mg).*

INSTANT AND FLAVORED HOT CEREAL

	Cal	Fat	Sat	Chol	Carb	Fib	Sug	Sod
Arrowhead Mills *Instant Oatmeal* Orig Plain	110	2	0	0	19	2	0	0
Instant Oatmeal Maple Apple Spice	140	2	0	0	26	3	5	45
Instant Oatmeal w/Flax	140	3	1	0	24	4	4	70
Country Choice Instant Oatmeal, Original	110	2	0	0	19	3	1	0
Instant Oatmeal, Maple	170	2	0	0	32	3	9	60
Instant Oatmeal, Apple Cinnamon	140	2	0	0	22	3	11	60
Fit Kids Choc Chip	150	3	1	0	28	3	13	100
Fit Kids Cinnamon Toast	130	2	0	0	26	3	11	100
Erewhon *Organic* Instant Oatmeal w/Oat Bran	130	3	1	0	25	4	1	0
Organic Brown Rice Cream	170	1	0	0	36	1	0	30

	Cal	Fat	Sat	Chol	Carb	Fib	Sug	Sod
Organic Instant Oatmeal Maple Spice............	130	2	1	0	25	3	4	100
Organic Instant Oatmeal Apple Cinnamon......	130	2	1	0	24	3	4	100
Organic Instant Oatmeal Cinnamon Raisin/Flax .	130	3	1	0	24	4	6	100
Food Club Instant Oatmeal............................	100	2	0	0	19	3	0	80
Glutenfreeda *Instant Oatmeal* Natural...........	190	3	1	0	34	5	1	0
Instant Oatmeal Banana Maple w/Flax	160	2	0	0	30	4	6	90
Instant Oatmeal Apple Cinnamon w/Flax	170	2	0	0	34	4	12	95
Instant Oatmeal Maple Raisin w/Flax	210	2	0	0	42	4	14	100
Kashi Go Lean Creamy, Truly Vanilla, 1 pkt	150	2	0	0	25	7	6	100
Go Lean Hearty, Honey & Cinnamon, 1 pkt.....	150	2	0	0	26	5	7	100
Heart to Heart Golden Brown Maple, 1 pkt	160	2	0	0	33	5	12	100
Heart to Heart Raisin Spice, 1 pkt	150	2	0	0	33	4	16	100
McCann's Instant Irish Oatmeal, Regular........	100	2	0	0	18	3	1	80
Mother's Instant Oatmeal or Rolled Oats........	150	3	1	0	27	4	2	0
Quick Cooking Barley..................................	160	1	0	0	37	5	2	0
Oat Bran or Whole Wheat (avg)	180	1	0	0	28	5	2	0
Nu-World Foods Amaranth Hot Cereal								
Berry Delicious or Cinnamon Delight.............	91	1	0	0	16	3	2	9
Quaker *Organic* Instant Oatmeal	100	2	0	0	19	3	1	0
Simple Harvest Vanilla/Almond/Honey	160	3	0	0	31	4	9	75
Simple Harvest Maple Brown Sugar w/Pecans...	160	4	1	0	30	4	9	75
Instant Oatmeal, Original..........................	100	2	0	0	19	3	0	80
Simple Harvest Apples w/Cinnamon..............	150	2	0	0	33	4	12	90
Organic Maple Brown Sugar Instant..............	150	2	0	0	31	3	12	95
Take Heart Blueberry Instant	160	3	1	0	33	6	9	105
Take Heart Golden Maple Instant	160	3	1	0	33	5	9	110
Roman Meal Maple Whole Grain..................	130	2	0	0	31	5	9	80
Original Whole Grain..................................	130	1	0	0	28	5	5	105
Raisin or Honey Whole Grain (avg)	135	1	0	0	31	4	10	120
Apple Whole Grain....................................	140	1	0	0	32	5	10	125
Village Farm Whole Grain Oatmeal, Blueberry...	120	3	0	0	21	6	1	90
Wild Harvest Original Instant Oatmeal	150	3	0	0	27	4	1	0
Willow Creek Mill Fitness Blend, 1/4 cup.......	220	2	0	0	21	4	0	0

CEREAL BARS

(see Granola/Cereal/Breakfast Bars, pg 69)

COFFEECAKE

(see Pastries/Other Breakfast Sweets, pg 72)

DIET/NUTRITIONAL DRINKS

(see Diet/Meal Replacement/Nutrition Drinks, pg 39)

DONUTS

	Cal	Fat	Sat	Chol	Carb	Fib	Sug	Sod
French cruller, glazed, 3", 1.5 oz.....................	175	8	2	5	25	1	15	147
Yeast, glazed, 3", 1.5 oz...............................	170	8	2	13	22	1	8	165
Jelly-filled, 3 oz	289	16	4	22	33	1	18	249
Creme-filled, 3 oz	307	21	5	20	26	1	12	263
Cake, plain, 3", 1.5 oz.................................	178	10	3	4	19	1	7	237
Sugar or glazed, 3", 1.5 oz........................	181	10	3	14	22	1	10	171
Choc-coated or frosted, 3", 1.5 oz	192	11	6	8	22	1	11	176

Brands . . . *(1.5 oz unless noted)*
MIXES

	Cal	Fat	Sat	Chol	Carb	Fib	Sug	Sod
Dixie Carb Counter Dough (Not!) Holes, 1.....	43	1	0	0	10	0	5	43

	Cal	Fat	Sat	Chol	Carb	Fib	Sug	Sod
King Arthur Flour Buttermilk Doughnut	140	0	0	0	32	1	15	70

SHELF-STABLE (READY-TO-EAT)

	Cal	Fat	Sat	Chol	Carb	Fib	Sug	Sod
Chatila's Bakery Boston Cream Doughnut	100	3	0	0	16	2	0	10
Vanilla w/Vanilla Cream or Choc Cream	100	1	0	0	16	7	1	55
Vanilla w/Raspberry or Strawberry................	100	2	0	0	16	7	1	55
Vanilla Frosted..	110	2	1	0	23	7	0	55
Choc w/Vanilla Cream or Choc Cream	100	1	0	0	16	7	1	55
Vanilla w/Blueberry	100	1	0	0	16	7	1	60
Choc w/Raspberry..	90	2	0	0	15	8	0	130
Entemann's Frosted Minis, 1.1 oz	160	11	7	5	15	1	9	90
Pop'ettes Glazed Cruller, 1.6 oz	210	12	6	10	25	0	17	140

FRENCH TOAST

(see Pancakes/Waffles/French Toast, pg 70)

GRANOLA , CEREAL AND BREAKFAST BARS

(also see Diet/Energy/Snack Bars, pg 217)

	Cal	Fat	Sat	Chol	Carb	Fib	Sug	Sod
Granola bar, soft, choc chip, 1 oz bar	117	5	20	0	20	1	8	50
Granola bar, soft choc coated, 1 oz bar........	130	7	0	0	18	1	10	56
Granola bar, hard, peanut butter, 0.9 oz bar......	116	6	2	0	15	1	9	68
Granola bar, oats, fruits and nuts, 1 oz bar	113	2	0	0	22	2	12	71
Granola bar, hard, choc chip, 0.9 oz bar	105	4	3	0	17	1	9	83
Granola bar, soft, peanut butter, 1 oz bar........	119	4	1	0	18	1	9	115
Cereal bar, mixed fruit, 1.3 oz bar	139	3	0	0	27	1	13	110
Breakfast cookie, oatmeal and raisin, 1.7 oz	170	5	1	5	33	5	15	190

Brands . . . *(1 bar unless noted)*
There are many low-sodium granola and cereal bars, the following have 75mg or less. NOTE: Bar sizes vary from 0.8 ounces to 2.2 ounces.

	Cal	Fat	Sat	Chol	Carb	Fib	Sug	Sod
18 Rabbits Bunny Bars, 1 oz (avg)................	120	4	0	0	19	2	8	0
Granola Bars, 1.9 oz (avg)	220	9	4	0	32	4	11	10
Bakery on Main Gluten Free Granola Bars								
Soft & Chewy all, 1.3 oz (avg)	140	5	1	0	22	2	1	70
Barbara's Bakery Peanut Butter Granola	200	9	1	0	26	3	9	55
Oats & Honey Granola, 1.3 oz	190	8	1	0	27	3	10	60
Bear Naked Fruit & Nut Granola, 2 oz	240	9	2	0	35	4	15	55
Chocolaty Cherry Granola, 2 oz....................	230	10	2	0	33	4	14	60
Tropical Fruit Granola, 2 oz..........................	220	7	2	0	38	4	18	60
Carb Counters SmartBreak 0.8 oz	65	3	2	0	5	3	1	4
Eating Right 100 Calorie Chewy Bars w/Yogurt								
Raspberry & Vanilla, 1.1 oz..........................	100	3	2	0	18	1	9	60
Apricot, 1.1 oz...	100	3	1	0	18	1	10	70
Enjoy Life Chewy Bars Caramel Apple, 1 oz	120	3	0	0	24	3	7	60
Chewy Bars Very Berry, 1 oz	120	2	0	0	24	2	7	70
EnviroKidz Crispy Rice Fruity Burst, 1 oz.........	110	3	1	0	21	1	8	65
Fi-Bar Chewy & Nutty Granola Bars								
Almond Crunch, Milk Choc or White Choc	140	5	3	0	23	1	11	20
Peanut Butter, Milk Choc or White Choc........	140	5	2	0	23	1	11	25
White Choc, Raspberry or Strawberry, 1.2 oz ...	120	2	2	0	26	3	13	25
Full Circle Fruit & Cereal Bars, 1.3 oz								
Apple Cobbler, Strawberry, or Blueberry	130	2	0	0	27	1	13	50
Glutino Blueberry Breakfast Bars, 1.4 oz	130	2	0	0	27	3	11	0
Apple, 1.4 oz...	130	2	0	0	28	3	11	5
Choc & Banana, 1 oz	100	2	0	0	21	1	9	35
Strawberry or Cherry....................................	160	3	0	0	30	3	13	50

69

BREAKFAST FOODS
Pancakes, Waffles and French Toast

	Cal	Fat	Sat	Chol	Carb	Fib	Sug	Sod
Wildberry, 1 oz	100	1	0	0	21	1	8	65
Gorge Delights *Just Fruit Bar*, all (avg)	145	0	0	0	35	5	22	10
Acai Fruit Bar, all (avg)	145	0	0	0	35	5	23	10
Great Value 90 Calorie Choc Chunk Chewy Granola	90	2	1	0	18	1	7	65
Health Valley *Organic Chewy Granola*								
Dutch Apple, Wild Berry, or Blueberry (avg)...	110	2	1	0	23	2	11	15
Choc Chip or Double Choc Chip, 1 oz (avg)....	110	3	2	0	22	3	10	15
Kashi *TLC Fruit & Grain Bars* Dark Choc Coconut	120	4	2	0	21	4	7	50
TLC Fruit & Grain Bars Pumpkin Pie, 1.1 oz ...	120	3	0	0	22	4	8	50
TLC Fruit & Grain Bars Raspberry Choc, 1.1 oz	120	3	1	0	21	4	7	50
TLC Chewy Granola Cherry Dark Choc, 1.3 oz ..	120	2	1	0	24	4	8	75
Kellogg's *Fiber Plus* Dark Chocolate, 1.3 oz	130	5	3	0	24	9	7	50
Fiber Plus Chocolate Chip, 1.3 oz..................	120	4	2	0	26	9	7	55
Nature's Path Chococonut Granola, 1.3 oz.....	140	5	2	0	24	2	11	35
Lotta Apricotta Granola, 1.3 oz	140	5	2	0	23	2	12	70
Nutlettes Apple Berry Granola Bar, 1.3 oz	87	2	1	0	16	10	2	3
Quaker Granola Bars								
Fiber & Omega 3 Peanut Butter Choc, 1.3 oz...	150	5	2	0	25	9	7	35
Fiber & Omega 3 Dark Choc Chunk, 1.3 oz	150	4	2	0	26	9	7	35
Chewy Dipps Caramel Nut, 1.1 oz	140	6	4	0	21	1	13	65
True Delights Dark Choc Raspberry Almond....	140	5	2	0	23	3	8	55
Chewy Choc Chip, 0.9 oz.............................	100	3	2	0	18	1	7	75
Chewy 90 Calorie, Strawberry Vanilla, 0.9 oz .	90	2	0	0	19	1	7	75
Chewy 90 Calorie, Dark Choc Cherry, 0.9 oz ..	90	2	1	0	19	1	7	75
Chewy 25% Less Sugar, Choc Chip, 0.9 oz	100	4	1	0	17	3	5	75
Russel Stover *Sugar Free* Chewy Granola	100	5	3	0	19	7	0	45
Spencer's *Crunchy* Granola Bars								
Peanut Butter or Roasted Almond, 2 bars	200	8	1	0	26	3	9	50
Oats 'N' Honey, 2 bars (1.5 oz)	200	7	1	0	27	3	9	55
Sunbelt Banana or Blueberry Granola (avg)....	130	5	3	0	19	1	8	50
Choc Chip Granola Bar, 1.3 oz......................	170	7	4	0	24	1	12	60
Oats & Honey Granola Bar, 1 oz	130	5	3	0	19	1	8	65
Fudge Dipped Coconut Granola Bar, 1.4 oz	200	11	8	0	23	2	13	65
Fudge Dipped Choc Chip Granola Bar, 1.5 oz..	210	10	6	0	29	2	16	70
Fruit & Grain Cereal Bars, all, 1.4 oz (avg).....	140	3	1	0	28	1	17	70

(MUFFINS AND SCONES)

(see Muffins/Scones, pg 56)

(PANCAKES, WAFFLES AND FRENCH TOAST)

(also see Breakfast Meals–Frozen, pg 63; Blintzes/Crepes, pg 138)

	Cal	Fat	Sat	Chol	Carb	Fib	Sug	Sod
Pancake, plain, frozen, 2.7 oz (2)	182	4	1	15	33	2	5	430
Pancake or waffle mix, plain, 2.7 oz...............	147	2	0	9	28	2	8	477
Waffle, plain, frozen, 2.7 oz (2)......................	217	7	1	11	33	2	4	485
Potato pancake, med, 2.6 oz..........................	199	11	2	70	21	5	2	565
French toast, ready-to-heat, 2 slices, 4.2 oz	251	7	2	96	38	1	10	584

Brands . . . *(2 pancakes, waffles, or French toast unless noted)*

PANCAKES AND WAFFLES
FROZEN/REFRIGERATED

	Cal	Fat	Sat	Chol	Carb	Fib	Sug	Sod
De Wafelbakkers A+ Cinn Waffles, Swt Potato	190	9	1	0	24	3	10	135
Oat Bran Spelt Whole Grain Waffles, 3	220	9	1	0	28	4	16	140
Lil' Joey *Pancake Pockets* Strawberry or Maple .	140	3	1	50	26	0	12	30
Pancake Pockets Chocolate, 1	140	3	1	50	26	0	12	35
Market Day Pancake Pods, Strawberry, 2 oz ..	140	3	1	45	25	0	14	30

	Cal	Fat	Sat	Chol	Carb	Fib	Sug	Sod
Tio Pepe's Churro Waffle Sticks, 1 oz	110	5	2	15	14	2	5	100

REDUCED SODIUM (LESS THAN GENERIC):

	Cal	Fat	Sat	Chol	Carb	Fib	Sug	Sod
De Wafelbakkers								
A+ Cinn Pancake, Sweet Potato	180	4	0	0	32	4	11	200
Buckwheat Berry Pancakes	140	4	0	0	31	6	11	210
Blueberry Whole Grain Waffles, 3	210	10	1	0	26	3	10	230
Blueberry Whole Grain Pancakes, 3	170	4	0	0	31	4	10	290
Eggo French Toast Waffle, 1.6 oz	140	6	2	10	19	1	5	240
Great Day Buttermilk Pancakes	140	2	0	10	28	0	6	260
Blueberry Pancakes, 3.8 oz (3)	230	5	2	5	43	1	10	290
Kashi GoLean Blueberry Waffles	170	3	0	0	33	6	4	300
GoLean Strawberry Flax Waffles	160	3	0	0	31	6	5	300
Market Day Waffle Sticks, Maple, 2.3 oz	190	7	2	20	22	3	9	210
Nature's Path Hemp Plus	200	8	1	0	30	5	5	290
Organic Batter Blaster Original or Whole								
Wheat Pancake Batter, 1/4 cup (avg)	85	1	0	15	17	1	5	280
Double Choc Pancake Batter, 1/4 cup	90	1	0	15	20	1	11	290

MIXES

	Cal	Fat	Sat	Chol	Carb	Fib	Sug	Sod
Arrowhead Mills Oat Bran Pancake/Waffle	120	2	0	0	21	6	1	75
Dixie Carb Counters								
Blueberry Cream, 1	19	0	0	0	4	3	0	137
Banana Supreme Pancake Mix, 1 pancake	22	0	0	0	5	3	0	139
Heidi's FF Cottage Cheese Pancake Mix	150	0	0	0	34	1	10	0
Sweet N'Low Pancake Mix	150	0	0	0	36	1	0	20
Toro Waffle & Pancake Celiac-Safe Mix, 1	120	1	0	31	24	1	5	59

REDUCED SODIUM (LESS THAN GENERIC):

	Cal	Fat	Sat	Chol	Carb	Fib	Sug	Sod
Arrowhead Mills Kamut Pancake/Waffle	140	2	0	0	24	4	0	200
Choc Chip Multigrain Pancake Mix	140	3	1	5	26	3	4	240
Multigrain Pancake & Waffle Mix	130	1	0	5	27	3	2	260
Authentic Foods Pancake & Baking Mix	130	2	0	0	24	2	1	170
Cherrybrook Kitchen Orig Pancake Mix	80	0	0	0	17	0	2	190
Classique Fare Apple Pancake Mix	105	2	0	24	19	1	3	150
Belgian Waffle Mix	70	1	0	40	13	0	5	160
Wild Blueberry Waffle Mix	170	1	0	41	36	3	13	165
Dixie Carb Counters Pancake/Waffle, 1	170	0	0	0	3	2	0	158
Fiddler's Green Farm Fiddle Cakes, 1/4 c	120	1	0	0	25	4	0	170
Heidi's Oats 'n Apple Pancake Mix	210	2	0	0	43	3	14	180
Hodgson Mill Gluten-Free Pancake/Waffle	140	2	0	0	30	3	0	199
Kungsornen Swedish Pancake/Waffle Mix	140	2	0	15	27	1	2	210
Maple Grove Farms								
Sugar Free Pancake/Waffle	120	3	2	0	11	5	0	210
Market Day Choc Chip Mini Pancakes, 6	130	3	1	5	22	1	8	240
Nature's Path Flax Plus Multigrain Pancake	140	1	0	0	27	2	5	240
Panni Bavarian Potato Pancake	50	0	0	0	12	1	0	230

FRENCH TOAST

FROZEN/REFRIGERATED

	Cal	Fat	Sat	Chol	Carb	Fib	Sug	Sod
Ian's Toast Sticks Wheat Free, 2 oz	210	9	5	0	29	0	4	70
Market Day Choc Chip Mini Pancakes, 6	130	3	1	5	22	1	8	240

PANCAKE AND WAFFLE SYRUP

	Cal	Fat	Sat	Chol	Carb	Fib	Sug	Sod
Maple syrup, 1/4 cup	210	0	0	0	54	0	48	7
Fruit syrup, 1/4 cup	210	0	0	0	52	0	50	10
Pancake syrup, 1/4 cup	184	0	0	0	48	0	26	64
Sugar free pancake syrup, 1/4 cup	30	0	0	0	12	0	0	115

BREAKFAST FOODS
Pastries and Other Breakfast Sweets

	Cal	Fat	Sat	Chol	Carb	Fib	Sug	Sod

Brands . . . *(1/4 cup unless noted)*
Maple syrup – *Most brands within generic range (7mg).*
Fruit syrup – *Most brands within generic range (10mg).*

	Cal	Fat	Sat	Chol	Carb	Fib	Sug	Sod
DaVinci Sugar Free Pancake	0	0	0	0	0	0	0	35
Griffin's Pancake Syrup	240	0	0	0	60	0	29	40
Sohgave Maple or Blueberry Syrup, 1 tbsp	60	0	0	0	16	0	16	0
Steel's All Natural Maple Flavor Syrup, 3 tbsp.	64	0	0	0	16	0	0	10

PASTRIES AND OTHER BREAKFAST SWEETS

(also see Muffins/Scones, pg 56; Donuts, pg 68; Blintzes/Crepes, pg 138)

	Cal	Fat	Sat	Chol	Carb	Fib	Sug	Sod
Strudel, apple, 1 oz	78	3	1	2	12	1	7	76
Coffeecake, creme-filled w/choc frosting, 1 oz	94	3	1	20	15	1	8	92
Cheese, 1 oz	96	4	2	24	13	0	6	96
Cinnamon w/crumb topping, 1 oz	119	7	2	9	13	1	6	100
Fruit, 1 oz	88	3	1	2	15	1	7	109
Eclair, custard-filled w/choc glaze, 1 oz	74	5	1	36	7	0	2	96
Cream puff, custard-filled, 1 oz	73	4	1	38	6	0	3	97
Danish pastry, fruit, 1 oz	105	5	1	32	16	1	8	100
Cinnamon, 1 oz	114	6	2	6	13	0	6	105
Cheese, 1 oz	106	6	2	5	11	0	2	128
Sweet roll, cheese, 1 oz	102	5	2	22	12	0	6	101
Cinnamon w/raisins, 1 oz	106	5	1	19	14	1	9	109
Cinnamon roll w/frosting, 1 oz	94	3	1	0	15	0	5	217

Brands . . . *(2 oz unless noted)*
FROZEN/REFRIGERATED

	Cal	Fat	Sat	Chol	Carb	Fib	Sug	Sod
Apollo or **Athens** Baklava, 2 oz (2)	230	11	2	0	30	1	17	75
Aunt Trudy's Maple Walnut Baklava, 1.7 oz	190	10	1	0	24	1	24	45
Apple Cinnamon Pocket Pastry, 5.6 oz	340	7	1	0	65	3	27	140
Delizza Choc Dipped Cream Puffs, 3.6 oz	375	25	16	130	34	1	26	68
Mini Cream Puffs, 2.7 oz	291	24	14	111	15	1	10	77
Mini Eclairs, 3.6 oz	333	21	13	63	32	1	20	128
Fillo Factory Organic Apple Turnover, 3 oz	170	5	1	0	30	1	8	90
Raspberry or Walnut Baklava, 2 oz	220	9	3	5	34	0	20	90
Choc Baklava	210	8	3	5	35	1	21	95
Market Day Trail Mix Breakfast Cookie, 2 oz	210	7	3	10	36	5	17	110
Rich's Bavarian Creme Eclair, 2 oz	220	12	10	40	25	0	19	90
REDUCED SODIUM (LESS THAN GENERIC)								
Sara Lee Crumb Coffee Cake, 1/10	200	8	2	20	30	1	18	150
MIXES								
Chébé Cinnamon Roll-ups	70	0	0	0	18	0	0	100
Cravings Place Cinnamon Crumble Coffee Cake	100	0	0	0	24	1	13	60
Dixie Carb Counters Sugar (Not!) Sticky Buns	51	0	0	0	12	1	6	17
Almond Cream Coffee Cake Mix, 1/12	46	1	0	0	5	1	3	140
SHELF-STABLE								
Chatila's Bakery Choc Eclair, 3 oz	190	14	3	40	14	2	4	15
Mini Eclair, 2.1 oz	90	5	1	50	8	0	2	30
Choc E'Toile, 2 (2.7 oz)	80	4	2	10	22	6	1	40
Vanilla Chip or Choc Chip Sandwich, 1.8 oz	150	7	1	0	16	7	0	45
Vanilla Swiss Roll, 3.9 oz	140	5	1	45	19	5	0	90
Gluten Free Strawberry Swiss Roll, 3.8 oz	120	1	0	35	30	2	1	95
French Napoleon, 2.5 oz	190	12	3	0	20	1	4	95
Coconut Truffle, 4.5 oz	160	3	2	0	41	13	1	105
Boston Napoleon, 3.9 oz	220	14	5	20	30	0	2	110
Pumpkin Swiss Roll, 3 oz	130	4	2	40	19	7	0	130

	Cal	Fat	Sat	Chol	Carb	Fib	Sug	Sod
Drake's Coffee Cake	140	6	2	5	20	0	11	100
LF Coffee Cake	100	2	1	10	21	0	12	110
Ferrara Apricot Glazed Pastry Puffs, 3	150	7	4	0	19	1	9	75
The Fillo Factory *Gourmet Pastries*								
Walnut or Raspberry Baklava, 2 oz	220	9	3	5	34	1	20	90
Choc Baklava, 2 oz	210	8	3	5	35	1	21	95
Heinemann's Apple Strip Coffee Cake	150	7	1	15	18	1	7	125
Cherry Strip Coffee Cake	160	7	1	10	18	0	8	130
Butter Pecan Coffee Cake	170	10	3	0	18	1	10	130
Hostess Cinnamon Coffee Cakes, 3	100	3	1	10	21	5	7	135
Market Day Apple Berry Breakfast Bowl, 6 oz	200	3	1	5	50	7	34	140
Nickles Angel Food Raspberry Jelly Roll, 1/8	140	0	0	0	33	0	-	135
Racine *Danish Kringles* Cranberry, 1.8 oz	180	8	2	10	25	0	16	135
Kringles Cherry or Strawberry Cheesecake	180	9	2	10	24	0	15	140
Kringles Raspberry or Blueberry Cheesecake	180	9	2	10	24	0	15	140
Choc Eclair, 1.8 oz	180	9	2	10	24	0	15	140
Svenhard's Cinnamon Roll	160	6	3	5	24	0	17	130
Walnut Cinnamon Roll	190	9	3	5	25	1	17	135
REDUCED SODIUM (LESS THAN GENERIC):								
Entenmann's Pecan Danish Ring, 1/8	240	15	4	20	24	1	11	150
Walnut Danish Ring, 1/8	240	14	4	20	24	2	11	150
Heinemann's Turtle Coffee Cake	160	8	2	0	21	1	13	150
Raspberry Alligator Coffee Cake	140	7	2	0	19	0	10	150
Cheese Strip Coffee Cake	160	10	2	25	16	0	5	150
Almond Strip Coffee Cake	160	9	1	15	18	1	6	150
Pepperidge Farm Peach Dumplings	320	11	3	0	50	4	15	150

TOASTER FOODS

	Cal	Fat	Sat	Chol	Carb	Fib	Sug	Sod
Toaster pastry, fruit, frosted, 2 oz	215	6	1	0	39	0	20	172
Toaster pastry, cinnamon, 2 oz	234	8	2	0	39	1	11	240
Brands . . . *(1 serving unless noted)*								
Amy's Toaster Pops Apple or Strawberry	150	4	0	0	27	1	10	110
Awrey's *Toaster Rounds*								
Cranberry Orange or Blueberry	150	7	1	20	19	0	9	110
Fiber One Blueberry or Strawberry	190	4	1	0	36	5	15	135
Brown Sugar Cinnamon	190	4	1	0	35	5	16	140
Great Value Toaster Pastries Frosted Strawberry	200	5	2	0	37	1	16	140
Frosted Brown Sugar Cinnamon	200	5	2	0	37	1	17	140
Health Valley *Organic* Toaster Tarts Choc	140	3	0	0	28	3	15	90
Strawberry or Baked Apple Toaster Tarts (avg)	145	3	0	0	28	1	16	95
Red Cherry, Blueberry or Raspberry (avg)	150	3	0	0	30	3	17	95
Nature's Path Blueberry Frosted	200	4	2	0	8	1	20	125
Brown Sugar Maple Cinnamon Frosted	210	5	3	0	39	1	20	125
Cherry Choc Stripes Frosted	200	5	3	0	38	1	19	125
Choc Frosted or Wild Berry Acai	210	5	3	0	38	1	18	130
Apple Cinnamon Frosted	210	5	2	0	39	1	21	130
Brown Sugar Maple Cinnamon	210	5	3	0	37	1	16	135
Strawberry Frosted	210	4	2	0	40	1	19	140
REDUCED SODIUM (LESS THAN GENERIC):								
Awrey's Toaster Rounds, Cornbread	180	9	2	30	22	0	11	150
Fiber One Choc Fudge	190	4	2	0	35	3	16	150
Kellogg's *Pop Tarts* Fiber Frosted Strawberry	190	5	2	0	35	5	13	150
Nature's Path Apple Cinn or Blueberry	210	5	2	0	40	1	18	150
Strawberry or Frosted Raspberry	210	5	2	0	40	1	18	150
Cherry Pomegran	200	5	3	0	37	1	17	150

73

CONDIMENTS AND SAUCES

*See RESOURCES, page 305, for a partial list of manufacturers and retailers offering low-salt products online or visit **LowSaltFoods.com** for additional sources.*

	Cal	Fat	Sat	Chol	Carb	Fib	Sug	Sod

CONDIMENTS AND SAUCES

CAPERS

	Cal	Fat	Sat	Chol	Carb	Fib	Sug	Sod
Capers, 1 tsp	2	0	0	0	0	0	0	105
Brands . . . *(1 tsp unless noted)*								
Delallo Nonpareil or Capote Capers	0	0	0	0	0	0	0	85
Roland Capers, all varieties	0	0	0	0	0	0	0	85

CHUTNEY, RELISHES AND OTHER ACCOMPANIMENTS

(also see Pickle Relish, pg 82; Vegetable Spreads, pg 95; Vegetables–Pickled/ Specialty, pg 96; Salsa, pg 164)

	Cal	Fat	Sat	Chol	Carb	Fib	Sug	Sod
Fruit varieties:								
Cranberry sauce, jellied, 1/2" slice	86	0	0	0	22	1	22	17
Cranberry sauce, whole, 1/4 cup	105	0	0	0	27	1	26	20
Cranberry/orange relish, 1/4 cup	122	0	0	0	32	0	27	22
Major Grey chutney, 1 tbsp	60	0	0	0	14	0	9	170

NOTE: Some Major Grey brands have up to 900mg of sodium per tbsp.

	Cal	Fat	Sat	Chol	Carb	Fib	Sug	Sod
Vegetable varieties:								
Chow chow, 1 tbsp	10	0	0	0	1	0	0	45
Corn relish, 2 tbsp	40	0	0	0	10	0	4	80

Brands . . . *(1 tbsp unless noted)*

FRUIT VARIETIES

Cranberry sauce/relish – *Most brands within generic average (17-22mg).*

	Cal	Fat	Sat	Chol	Carb	Fib	Sug	Sod
American Spoon Roast Apple/Onion Relish	40	0	0	0	11	1	10	40
Bombay Authentics Luxury Mango Chutney	60	1	0	0	11	1	3	115
Busha Browne's Banana or Spicy Fruit Chutney	40	0	0	0	10	0	9	0
Crosse & Blackwell Cranberry Chutney	40	0	0	0	10	0	9	0
Pear Cardamom Chutney	25	0	0	0	6	0	5	10
Peach Zinfandel Chutney	20	0	0	0	5	0	5	15
Apricot Chardonnay Chutney	25	0	0	0	6	0	5	20
Apple Curry Chutney	25	0	0	0	7	0	5	25
Delicae Gourmet Key Lime Mango Relish	25	0	0	0	7	0	5	0
Cranberry Orange Liqueur Chutney	20	0	0	0	6	0	5	0
Key Lime Mango Chutney	20	0	0	0	5	0	5	0
Durbar Katki Diced Mango Chutney	61	0	0	0	15	0	15	124
Fanci Food Mango Raisin Chutney	60	0	0	0	14	0	13	100
Mango Pomegranate Chutney	50	0	0	0	13	0	2	100
Major Grey Chutney	60	0	0	0	14	0	2	105
Pineapple Chutney	60	0	0	0	16	0	2	115
Gloria's Depoe Bay Cranberry Chutney	50	0	0	0	14	0	12	0
Shady Grove Apple Chutney	30	0	0	0	7	0	5	15
Happy Valley Apple Salsa	20	0	0	0	4	0	3	45
Hannaford *Inspirations* Cranberry Apple Chutney	25	0	0	0	7	0	6	0
Inspirations Mango Chutney	25	0	0	0	6	0	6	35
Island Grove Tropical Salsa	16	0	0	0	4	0	4	51
Laxmi Brand Date Chutney	4	0	0	0	3	0	0	60
Kozlowski Farms Peach Chutney	30	0	0	0	7	0	3	0
Lost Acres Country Cranberry Relish, 1/4 cup	200	4	0	0	43	1	40	0
Native Forest Organic Pineapple Chutney	35	0	0	0	9	0	9	40
Organic Papaya Chutney	35	0	0	0	9	0	8	45
Organic Chutney, Hot Mango or Mango Passion	35	0	0	0	9	0	9	60
Neera's Pear Cardamom Chutney	30	0	0	0	7	1	3	23
Mango Chutney	20	0	0	0	2	0	1	26

75

CONDIMENTS AND SAUCES
Chutney, Relishes and Other Accompaniments

	Cal	Fat	Sat	Chol	Carb	Fib	Sug	Sod
Peach Chutney	22	0	0	0	6	0	2	30
Ginger Pineapple Chutney	31	0	0	0	7	0	6	54
Caribbean Salsa	25	0	0	0	7	0	6	60
Robert Rothschild Farm								
Roasted Pepper & Habanero Dip	0	0	0	0	14	0	14	0
Hot Pepper Raspberry Spread	70	0	0	0	16	1	15	0
Roasted Garlic & Fig Spread	60	0	0	0	14	0	12	25
Roland Major Grey's Mango Chutney, all	40	0	0	0	11	0	9	40
Peach Chutney	30	0	0	0	8	0	7	53
Steel's Natural Spiced Cranberry Sauce	30	0	0	0	8	1	7	0
Stonewall Kitchen Old Farmhouse Chutney	35	0	0	0	8	0	8	0
New England Cranberry Relish	25	0	0	0	7	0	6	0
Apple Cranberry Chutney	30	0	0	0	8	0	8	5
Major Grey Chutney	25	0	0	0	6	0	5	10
Mango or Fig Raisin Chutney (avg)	25	0	0	0	7	0	6	35
Taaza Tamarind Chutney	30	0	0	0	8	0	7	25
Sweet & Spicy Mango Chutney	20	0	0	0	4	0	3	40
Cilantro Mint Chutney	5	0	0	0	1	0	0	75
Major Grey Mango Chutney	25	0	0	0	6	0	5	90
Wild Thymes Mango Papaya Chutney	15	0	0	0	4	0	3	0
Cranberry Chutney, all varieties (avg)	21	0	0	0	5	0	4	0
Plum Ginger Chutney	20	0	0	0	5	0	4	1
Caribbean Peach Lime Chutney	15	0	0	0	4	0	3	5
VEGETABLE VARIETIES								
FROZEN/REFRIGERATED								
Cantare Moroccan Olive Salsa	35	3	1	0	3	1	1	100
Chipotle Olive Salsa	35	4	0	0	1	0	0	105
Sabra Caponata	55	5	1	0	2	1	0	65
SHELF-STABLE								
Alberto's Sweet Zucchini Relish	30	0	0	0	7	0	0	0
Am Spoon Red Spoon Peppers Relish	30	0	0	0	7	0	6	50
Sweet Tomato Relish, 2 tbsp	15	0	0	0	3	0	3	65
Portabello Mushroom Relish	20	1	0	0	2	1	1	105
Ripe Olive Relish	15	2	0	0	1	0	0	125
Braswell's Sweet Vidalia Onion Relish	15	0	0	0	3	0	3	45
Green Tomato Relish	20	0	0	0	5	0	4	115
Delicae Gourmet								
Roasted Garlic Tomato Chutney	10	0	0	0	5	0	2	50
Kalamata Sun-Dried Tomato Relish	15	0	0	0	3	1	2	70
Roasted Red Pepper Relish	15	0	0	0	4	1	3	85
Fischer & Wieser Sweet Onion/Pepper Relish	30	0	0	0	9	0	8	50
Gloria's Roasted Red Pepper/Ginger/Garlic	10	0	0	0	2	0	1	45
Howard's Hot or Sweet Pepper Relish	20	0	0	0	5	0	5	55
Green Tomato Piccalilli	15	0	0	0	4	1	3	90
Jok 'n' Al Tomato Relish	17	0	0	0	4	0	2	105
Piccalilli	15	1	0	3	3	0	2	110
Mezzetta Sweet Bell Pepper Relish	25	0	0	0	6	0	5	55
Deli-Style Hot Bell Pepper Relish	25	0	0	0	6	0	5	60
Mrs Campbells								
Chow Chow Relish, Sweet or Hot	10	0	0	0	3	0	2	20
Mrs Renfro's Tomato Relish, Mild or Hot	10	0	0	0	3	0	2	40
Chow Chow, Mild or Hot	10	0	0	0	3	0	2	45
Corn Relish	15	0	0	0	4	0	3	45
Nance's Corn Relish	20	0	0	0	5	0	3	75

	Cal	Fat	Sat	Chol	Carb	Fib	Sug	Sod
Neera's Hot Vegetable Chutney	21	2	0	0	2	0	1	49
Tomato Mint Chutney	30	2	0	0	5	1	5	54
Peloponnese Sweet Pepper Spread	15	2	0	0	0	0	0	90
Prairie Thyme Roasted Tomato Chutney	40	0	0	0	10	0	9	75
Roland Tomato Chutney	60	0	0	0	16	0	14	115
Robert Rothschild Farm								
Caramelized Onion Balsamic Spread	60	1	0	0	14	0	12	0
Roasted Red Pepper & Onion Dip & Relish	20	0	0	0	5	0	5	15
Stonewall Kitchen Artichoke & Caper Relish	10	1	0	0	1	0	0	15
Dried Tomato/Olive Relish	45	2	0	0	7	0	6	120
Farmhouse Red Relish	20	0	0	0	6	0	5	130
Spicy Corn Relish	35	0	0	0	8	0	6	140
Sunshine Specialty Foods Relishes								
Sweet Corn or Spicy Corn & Black Bean	15	0	0	0	3	0	2	20
Tomatillo Relish	10	0	0	0	2	0	1	40
Relish This! Sweet & Tangy	20	0	0	0	5	0	4	40
Relish This! Hot & Spicy or Sweet & Spicy	20	0	0	0	5	0	4	55
Taaza Tomato Garlic Chutney	25	3	0	0	1	0	3	55
Texas Sassy								
Hotter Than Hell or Hell or a Relish	25	0	0	0	7	0	6	25

COOKING WINE

Mirin sweet cooking wine, 1 fl oz	40	0	0	0	10	0	6	70
Cooking wine, 1 fl oz	14	0	0	0	2	0	0	182

Brands... *Most brands within generic average.*
NOTE: Instead of cooking wines, use madeira, sherry, etc. from the wine section, which have little or no sodium (see Wine/Champagne, pg 35).

HOLLANDAISE SAUCE

(see Hollandaise/Bearnaise Sauce, pg 93)

HORSERADISH

Horseradish sauce, 1 tsp	15	1	0	0	1	0	0	40
Brands...(1 tsp unless noted)								
Abeles & Haymann Horseradish Sauce	20	2	0	5	1	0	1	30
Ba-Tampte Horseradish or Horseradish/Beets	0	0	0	0	0	0	0	30
Beano's Horseradish Sauce	20	2	1	0	1	0	1	30
Beaver Cream or Wasabi Horseradish	10	1	0	0	1	0	1	20
Bell-View Cranberry Horseradish, Squeezable	10	1	0	0	1	0	1	5
Fancy Horseradish Sauce	20	2	0	0	1	0	1	30
Gold's Prepared Horseradish & Beets	0	0	0	0	0	0	0	30
Heluva Good Prepared Horseradish	0	0	0	0	1	0	0	5
Inglehoffer Cream Style or Wasabi	10	1	0	0	1	0	0	20
Extra Hot	10	1	0	0	1	0	0	30
Manischewitz Original or Wasabi (avg)	15	1	0	0	1	0	1	22
Lemon Horseradish Sauce	20	2	0	0	1	0	1	30
Noam Gourmet Prep Beets w/Horseradish	15	0	0	0	4	0	3	0
Prepared Beets w/Horseradish, no sugar	5	0	0	0	2	0	0	35
Robt Rothschild Farm Raspberry Cranberry	10	0	0	0	2	0	2	0
Roller's Prepared Horseradish	0	0	0	0	0	0	0	0
ShopRite Horseradish Sauce	15	2	0	5	1	0	0	15
Prepared Horseradish Full Strength	0	0	0	0	0	0	0	25
Silver Spring Cranberry Horseradish	10	0	0	0	2	0	1	10
Cream Style or Prepared Horseradish	0	0	0	0	0	0	0	10

	Cal	Fat	Sat	Chol	Carb	Fib	Sug	Sod
Pineapple Apricot Horseradish	10	0	0	0	2	0	1	25
Tulelake Old Fashioned Horseradish	0	0	0	0	0	0	0	0
Cream Style Horseradish	20	2	0	0	1	0	0	25
Wegmans Prepared Horseradish	0	0	0	0	0	0	0	0
Woeber's Sandwich Pal or Reserve Smoky Sauce	20	2	0	0	5	1	1	30
Zatarain's Prepared Horseradish	5	0	0	0	1	0	0	30

JAMS, JELLIES AND FRUIT SPREADS

	Cal	Fat	Sat	Chol	Carb	Fib	Sug	Sod
Fruit butter, 1 tbsp	29	0	0	0	7	0	6	3
Jam or jelly, 1 tbsp	56	0	0	0	14	0	10	6
Lemon curd, 1 tbsp	20	2	1	40	7	0	6	10

Brands . . . *Most brands within generic average.*

KETCHUP AND KETCHUP-LIKE SAUCES

	Cal	Fat	Sat	Chol	Carb	Fib	Sug	Sod
Ketchup, 1 tbsp	15	0	0	0	4	0	4	190

Brands . . . *(1 tbsp unless noted)*

	Cal	Fat	Sat	Chol	Carb	Fib	Sug	Sod
Chef Allen Mango Ketchup	20	0	0	0	5	0	4	25
Dickinson's Premium Tomato Ketchup	25	0	0	0	5	0	4	120
Heinz No Salt Ketchup	20	0	0	0	5	0	4	0
Hunt's NSA Ketchup	20	0	0	0	5	0	4	0
Montebello Kitchens Curry Ketchup	10	0	0	0	2	0	1	90
Robbie's Sweet & Tangy Ketchup	15	0	0	0	3	0	3	5
Savion Spicy Ketchup w/Horseradish	15	0	0	0	4	0	3	80
Steels All Natural Ketchup	5	0	0	0	2	0	1	20
Texas Sassy Tequila Ketchup	20	0	0	0	5	0	5	5
Westbrae Natural Unsweetened Un-Ketchup	5	0	0	0	1	0	0	60

MARASCHINO CHERRIES

	Cal	Fat	Sat	Chol	Carb	Fib	Sug	Sod
Maraschino cherries, 1	8	0	0	0	2	0	2	0

Brands . . . *Most brands within generic average.*

MARINATED VEGETABLES

(see Vegetables–Pickled/Specialty, pg 96)

MAYONNAISE AND SANDWICH SPREADS

	Cal	Fat	Sat	Chol	Carb	Fib	Sug	Sod
Mayonnaise, 1 tbsp	103	12	2	0	0	0	0	85
Light, 1 tbsp	49	5	1	0	1	0	1	120
Mayonnaise-type salad dressing, 1 tbsp	57	5	1	4	4	0	1	105
FF, 1 tbsp	13	0	0	0	2	0	2	126
Sandwich Spread, 1 tbsp	58	5	1	11	3	0	2	150

Brands . . . *(1 tbsp unless noted)*

MAYONNAISE AND MAYO-TYPE SPREADS
The following have 75mg or less sodium; light or fat free have 95mg or less.

	Cal	Fat	Sat	Chol	Carb	Fib	Sug	Sod
Agrosik Mayonnaise	90	10	2	5	0	0	0	50
Bama Real Mayonnaise	100	11	2	10	0	0	0	65
Best Made Mayonnaise	100	11	1	5	1	0	1	70
Cains All Natural Mayonnaise	100	11	2	5	0	0	0	75
Naturally Delicious Mayonnaise	90	10	1	10	0	0	0	75
Duke's Real Mayonnaise	100	12	2	10	0	0	0	75
Dynasty Wasabi Mayonnaise	100	11	2	10	0	0	0	70
Giant Real Mayonnaise	90	10	2	5	0	0	0	75
Hain Canola Mayonnaise	100	11	1	5	0	0	0	75
Hannaford Real Mayonnaise	100	11	2	5	0	0	0	75

	Cal	Fat	Sat	Chol	Carb	Fib	Sug	Sod
Hy-Vee Mayonnaise	100	11	2	5	0	0	0	75
JFG Real Mayonnaise	100	11	2	10	0	0	0	70
Kewpie Mayonnaise	100	10	1	3	0	0	0	14
Kraft Real Mayo or Mayo	90	10	2	5	0	0	0	70
La Costena Mayonnaise	100	12	2	15	0	0	0	65
Meijer Real Mayonnaise	100	11	2	5	0	0	0	75
Mrs Filbert's Real Mayonnaise Mayonesa	100	12	2	10	0	0	0	70
Nalley Real Mayonnaise	90	10	1	5	0	0	0	75
The Ojai Cook Latin Lemonaise	100	11	1	20	0	0	0	40
Fire & Spice Lemonaise	100	11	1	15	0	0	0	75
Saffola Mayonnaise	100	11	1	10	0	0	0	70
Sauer's Real Mayonnaise	100	11	2	10	0	0	0	75
Silver Palate *Organic* Roasted Garlic Mayonnaise	100	11	2	10	0	0	0	30
Organic Wasabi Mayonnaise	100	11	2	10	0	0	0	65
Spectrum Roasted Garlic Mayonnaise	100	11	2	10	0	0	0	30
Organic or Wasabi Mayonnaise	100	11	2	10	0	0	0	65
Roasted Garlic Mayonnaise	100	10	2	10	1	0	0	75
Olive Oil Mayonnaise	100	11	2	5	0	0	0	75
LIGHT MAYONNAISE								
Best Foods Canola Mayonnaise	45	5	0	0	1	0	0	95
Giant Light Mayonnaise	35	4	1	0	0	0	0	60
Follow Your Heart *Vegenaise* Reduced Fat	45	5	0	0	1	0	0	90
Hellmann's Canola Mayonnaise	45	5	0	0	1	0	0	95
Kraft Light Mayo or Mayo w/Olive Oil	45	4	0	5	0	0	0	95
Nalley Light Mayonnaise Dressing	50	5	1	10	1	0	0	95
Spectrum Lite Canola Eggless Mayonnaise	35	4	0	0	0	0	0	65
Walden Farms Mayo	0	0	0	0	0	0	0	90
SANDWICH SPREADS AND SAUCES								
Beano's All American Sandwich Spread	50	4	1	5	3	0	2	105
Wasabi Sandwich Sauce, 1 tsp	20	2	0	5	1	0	1	35
Bell-View Sandwich Spread	50	4	0	5	2	0	2	105
Blue Plate Sandwich Spread	75	7	1	5	3	0	2	105
Cain's Sandwich Spread	70	1	0	5	2	0	2	130
DiLusso Sweet Onion Sauce, 1 tsp	30	0	0	0	8	0	7	75
Mezzetta *Sandwich Spread* Jalapeno	40	4	1	0	1	0	0	55
Sandwich Spread Sun-Ripened Tomato	25	2	0	0	1	0	1	65
The Ojai Cook Latin Lemonaise	100	11	1	20	0	0	0	40
RC Fine Foods Ancho Chipotle Sandwich Sauce	10	0	0	0	3	0	2	5
Mango Habanero Mix Sandwich Sauce	15	0	0	0	4	0	3	15

MUSTARD

	Cal	Fat	Sat	Chol	Carb	Fib	Sug	Sod
Honey mustard, 1 tsp	10	0	0	0	2	0	1	25
Honey dijon, 1 tsp	10	0	0	0	2	0	2	50
Yellow mustard, 1 tsp	3	0	0	0	0	0	0	57
Dijon-type mustard, 1 tsp	5	0	0	0	0	0	0	120

Brands . . . *(1 tsp unless noted)*

Honey mustard – Most brands within generic average (25mg).

	Cal	Fat	Sat	Chol	Carb	Fib	Sug	Sod
A Perfect Pear Spicy Ginger Pear Mustard	5	0	0	0	1	0	0	0
Cherchies Champagne Mustard	10	0	0	5	2	0	2	0
East Shore, all varieties	15	0	0	0	2	0	0	0
Fischer & Wieser Smokey Mesquite	20	0	0	0	13	0	13	0
Brat Haus Beer Mustard	20	1	0	0	3	0	2	15
Pretzel Dipping Mustard	35	0	0	0	8	0	8	35
Haus Barhyte Sweet & Sour Mustard	15	0	0	0	3	0	3	20
HoneyCup Uniquely Sharp Stone Ground	15	1	0	0	3	0	1	0

CONDIMENTS AND SAUCES
Nut Butters

	Cal	Fat	Sat	Chol	Carb	Fib	Sug	Sod
Uniquely Sharp Mustard	20	1	0	0	2	0	2	5
Inglehoffer Sweet Hot Mustard	15	1	0	0	2	0	0	30
Raye's Hot & Spicy or Sweet & Spicy	5	0	0	0	0	0	0	10
Robt Rothschild Farm Raspberry Wasabi Dipping	10	1	0	0	1	0	0	15
Westbrae Natural Stone Ground NSA	0	0	0	0	0	0	0	0

DIJON-TYPE MUSTARDS
	Cal	Fat	Sat	Chol	Carb	Fib	Sug	Sod
Bell-View Creamy Dijon	15	1	0	5	1	0	1	55
Gold's Dijon	0	0	0	0	0	0	0	40
Grey Poupon Savory Honey Dijon	10	0	0	0	1	0	0	5
Laurent du Clos Walnut Dijon	10	1	0	0	0	0	0	80
Musette NSA Dijon Mustard	10	1	0	0	0	0	0	7
O Organics Dijon	0	0	0	0	0	0	0	65
Plochman's Honey Dijon	10	0	0	0	2	0	2	0
Temeraine NSA Dijon	7	1	0	0	0	0	0	7
Tree of Life Organic Dijon	0	0	0	0	0	0	0	65
True Natural Taste Dijon	0	0	0	0	0	0	0	55
Vineyard Pantry Blue Cheese Dijon	10	0	0	0	0	0	0	70
Westbrae Natural Dijon Style	0	0	0	0	0	0	0	65
Woodstock Farms Organic Dijon	0	0	0	0	0	0	0	60

MISC MUSTARDS
	Cal	Fat	Sat	Chol	Carb	Fib	Sug	Sod
Backyard Gardens Jalapeno Pepper Mustard	5	0	0	0	2	0	2	10
Banana Pepper Mustard, Sweet or Hot	5	0	0	0	2	0	2	10
Bell-View Onion Mustard	5	0	0	0	1	0	1	45
Mustard Relish	0	0	0	0	1	0	0	65

⬛ NUT BUTTERS

	Cal	Fat	Sat	Chol	Carb	Fib	Sug	Sod
Tahini, 2 tbsp	179	16	2	0	6	3	0	35
Almond butter, 2 tbsp	203	19	2	0	7	1	2	144
Peanut butter, 2 tbsp	188	16	3	0	6	2	3	147
Cashew butter, 2 tbsp	188	16	3	0	9	1	2	196

Brands . . . *(2 tbsp unless noted)*
The following have 80mg or less per serving.

PEANUT BUTTER
	Cal	Fat	Sat	Chol	Carb	Fib	Sug	Sod
Adams 100% Natural, Unsalted	210	16	3	0	6	2	1	0
Organic Peanut Butter	210	16	3	0	6	2	1	50
Arrowhead Mills Valencia or Organic Valencia	190	17	3	0	6	2	1	0
Crazy Richard's Natural Creamy or Crunchy	200	17	2	0	6	0	2	0
Das Dutchmen Essenhaus Amish PB, 1 tbsp	70	3	1	0	11	1	9	30
Fifty50 w/o Sugar, Creamy or Crunchy Peanut	190	16	2	0	7	3	1	0
Full Circle Organic Peanut Butter	190	15	4	0	7	2	2	55
Justin's Classic Peanut Butter	190	17	3	0	7	2	1	0
Honey Peanut Butter	180	15	2	0	8	2	2	65
Kettle Organic Peanut Butter, Unsalted	160	14	3	0	5	2	3	0
Koeze Co Cream Nut Natural Peanut Butter	190	16	3	0	6	2	1	35
Krema Natural Peanut Butter	190	16	2	0	7	3	2	0
Laura Scudder's Smooth Unsalted Peanut	210	16	3	0	6	2	1	0
Organic Nutty or Smooth	210	16	3	0	6	2	1	50
Maple Grove Farm Smooth or Crunchy	190	15	2	0	6	2	2	15
MaraNatha NSA Peanut Butter	190	16	2	0	7	4	2	0
Dark Choc Peanut Spread	180	13	2	0	12	1	8	30
Peanut Butter w/Salt	190	16	2	0	7	3	1	80
Natural Value NSA, all varieties (avg)	200	15	3	0	6	1	2	0
Nutella	200	11	4	0	22	1	21	15
Once Again NSA Peanut Butter	180	15	3	0	6	2	1	0

	Cal	Fat	Sat	Chol	Carb	Fib	Sug	Sod
Peanut Butter & Co White Choc Wonderful	180	14	3	0	11	1	7	35
Dark Choc Dreams or Cinnamon Raisin (avg) ..	165	12	3	0	12	2	8	35
The Heat is On...	190	16	3	0	6	2	1	40
Old Fashioned Smooth or Crunch Time..........	190	16	2	0	6	2	1	40
The Bee's Knees or Mighty Maple..................	180	14	3	0	12	1	8	60
Santa Cruz Organic Peanut Butter, all	210	16	3	0	6	2	1	50
Simply Jif	190	16	3	0	6	2	2	65
Smucker's Natural NSA...............................	210	16	3	0	6	2	7	0
Teddie Unsalted Peanut Butter	190	16	2	0	7	3	1	0
Tree of Life NSA Peanut Butter	190	16	4	0	7	1	0	0
Wegmans *Food Feel Good About* Natural........	200	16	3	0	6	2	1	10
Wild Harvest Organic Creamy	210	17	3	0	7	2	2	0
Woodstock Farms Organic Peanut Butter	180	15	3	0	6	2	1	40
Organic Classic Peanut Butter	190	15	4	0	7	2	2	55

OTHER NUT BUTTERS

	Cal	Fat	Sat	Chol	Carb	Fib	Sug	Sod
Arrowhead Mills Cashew, Creamy or Crunchy ..	160	13	3	0	9	1	2	0
Almond Butter, Creamy or Crunchy..............	200	17	2	0	6	4	2	0
Sesame Tahini	190	18	3	0	3	1	1	10
Blue Diamond Creamy or Crunchy (avg)........	190	17	3	0	7	3	2	75
Almond Butter w/Honey (avg).......................	180	14	2	0	10	3	3	75
Dan-D-Pak Almond Butter...........................	210	18	2	0	5	0	3	35
Eastwind, all nut butters (avg)	210	16	3	0	10	2	3	10
Full Circle Organic Almond Butter...............	180	16	2	0	7	4	2	0
Futters Natural Cashew or Organic Cashew.....	172	14	3	0	10	2	0	0
Natural or Organic Almond or Almond Haze......	170	15	1	0	5	4	0	0
Natural Hazelnut or Sunflower (avg)	185	17	1	0	5	3	0	0
Natural or Organic Pistachio........................	180	13	2	0	9	3	0	0
Natural Brazil Nut....................................	190	19	5	0	4	2	0	0
Natural & Organic Macadamia	230	24	4	0	5	3	0	0
Natural & Organic, Pecan or Walnut (avg)......	200	20	2	0	4	3	0	0
Natural or Organic Choc Almond (avg)	187	15	3	0	11	4	4	0
Natural Choc Haze or Choc Cherry Haze...........	210	19	2	0	8	2	3	0
Organic Choc Cherry Almond Haze	190	17	3	0	7	3	3	0
Organic & Natural Choc Almond Bliss	205	17	3	0	11	4	5	0
Justin's Classic Almond Butter	200	18	2	0	6	4	1	0
Honey Almond or Maple Almond (avg)	190	17	2	0	8	3	3	65
Kettle Cashew Butter, Unsalted	160	14	3	0	8	1	0	0
Hazelnut or Almond Butter, Unsalted (avg)	180	17	2	0	6	3	1	0
Almond Butter, Lightly Salted......................	180	17	2	0	6	2	0	55
Landau Tahini	180	15	2	0	8	5	0	10
MaraNatha NSA Cashew Macadamia Butter	200	18	3	0	8	1	2	0
NSA Macadamia Butter	230	24	4	0	4	3	1	0
NSA Almond or NSA Cashew Butter	190	16	3	0	9	3	2	0
Honey Almond Butter	180	14	1	0	9	3	5	70
Once Again Tahini	180	17	2	0	4	4	0	0
Almond Butter or Cashew Butter (avg)..........	180	16	3	0	8	3	2	0
Sunbutter NSA Sunflower Seed....................	220	20	2	0	5	2	1	30
Woodstock Farms Sesame Tahini, Unsalted ...	180	17	2	0	4	4	0	0
Cashew Butter, Unsalted	180	15	3	0	9	1	2	0
Almond Butter, Unsalted or Raw	180	16	2	0	7	4	2	0
Zinke Orchards Natural Almond Butter..........	182	16	2	0	6	1	0	4

OLIVES

	Cal	Fat	Sat	Chol	Carb	Fib	Sug	Sod
Black (Ripe), 0.5 oz	16	2	0	0	1	0	0	122
Green, 0.5 oz...	20	2	0	0	1	1	0	218

CONDIMENTS AND SAUCES
Pickles and Pickle Relish

	Cal	Fat	Sat	Chol	Carb	Fib	Sug	Sod
Kalamata, 0.5 oz	40	4	0	0	1	0	0	240
Brands . . . *(0.5 oz unless noted)*								
Bella Hot Jalapeno Stuffed Olives...................	25	2	0	0	0	0	0	95
Bell-View Extra Large Pitted Ripe Olives.........	25	3	0	0	1	0	0	110
Small Pitted Ripe Olives	25	3	0	0	1	0	0	115
Black Pearls Black, whole, sliced, or chopped .	25	2	0	0	1	0	0	95
Cento Jumbo Whole Calif Ripe Olives, 2..........	15	2	0	0	1	0	0	90
Graber Olives Tree Ripened, 0.7 oz (3)..........	25	2	1	0	1	1	0	95
Kalamata Gold Organic Kalamata	45	4	1	0	2	0	0	100
Lindsay LS, med	25	3	2	0	1	0	0	40
Mario LS Olives..	25	3	2	0	1	0	0	40
Kalamata	45	5	9	9	1	9	9	140
Mezzetta Garlic Stuffed Olives	20	1	0	0	2	1	0	125
Napa Valley Bistro Garlic Stuffed Olives.........	15	1	0	0	1	0	0	140
Napoleon Alfonso Olives	25	3	0	0	1	0	0	115
Pearls Reduced Salt Pimiento Stuffed.............	25	3	1	0	0	0	0	70
Santa Barbara Olive Co Pitted Green or Black	25	3	0	0	1	1	0	77
Tassos Kalamata Greek Olives	25	2	2	0	1	0	0	115
Blonde Olives or Stuffed Pimiento Evian Olives	25	2	2	0	1	0	0	115
Evian Olives or Stuffed Almond Evian Olives ..	25	2	0	0	1	1	0	115
Garlic Stuffed Collosal.................................	25	3	0	0	1	1	0	115
Vigo Jalapeno Stuffed Olives	25	2	0	0	0	0	0	95

PATÉ

(see Patés, pg 201; Sandwich Spreads, pg 201)

PICKLED AND SPECIALTY VEGETABLES

(see Vegetables–Pickled/Specialty, pg 96)

PICKLES AND PICKLE RELISH

(also see Vegetable Chutneys/Relishes, pg 76)

	Cal	Fat	Sat	Chol	Carb	Fib	Sug	Sod
Pickles:								
Bread and butter pickles, 1 oz......................	25	0	0	0	6	0	5	190
Sweet pickles, 1 oz.....................................	33	0	0	0	9	0	4	263
Sweet gherkin, 1 oz	35	0	0	0	10	0	4	282
Dill pickles, 1 oz...	5	0	0	0	1	0	1	359
Pickle relish:								
Sweet pickle relish, 1 tbsp...........................	20	0	0	0	5	0	2	122
Hamburger or hot dog relish, 1 tbsp	17	0	0	0	4	0	3	164
Dill pickle relish, 1 tbsp...............................	5	0	0	0	1	0	1	240
Brands . . . *(1 oz unless noted)*								
BREAD AND BUTTER PICKLES								
B&G Bread & Butter Topper...........................	30	0	0	0	7	0	6	120
Ba-Tampte Bread & Butter...........................	20	0	0	0	5	0	5	120
Cains Sweet Bread & Butter Chips, 4 slices	25	0	0	0	7	0	6	110
Full Circle Bread & Butter.............................	30	0	0	0	7	0	7	90
Meijer Sugar Free Bread & Butter Chips	0	0	0	0	1	0	0	120
Mt Olive Sandwich Stuffers or Spears.............	20	0	0	0	6	0	4	105
No Sugar Added, Sandwich Stuffers or Spears ...	0	0	0	0	1	0	0	105
Nalley Sugar Free Bread & Butter	0	0	0	0	1	0	0	120
Bread & Butter Cucumber Chips	35	0	0	0	9	0	8	135
ShopRite NSA Bread & Butter Chips...............	25	0	0	0	6	0	6	0
Bread & Butter - Sandwich or Chips...............	30	0	0	0	6	0	6	120
Steinfeld's Bread & Butter Chips....................	40	0	0	0	11	0	10	110

	Cal	Tot	Sat	Chol	Carb	Fib	Sug	Sod
Tony Packo's Bread & Butter	30	0	0	0	8	0	7	70
Vlasic Zesty Bread & Butter	40	0	0	0	10	0	9	110
Wegmans NSA Bread & Butter Chips	30	0	0	0	7	0	7	0

DILL PICKLES

	Cal	Tot	Sat	Chol	Carb	Fib	Sug	Sod
Mt Olive Reduced Sodium Kosher Dills, all	0	0	0	0	1	0	0	135
Wegmans Reduced Sodium Kosher Dill Spears	0	0	0	0	1	0	0	140

REDUCED SODIUM (LESS THAN GENERIC):

	Cal	Tot	Sat	Chol	Carb	Fib	Sug	Sod
Ba-Tampte Garlic Dill	0	0	0	0	1	0	0	180
Bessinger Baby Dill Pickles	5	0	0	0	1	0	0	180
Grundelsheim Crunchy Dills	10	0	0	0	2	0	1	150
Marco Polo Dill Pickles	15	0	0	0	3	0	3	176
Vlasic Reduced Sodium Dill Spears	0	0	0	0	1	0	0	150

SWEET PICKLES

	Cal	Tot	Sat	Chol	Carb	Fib	Sug	Sod
B&G Sweet Gherkins or Sweet Mixed Pickles	35	0	0	0	9	0	7	115
Bell-View Candied Chips, Sweet or Raisin	50	0	0	0	12	0	11	140
Branch Ranch Sweet Cucumber Pickles	50	0	0	0	13	0	10	100
Hengstenberg Cornichons	10	0	0	0	2	0	1	140
Meijer Sugar Free Sweet Pickles	0	0	0	0	0	0	0	120
Mt Olive Sweet, Sweet Gerkins, or Midgets	35	0	0	0	8	0	7	100
Sweet Gherkins, No Sugar Added	0	0	0	0	1	0	0	100
Nathan's Sweet Horseradish Pickles	28	0	0	0	1	0	8	90
Sechler's Candied Sweet Dill Chunks	45	0	0	0	11	0	9	130
Candied Sweet Orange Strips	45	0	0	0	11	0	9	130
ShopRite Sweet Gherkins or Sweet Mixed	35	0	0	0	7	0	7	115

MISC PICKLES

	Cal	Tot	Sat	Chol	Carb	Fib	Sug	Sod
Frog Ranch Peppered Pickles	30	0	0	0	8	0	7	100

PICKLE RELISH *(1 tbsp unless noted)*

	Cal	Tot	Sat	Chol	Carb	Fib	Sug	Sod
B&G Sweet Relish, Unsalted	20	0	0	0	5	0	4	0
Hot Dog Relish	20	0	0	0	3	0	3	75
Cascadian Farm Sweet Pickle Relish	15	0	0	0	4	0	4	65
Claussen Sweet Pickle Relish	10	0	0	0	3	0	2	85
Farman's Sweet Pickle Relish	15	0	0	0	3	0	2	90
Full Circle Organic Sweet Relish	15	0	0	0	4	0	4	60
Gedney Hot Dog Pickle Relish	18	0	0	0	4	0	3	100
Gold's Sweet Hot Dog Relish	15	0	0	0	3	0	3	90
Heinz Sweet Relish	20	0	0	0	5	0	3	95
Hot Dog or India Relish (avg)	18	0	0	0	4	0	3	100
Meijer Sugar Free Sweet Relish	0	0	0	0	0	0	0	90
Mt Olive Reduced Sodium Sweet Relish	20	0	0	0	4	0	2	50
Sweet Relish or Sweet India	20	0	0	0	4	0	2	90
Natural Valley Sweet Pickle Relish	20	0	0	0	5	0	4	75
Safeway Squeeze Pickle Relish	20	0	0	0	4	0	4	80
ShopRight Sweet Pickle Relish	20	0	0	0	4	0	2	90
Steinfeld's Sweet Pickle Relish	20	0	0	0	5	0	4	105

(PIMENTO)

	Cal	Tot	Sat	Chol	Carb	Fib	Sug	Sod
Pimento, 1 oz	6	0	0	0	1	0	1	3

Brands . . . *Most brands within generic average.*

(SALAD DRESSING)

	Cal	Tot	Sat	Chol	Carb	Fib	Sug	Sod
Vinegar and oil, 2 tbsp	144	16	3	0	1	0	0	0
Ranch dressing, ready-to-use, 2 tbsp	145	15	2	10	2	0	1	245
Mix, to make 2 tbsp	120	0	0	0	1	0	0	135
FF, ready-to-use, 2 tbsp	33	0	0	0	7	0	2	211

CONDIMENTS AND SAUCES
Salad Dressing

	Cal	Fat	Sat	Chol	Carb	Fib	Sug	Sod
LF, ready-to-use, 2 tbsp	59	4	0	5	6	0	1	273
Thousand island dressing, ready-to-use, 2 tbsp	111	11	2	8	4	0	4	259
FF, ready-to-use, 2 tbsp	42	0	0	2	9	1	5	233
Green goddess dressing, ready-to-use, 2 tbsp..	128	13	2	12	2	0	2	260
French dressing, ready-to-use, 2 tbsp	146	14	2	0	5	0	5	268
LF, ready-to-use, 2 tbsp	67	3	0	0	9	0	5	236
Blue cheese or roquefort, ready-to-use, 2 tbsp.	143	15	2	9	1	0	1	279
FF, ready-to-use, 2 tbsp	39	0	0	1	9	1	3	277
Russian dressing, ready-to-use, 2 tbsp	107	8	1	0	10	0	5	298
Caesar dressing, ready-to-use, 2 tbsp	163	17	3	1	1	0	1	323
Cole slaw dressing, ready-to-use, 2 tbsp	140	13	2	15	6	0	5	340
Italian dressing, ready-to-use, 2 tbsp	86	8	1	0	3	0	2	486
FF, ready-to-use, 2 tbsp	13	0	0	0	2	0	2	316
Mix, to make 2 tbsp	5	0	0	0	1	0	1	320
LF, ready-to-use, 2 tbsp	23	2	0	2	1	0	1	410
Zesty Italian, ready-to-use, 2 tbsp	109	11	1	0	2	0	1	505
Brands . . . *(2 tbsp unless noted)*								
MIXES								
Delicaé Pantry Coleslaw Dressing Base, 1 tbsp .	25	0	0	0	7	0	7	95
RC Fine Foods Honey Mustard	5	0	0	0	1	0	1	80
LF Honey Mustard	10	0	0	0	2	0	1	90
Caesar or Siena Vinaigrette	5	0	0	0	1	0	1	140
Simply Organic Apple-Basil	10	0	0	0	2	0	0	135
READY-TO-USE								
American Spoon Raspberry Vinaigrette	70	4	0	0	10	0	9	45
Cherry Vinaigrette	80	3	0	0	14	0	13	70
Annie's Naturals FF Mango Vinaigrette	20	0	0	0	5	0	5	5
FF Raspberry Vinaigrette	30	0	0	0	7	0	7	10
Lite Raspberry Vinaigrette	40	3	0	0	5	0	4	55
Balsamic or Organic Balsamic Vinaigrette (avg)..	100	10	1	0	2	0	1	55
Lite Honey Mustard	40	3	0	0	4	0	3	125
A Perfect Pear Ginger Pear Salad Dressing	20	0	0	0	6	0	2	0
Champagne Pear Vinaigrette	60	5	0	0	3	0	2	35
Bragg Organic Healthy Vinaigrette	90	9	2	0	3	0	2	60
Braswell's Creamy Vidalia Onion Dressing	120	9	2	0	10	0	9	95
Brianna's Champagne Caper Vinaigrette	160	15	1	0	5	0	4	105
Cain's Light Raspberry Vinaigrette	80	4	1	0	11	0	6	20
Raspberry Vinaigrette	80	6	1	0	6	0	4	130
Consorzio Strawberry & Balsamic FF	20	0	0	0	4	0	4	0
FF Mango or FF Raspberry & Balsamic (avg) ..	25	0	0	0	7	0	6	20
Delicae Gourmet Key Lime Mango Rum	50	0	0	0	14	0	12	0
Orange Lavendar Horseradish Salad Dressing	50	0	0	0	12	0	12	20
Peach Honey Mustard	30	0	0	0	8	0	6	50
Greek Mediterranean Salad Dressing	30	0	0	0	6	0	4	80
Cherry Balsamic Salad Dressing	30	0	0	0	6	0	6	90
Strawberry Balsamic Salad Dressing	30	0	0	0	6	0	4	110
Drew's Greek Olive Dressing	120	12	2	0	6	0	0	130
Smoked Tomato Dressing	100	10	0	0	4	0	0	138
Roasted Garlic Dressing	140	16	2	0	0	0	0	138
Shiitake Ginger Dressing	160	16	2	0	0	0	0	140
Emeril's Balsamic Vinaigrette	30	3	0	0	2	0	1	85
Farmer Boy Restaurant Lite Greek Dressing	40	3	0	0	4	0	3	0
Fischer & Wieser Sweet Corn/Shallots Dressing	70	5	0	0	4	0	0	70
Roasted Raspberry Vinaigrette	100	4	0	0	16	0	14	100

	Cal	Fat	Sat	Chol	Carb	Fib	Sug	Sod
Follow Your Heart Vegan Honey Mustard	117	10	1	0	6	0	6	129
Foods Alive Flax or Hemp Oil Dressing								
Sweet & Sassy	160	15	2	0	6	0	6	70
Mike's Special	150	15	2	0	2	0	2	120
Full Circle *Organic* Raspberry Vinaigrette	50	0	0	0	1	0	1	10
Organic Ranch Salad Dressing	100	10	2	5	2	0	1	130
Galeo's Miso Dressing & Dip	44	4	0	0	1	1	1	70
Miso Dijonnaise Dressing & Dip	38	4	0	0	1	1	1	70
Miso Ginger Wasabi Dressing & Dip	28	2	0	0	1	1	1	84
Miso Caesar Dressing & Dip	28	2	0	0	1	1	1	112
Girard's Raspberry Vinaigrette	120	10	2	0	9	0	9	65
Apple Poppyseed	110	9	2	0	8	0	8	105
Light Raspberry Dressing	60	4	0	0	7	0	7	130
Peach Mimosa Vinaigrette	100	8	2	0	5	0	5	135
Gloria's Caribbean Sunshine	45	1	0	0	9	0	8	0
Raspberry Poppyseed	140	9	0	0	16	0	14	0
Raspberry Poppyseed, Oil Free	60	0	0	0	15	0	14	0
Marionberry, Cranberry, or Huckleberry Poppy Seed	60	0	0	0	15	0	14	0
Roasted Red Pepper Vinaigrette	65	7	0	0	2	0	0	70
Gunther's Vinaigrette & Marinade								
Roasted Garlic & Sundried Tomato	180	20	2	0	0	0	0	50
Lemon Oregano	160	18	3	0	0	0	0	70
Orange Balsamic	40	3	0	0	4	0	0	80
Island Grove								
Caribbean Garlic Dressing/Marinade	70	7	1	0	3	0	3	5
LF Raspberry Poppy Dressing & Marinade	40	3	0	0	5	0	5	40
LF Roasted Vadalia Onion Dressing & Marinade	35	2	0	0	5	0	5	55
Key Lime Honey Ginger Dressing & Marinade	125	10	1	0	9	0	8	90
Oriental Sweet Heat Dressing & Marinade	25	0	0	0	5	0	5	95
Lite Balsamic Vinaigrette	30	3	0	0	0	0	0	98
LF Mango Poppy Seed Dressing & Marinade	50	3	0	0	8	0	8	103
Lite Florida Keys' Key Lime Pepper	25	2	0	0	0	0	0	120
LF Florida Keys' Key Lime Pepper	50	3	0	0	8	0	8	130
LF Florida Orange Poppy Dressing & Marinade	55	3	0	0	7	0	6	130
Key Lime Honey Mustard	150	10	2	10	7	0	7	140
Lite Mango Poppy	30	3	0	0	0	0	0	140
Ken's Steak House								
Lite Accents Raspberry Walnut, 10 sprays	15	1	0	0	1	0	1	35
Lite Accents Asian Vinaigrette, 10 sprays	15	1	0	0	2	0	2	80
Lite Accents Honey Mustard, 10 sprays	10	0	0	0	2	0	2	95
Lite Accents Balsamic Vinaigrette, 10 sprays	10	1	0	0	1	0	1	95
Golden Vidalia Onion	120	9	2	0	10	0	9	95
Sweet Vidalia Onion	120	9	2	0	10	0	10	115
Lite Raspberry Walnut Vinaigrette	80	6	0	0	7	0	6	120
Lite Accents Italian Vinaigrette, 10 sprays	15	1	0	0	1	0	1	135
Kozlowski Farms								
Raspberry Poppy Seed	15	0	0	0	4	0	3	58
Roasted Garlic & Pepper	10	0	0	0	2	0	0	80
Honey Mustard	30	0	0	0	7	0	6	105
Lucini Cherry Balsamic & Rosemary Vinaigrette	120	12	1	0	3	0	3	105
Maple Grove Farms								
Balsamic Vinaigrette w/Maple Syrup	50	3	0	0	5	0	5	35
Ginger Pear	40	3	0	0	3	0	2	40
Italian White Balsamic, Sugar Free	100	11	1	0	1	0	0	70
Citrus Vinaigrette	80	6	0	0	6	0	5	70

CONDIMENTS AND SAUCES
Salad Dressing

	Cal	Fat	Sat	Chol	Carb	Fib	Sug	Sod
Balsamic Vinaigrette, Sugar Free..................	5	0	0	0	1	0	0	90
FF Balsamic Vinaigrette..............................	15	0	0	0	3	0	2	95
Creamy Ranch, Sugar Free	100	12	1	0	1	0	0	110
Champagne Vinaigrette..............................	100	11	1	0	2	0	1	130
FF Lime Basil Vinaigrette	25	0	0	0	6	0	5	130
FF Vidalia Onion.......................................	20	0	0	0	5	0	4	140
Raspberry Vinaigrette, Sugar Free	5	0	0	0	1	0	0	140
Marzetti *Organic* Raspberry Cranberry	100	8	1	0	6	0	6	65
Strawberry Chardonnay Vinaigrette	100	8	2	0	6	0	6	140
Strawberry Vinaigrette..............................	100	8	2	0	6	0	6	140
Matsos Greek Dressing & Marinade................	150	16	5	0	1	0	1	10
Naturally Delicious Light Raspberry	60	3	0	0	8	0	8	70
Organic Ville Pomegranate Vinaigrette	100	10	2	0	2	0	2	55
Robt Rothschild Farm Raspberry Dressing	60	2	0	0	11	0	9	0
Raspberry Wasabi	60	5	3	0	3	1	1	75
Peanut Ginger Dressing.............................	130	10	2	0	11	0	8	95
Seeds of Change Balsamic Vinaigrette	60	4	0	0	6	0	3	105
Silver Palate *Salad Splash* Balsamic Country	180	13	2	0	4	0	4	25
Salad Splash Really Raspberry	25	0	0	0	6	0	4	70
Salad Splash Raspberry Sun	80	8	8	0	4	0	3	120
Red Wine w/Olive Oil	150	17	3	0	0	0	0	135
Simply Natural								
Raspberry Vinaigrette	60	6	1	0	3	0	2	100
Roasted Red Pepper Vinaigrette	80	8	2	0	2	0	2	100
Smith & Wollensky Caesar Dressing.............	130	14	2	10	0	0	0	70
Steel's All Natural Ginger Lime Dressing	73	8	0	0	2	1	1	10
All Natural Honey Mustard Dressing	93	8	1	0	2	0	2	125
Stonewall Kitchen Olive Oil & Balsamic	160	18	3	0	2	0	2	0
Strawberry Balsamic Dressing.........................	80	5	0	0	8	0	7	55
Classic Italian Dressing	180	20	2	0	1	0	0	75
Maple Balsamic Dressing	90	7	1	0	8	0	7	95
Balsamic Fig Dressing	80	5	0	0	11	0	10	120
Teresa's Select Recipes								
Blueberry Pomegranate Vinaigrette..............	130	11	2	0	8	0	7	125
Melon Cucumber	100	9	2	0	5	0	5	130
Texas Sassy All Natural Vinaigrette	80	8	2	0	4	0	4	10
Wild Thymes Salad Refreshers, all (avg)........	70	5	0	0	6	0	6	9
Vinaigrettes, all (avg)...............................	86	8	1	0	4	0	2	14
Parmesan Walnut Caesar Vinaigrette.............	90	9	1	0	2	0	1	36
Tuscan Tomato Basil Vinaigrette	78	8	1	0	2	0	1	38
Toasted Sesame Wasabi Vinaigrette..............	84	8	1	9	2	9	1	111
REFRIGERATED								
Bolthouse Farms Raspberry Merlot Vinaigrette	30	1	0	0	6	0	5	50
Honey Mustard Yogurt Dressing	45	2	1	5	7	0	6	80
Tropical Mango Vinaigrette	30	2	0	0	5	0	4	95
Creamy Italian Yogurt Dressing	70	7	2	10	2	0	1	105
Chunky Blue Cheese Yogurt Dressing	50	5	2	10	1	0	1	140
Litehouse Organic Raspberry Lime Vinaigrette .	45	3	0	0	5	0	4	60
White Balsamic..	90	9	1	0	4	0	3	70
Raspberry Walnut Vinaigrette......................	100	9	1	0	5	0	5	75
Huckleberry Vinaigrette.............................	25	0	0	0	6	0	4	105
Harvest Cranberry Vinaigrette......................	25	0	0	0	6	0	6	110
Pomegranate Blueberry.............................	25	0	0	0	6	0	5	130
Red Wine & Olive Oil Vinaigrette..................	90	9	1	0	3	0	1	140
Marie's Raspberry Vinaigrette	40	1	0	0	8	0	6	60

	Cal	Fat	Sat	Chol	Carb	Fib	Sug	Sod
Caprese Dressing	110	11	2	0	2	0	2	85
Creamy Italian Garlic	180	19	3	15	1	0	0	135
Naturally Fresh Cranberry Walnut (seasonal)	90	10	3	10	6	0	5	30
Bleu or Bacon Bleu Cheese	170	18	3	15	1	0	0	120
Roasted Garlic Bleu Cheese	170	18	4	15	1	0	1	125
Lite Bleu Cheese	100	10	3	10	1	0	1	130
Riverhouse Cheddar and Chives	140	13	3	5	5	1	3	110
Wegmans Raspberry Cherry Vinaigrette	70	4	1	0	8	0	4	10

SALAD TOPPINGS

	Cal	Fat	Sat	Chol	Carb	Fib	Sug	Sod
Croutons, plain, 2 tbsp	58	0	0	0	10	0	0	99
Seasoned, 2 tbsp	66	1	0	1	9	1	0	155
Bacon bits, 1 tbsp	25	2	1	5	0	0	0	250
Imitation (meatless), 1 tbsp	33	2	0	0	2	1	0	124

Brands . . . *(2 tbsp unless noted)*

BACON BITS – *Most brands within generic average.*

CROUTONS

Most brands are low sodium, the following have 75mg or less sodium per serving.

	Cal	Fat	Sat	Chol	Carb	Fib	Sug	Sod
Albertsons Restaurant Style Cheese & Garlic	30	1	0	0	5	0	0	60
Aunt Millie's Plain Croutons, 1/3 cup	40	0	0	0	8	1	1	63
Cardini's Gourmet Cut Caesar	35	2	0	0	4	0	0	50
Gourmet Cut Garlic	35	2	0	0	4	0	0	55
Gourmet Cut Romano Cheese	40	3	0	0	3	0	0	60
Chatham Village Caesar	35	2	0	0	4	0	0	50
Large Cut - Caesar or Garlic & Butter	35	2	0	0	4	0	0	55
Garden Herb or Garlic & Butter	35	2	0	0	4	0	0	55
Cheese & Garlic, Large Cut	40	3	0	0	3	0	0	60
Edward & Sons Organic Onion Garlic	30	1	0	0	5	0	0	60
Organic Italian Herbs	30	1	0	10	5	0	0	75
Ener-G	25	1	0	0	3	0	0	25
Fresh Gourmet FF Garlic Caesar Premium	15	0	0	0	3	0	0	55
Sweet Butter Cornbread	30	1	0	0	4	0	0	60
Butter & Garlic or Cheese & Garlic	30	1	0	0	5	0	0	65
Cheese & Garlic Premium	30	1	0	0	5	0	0	65
Organic Seasoned	30	2	0	0	4	0	0	70
Marie Callender's Whole Grain Caesar	35	2	0	0	4	1	0	65
Cheese & Garlic	30	1	0	0	5	0	0	70
Ranch	30	1	0	0	5	0	0	75
Marzetti Caesar, large cut	35	2	0	0	4	0	1	50
Garlic & Butter, reg or large cut	35	2	0	0	4	0	1	55
Cheese & Garlic, large cut	40	3	0	0	3	0	0	60
Mrs Cubbison's Caesar Salad	35	2	0	0	4	0	1	65
Cool Herb Ranch	30	1	0	0	5	0	1	75
Musso's Garlic Croutons, 1/4 cup	30	1	1	0	5	0	0	55
New York Texas Toast Garlic & Butter	35	2	0	0	4	0	0	55
Texas Toast Cheese & Garlic	35	2	0	0	4	0	0	65
Texas Toast Caesar	35	2	0	0	4	0	0	70
Old London Restaurant Style Seasoned	30	1	0	0	5	0	0	65
Restaurant Style Italian	30	1	0	0	5	0	0	70
Olivia's Croutons								
Butter & Garlic or Parmesan Pepper	40	1	1	5	4	0	0	50
Osem Mediterranean Caesar	32	2	1	0	4	0	0	57
Mediterranean Tri-Color	32	2	1	0	4	0	0	62
Mediterranean Herbs	32	2	1	0	4	0	0	74

CONDIMENTS AND SAUCES
Sauces – BBQ/Grilling Sauces and Marinades

	Cal	Fat	Sat	Chol	Carb	Fib	Sug	Sod
Pepperidge Farm Whole Grain Caesar...........	35	1	0	0	5	0	1	50
Zesty Italian	30	1	0	0	5	0	1	55
Classic Caesar	30	1	0	0	5	0	1	60
Four Cheese & Garlic	30	1	0	0	5	0	1	65
Onion & Garlic	30	1	0	0	5	0	1	70
Seasoned	30	1	0	0	5	0	1	75
Reese Whole Grain Garlic & Cheese	30	1	0	0	5	1	0	60
Caesar	30	1	0	0	5	1	0	65
Italian Herb	30	1	0	0	5	1	0	70
Sami's Bakery Millet & Flax Croutons	8	0	0	0	4	1	0	50
Wegman's Caesar......................................	35	2	0	0	4	0	0	50
Lightly Seasoned or Garlic............................	35	2	0	0	4	0	0	55
Unseasoned	25	0	0	0	5	0	0	55
Seasoned..	25	0	0	0	5	0	0	60
Cheese & Garlic	40	3	0	0	3	0	0	60
Whole Wheat	35	2	0	0	4	1	0	70
Organic Italian Herbs....................................	30	1	0	10	5	0	0	75

OTHER SALAD TOPPINGS

	Cal	Fat	Sat	Chol	Carb	Fib	Sug	Sod
Durkee *Salad Sensations* Garden Style, 1 tbsp .	35	2	0	0	3	1	1	70
French's French Fried Onions, 2 tbsp	45	4	1	0	3	0	0	60
Cheddar French Fried Onions, 2 tbsp	45	4	1	0	3	0	0	65
Fresh Gourmet Tortilla Strips Tri-Color, 2 tbsp..	35	2	0	0	5	0	0	15
Tortilla Strips Lightly Salted, 2 tbsp	35	2	0	0	5	0	0	15
Tortilla Strips Santa Fee Style, 2 tbsp	30	2	0	0	4	0	0	25
Wonton Strips Garlic Ginger, 2 tbsp	35	2	0	0	4	0	0	35
Wonton Strips, 2 tbsp	20	0	0	0	4	0	0	45
Crispy Onions Lightly Salted, 1.5 tbsp..........	40	3	0	0	4	0	0	45
Crispy Onions Garlic Pepper, 1.5 tbsp...........	35	2	0	0	4	0	0	50
Garlic Gold Nuggets, 1 tsp	10	1	0	0	1	0	0	0
T. Marzetti's *Salad Accents* Fruit & Nut, 1 tbsp.	45	2	0	0	5	1	4	25
Salad Accents Asian Sesame, 1 tbsp.............	40	3	0	0	3	1	0	55
Salad Accents Bacon Almond Crunch, 1 tbsp..	35	2	0	0	3	1	0	60
McCormick *Salad Toppins* Garden Veg, 1.3 tbsp .	35	2	0	0	3	0	1	60
Naturally Fresh *Salad Toppings*								
Glazed Almond & Pecan Pieces, 0.5 tbsp........	40	3	0	0	3	1	2	0
Roasted & Glazed Pecan Pieces, 0.5 tbsp.......	45	5	0	0	2	1	1	15
Nuts & Fruit Mix, 0.5 tbsp............................	45	4	0	0	2	1	1	20
New York *Texas Toast* Tortilla Strips								
Chipotle Cheddar, 0.25 oz	35	2	0	0	4	0	0	45
Chile Lime, 0.25 oz	35	2	0	0	4	0	0	50
Rising Sun Farms *Salad Energizer*								
Cranberry, Hazelnut & Gorgonzola	110	7	2	5	13	1	10	100
Currants, Pecan & Parmesan........................	110	6	2	5	13	1	11	125
Figs, Sunflower Seeds & Feta.......................	70	4	1	5	8	2	5	135
Sargento *Salad Finishers* Cranberry Pecan......	140	10	3	10	9	1	6	120
Sunkist *Almond Accents* Butter Toffee Glazed..	40	3	0	0	2	1	1	30
Almond Accents Bacon Cheddar, 1 tbsp...........	45	4	0	0	1	1	0	55
Almond Accents Original, 1 tbsp..................	40	4	0	0	1	0	0	70

SAUCES – BBQ/GRILLING SAUCES AND MARINADES

(also see Dipping/Finishing Sauces/Glazes, pg 91; Asian Sauces, pg 159)

	Cal	Fat	Sat	Chol	Carb	Fib	Sug	Sod
Jerk sauce, 2 tbsp	20	0	0	0	3	0	3	210
Barbecue sauce, 2 tbsp................................	53	0	0	0	13	0	9	392
Marinade, 1 tbsp	10	1	0	0	1	0	1	380

There are many low-sodium barbecue/grilling sauces and marinades, the following have 100mg or less per serving.

Brands . . . *(2 tbsp unless noted)*

	Cal	Fat	Sat	Chol	Carb	Fib	Sug	Sod
MIXES								
Bernard LS Barbecue Sauce Mix, 2 tbsp	40	0	0	0	10	0	6	5
READY-TO-USE								
American Spoon Ginger Plum Grilling	70	0	0	0	18	0	15	5
Apple Cider Grilling	45	0	0	0	12	0	11	85
A Perfect Pear Ginger Pear Marinade	15	0	0	0	4	0	2	40
Pear Chipotle Grill	80	0	0	0	20	0	20	60
Blue Crab Bay Co Seafood Marinade/Grilling	120	12	2	0	6	0	6	40
Bob Evans Wildfire BBQ Sauce	60	0	0	0	14	1	-	95
Braswell's Smokey Rib Sauce	20	0	0	0	5	0	3	35
Bronco Bob's Roasted Raspberry Chipotle	30	0	0	0	7	0	7	40
Roasted Mango Chipotle Sauce	60	0	0	0	15	0	14	50
Tangy Apricot	45	0	0	0	11	1	10	100
Chef Allen Papaya Pineapple BBQ	30	0	0	0	8	0	2	50
Tamarind Chili Spicy Grill Sauce	30	0	0	0	8	0	2	80
Passion Fruit Mojo Marinade	20	0	0	0	4	0	4	90
Country Sweet Hot or Mild	50	0	0	0	13	0	13	36
Cunningham's Memphis Basting Sauce	10	0	0	0	1	0	0	30
Dave's Gourmet Badlands BBQ Sauce	40	1	0	0	8	0	7	100
Delicae Gourmet Ginger Peach Asian Grilling	60	0	0	0	14	0	14	0
Key Lime Mango Rum Dressing & Marinade	50	0	0	0	14	0	12	0
Mango Key Lime Tequilla Marinade	40	0	0	0	10	0	10	0
Papaya Key Lime Grilling Sauce	30	0	0	0	6	0	6	30
Roasted Red Pepper Grilling	20	0	0	0	6	0	4	30
Mango Curry BBQ	40	0	0	0	10	0	10	40
Key Lime Steak & Grilling Sauce	30	0	0	0	8	0	6	80
Diana's Grill Crazy Lime Wasabi	25	0	0	0	7	0	0	5
Earth & Vine Papaya Chipotle Pineapple	45	0	0	0	11	0	9	5
Raspberry Ancho Orange	45	0	0	0	11	1	8	15
Fischer & Wieser Papaya Lime Serrano Sauce	80	0	0	0	22	0	20	0
Charred Pineapple Bourbon	70	0	0	0	16	0	16	0
Mango Ginger Habanero	80	0	0	0	22	0	18	0
Plum Chipotle Grilling Sauce	80	0	0	0	20	0	20	30
Harvest Apple Cider Grilling	40	0	0	0	12	0	10	40
Asian Wasabi Plum Dipping Sauce	40	0	0	0	10	0	8	40
Sweet, Sour & Smokey Mustard	70	0	0	0	16	0	16	70
Sweet Corn/Shallots Dressing/Marinade	70	5	0	0	4	0	0	70
Black Raspberry Chipotle Sauce	70	0	0	0	22	0	20	80
Floribbean Mango Garlic or Key Lime w/Ginger	40	0	0	0	10	0	8	5
Garlic Survival Roasted Garlic Marinade	10	0	0	0	2	0	0	0
Garlic Lemon Marinade	10	0	0	0	2	0	2	10
44 Clove Garlic Cooking	10	0	0	0	2	1	1	70
Ginger People Ginger Wasabi Dressing/Dipping	40	4	0	0	1	0	1	35
Ginger Lemon Grass Dressing/Cooking	90	9	1	0	3	0	3	90
Gunther's Vinaigrette & Marinade								
Roasted Garlic & Sundried Tomato	180	20	2	0	0	0	0	50
Lemon Oregano	160	18	4	0	0	0	0	70
Orange Balsamic	40	4	0	0	4	0	0	80
Hook to Cook Tropic Sauce	73	0	0	0	18	0	16	9
Hot Rod Bob's Original All Natural BBQ Sauce	44	1	0	0	9	0	11	31
Thick & Spicy All Natural BBQ Sauce	44	1	0	0	9	0	11	31

89

CONDIMENTS AND SAUCES
Sauces – BBQ/Grilling Sauces and Marinades

	Cal	Fat	Sat	Chol	Carb	Fib	Sug	Sod
Hurricane Bay Florida Spice	25	0	0	0	6	0	6	45
Southwestern Marinade	47	0	0	0	12	0	12	47
Isaly's Original or Spicy BBQ Sauce	30	0	0	0	7	0	5	95
Island Grove Caribbean Garlic Dressing/Marinade	70	7	1	0	3	0	3	5
LF Raspberry Poppy	40	3	0	0	5	0	5	40
LF Vadalia Onion	35	2	0	0	5	0	5	55
Balsamic Vinaigrette	30	3	0	0	3	0	3	73
Key Lime Honey Ginger	125	10	1	0	9	0	8	90
Oriental Sweet Heat	25	0	0	0	5	0	5	95
Lite Balsamic Vinaigrette	30	3	0	0	0	0	0	98
Kelly's BBQ Sauce, Hickory or Hot & Spicy	25	0	0	0	6	0	5	85
Ken's Steak House NSA Honey Garlic	7	5	0	0	6	0	6	0
NSA Lemon Pepper or NSA Sesame Ginger (avg)	30	0	0	0	6	0	3	0
Kona Coast Aloha Sweet Onion Grilling/Dipping	60	0	0	0	14	1	11	90
Kozlowski Farms Grilling Sauce								
Mango & Apricot Roasted Chipotle	80	0	0	0	20	0	20	50
Lollipop Tree Mango Garlic	60	0	0	0	14	0	13	10
Lum Taylor's Barbeque Sauce	110	0	0	0	27	0	27	15
Marinade Bay Cooking & Grilling Sauce								
Cilantro & Lime, 1 tbsp	50	4	1	0	2	0	2	55
Rosemary Mint, 1 tbsp	50	5	1	0	3	0	3	55
Garlic & Herb, 1 tbsp	45	5	1	0	2	0	2	70
Lemon & Herb or Santa Fe, 1 tbsp (avg)	47	5	1	0	2	0	2	75
Lemon Pepper, 1 tbsp	25	1	0	0	4	0	4	80
Honey Bourbon, 1 tbsp	50	4	1	0	3	0	3	95
Miko Marinade/Sauce, Ginger or Wasabi Ginger	70	6	0	0	4	0	2	50
Key Lime Ginger Marinade & Sauce, 1 tbsp	70	6	0	0	2	0	2	50
Monty Smith's All Natural Barbecue Sauce	30	0	0	0	7	0	4	10
Mr. Spice Organic Salt Free Sauces								
Honey BBQ & Marinade	40	0	0	0	10	0	8	0
Honey Mustard Sauce & Marinade	35	0	0	0	8	0	7	0
Thai Peanut Sauce & Marinade	50	1	0	0	6	0	4	0
Ginger Stir-Fry Sauce & Marinade	30	0	0	0	8	0	6	0
Indian Curry Sauce & Marinade	30	0	0	0	6	0	4	0
Sweet & Sour Sauce & Marinade	45	0	0	0	10	1	9	0
Garlic Steak Sauce & Marinade	40	0	0	0	8	0	6	0
Mrs. Dash *10-Minute Marinades*, all (avg)	25	2	0	0	3	0	1	0
Olde Cape Cod Lemon Ginger BBQ/Grilling	25	0	0	0	5	0	4	10
Robbie's Barbecue Sauce, 1 tbsp	25	0	0	0	6	0	5	30
Robert Rothschild Farm								
Hot Pepper Raspberry Chipotle Sauce	60	0	0	0	16	1	15	0
Cherry Pomegranate Habanero Sauce	50	0	0	0	12	0	12	5
Ana Mae's Smoky Sweet Oven & Grill	30	0	0	0	7	0	5	25
Blackberry Chipotle Sauce	50	0	0	0	14	1	13	70
Anna Mae's Smoky Sweet Chipotle Sauce	35	0	0	0	9	0	8	80
Southern Delight NSA Mint Julep Marinade	25	0	0	0	5	0	4	30
NSA Classic Sweet & Spicy Marinade	20	0	0	0	5	0	4	30
NSA Smoky Pecan Peppercorn Marinade	30	1	0	0	6	0	4	30
NSA Classic Sweet & Spicy BBQ	35	0	0	0	8	0	7	35
NSA Smoky Pecan Peppercorn BBQ	40	1	0	0	8	0	6	35
NSA Mint Julep BBQ	35	0	0	0	8	0	6	35
NSA Sweet Bacon/Spice BBQ	40	0	0	0	8	0	6	65
NSA Sweet Bacon & Spice Marinade	25	0	0	0	5	0	4	65
Stonewall Kitchen Curried Mango Grille	60	0	0	0	15	0	14	15
Garlic Rosemary Citrus	50	0	0	0	13	0	12	55

	Cal	Fat	Sat	Chol	Carb	Fib	Sug	Sod
Honey Barbecue Sauce	70	0	0	0	17	0	15	85
Roasted Garlic Peanut Sauce	60	3	0	0	8	0	6	95
Mesquite Steak Sauce	50	0	0	0	12	0	10	95
Roasted Tomato Grille Sauce	30	0	0	0	6	0	5	100
Sunshine Specialty Foods Pina Colada								
Dessert & Cooking Sauce, 1 tbsp	45	3	2	0	5	0	4	0
Texas Sassy Salsa Marinade	30	0	0	0	6	0	6	90
Tony Chachere's Injectables								
Praline Honey Ham Marinade, 1 tbsp	35	0	0	0	9	0	7	0
Wild Thymes Chili Ginger Honey Marinade	64	0	0	0	17	0	15	24
Tropical Mango Lime Marinade	24	0	0	0	6	1	4	63
JERK AND WING SAUCE								
Island Grove Redneck Whisky Wing Sauce	0	0	0	0	0	0	0	18
JCS Boston Jerk Sauce, 1 tbsp	15	0	0	0	3	0	1	70
Mr Spice Organic SF Hot Wing Sauce/Marinade	30	0	0	0	6	0	4	0
Walkerswood Jerk Barbecue Sauce	45	1	0	0	10	0	10	125
Wing Time Buffalo Wing Sauce								
Medium, Hot, or Super Hot	45	4	1	0	2	0	1	40
Mild	45	5	1	0	1	0	1	50
Garlic	50	5	1	0	2	0	1	55

SAUCES – BEARNAISE SAUCE

(see Hollandaise/Bearnaise Sauce, pg 93)

SAUCES – BROWNING AND SEASONING SAUCE

	Cal	Fat	Sat	Chol	Carb	Fib	Sug	Sod
Browning and seasoning sauce, 1 tsp	15	0	0	0	3	0	0	10

Brands . . . *Most brands within generic average.*

SAUCES – CHEESE SAUCE

(also see Alfredo Sauce, pg 208)

	Cal	Fat	Sat	Chol	Carb	Fib	Sug	Sod
Cheese sauce, ready-to-serve, 1/4 cup	110	8	4	18	4	0	0	522
Mix, prep, 1/4 cup	60	3	2	4	8	0	1	685

Brands . . . *(1/4 cup prep unless noted)*
MIXES

	Cal	Fat	Sat	Chol	Carb	Fib	Sug	Sod
Bernard LS Cheese Sauce Mix	25	1	0	0	5	0	2	70
Med-Diet Cheddar Cheese	20	0	0	0	3	0	-	115
REDUCED SODIUM (LESS THAN GENERIC):								
Rico's Cheddar Cheese Sauce	70	6	3	5	4	0	1	280

SAUCES – CLAM SAUCE

(see Pasta Sauce, pg 205)

SAUCES – COCKTAIL SAUCE

(see Seafood Sauces, pg 94)

SAUCES – COOKING SAUCE

(see BBQ/Grilling Sauces/Marinades, pg 88; Asian Sauces, pg 159; Mediterranean/Middle Eastern–Sauces, pg 170)

SAUCES – DIPPING/FINISHING SAUCES AND GLAZES

(also see BBQ/Grilling/Marinades, pg 88; Seafood Sauces, pg 94)
Brands . . . *(1 tbsp unless noted)*

	Cal	Fat	Sat	Chol	Carb	Fib	Sug	Sod
Crosse & Blackwell Ham Glaze	30	0	0	0	7	0	5	25

CONDIMENTS AND SAUCES
Sauces – Gravy and Cream Sauces

	Cal	Fat	Sat	Chol	Carb	Fib	Sug	Sod
Delicae Gourmet Key Lime Ginger Mango	15	0	0	0	4	0	3	0
Orange Marmalade Coconut Dipping	30	0	0	0	7	0	6	0
Raspberry Chipotle Sauce....................	25	0	0	0	6	0	6	0
Indian Curry Finishing Sauce	20	0	0	0	6	0	5	0
Sweet Onion Balsamic Finishing Sauce	15	0	0	0	4	0	3	0
Pomegranate Orange Dipping Sauce	35	0	0	0	9	0	8	10
Mexican Mole Finishing	10	0	0	0	2	0	1	40
Key Lime Mustard Seafood Sauce	35	3	0	0	3	0	2	55
Sweet Honey Mustard Dipping Sauce	30	2	0	0	4	0	4	70
Asian Finishing Sauce	25	0	0	0	6	0	5	95
Fischer & Wieser Sweet & Savory Onion Glaze .	45	0	0	0	11	0	11	5
Raspberry Chipotle Sauce, 1 tbsp....................	40	0	0	0	10	1	9	60
Pasilla Chile Finishing Sauce	10	1	0	0	1	0	1	85
Ginger People Sweet Ginger Chili Sauce, 2 tbsp	70	0	0	0	16	0	14	5
Hot Ginger Jalapeno, 2 tbsp.........................	15	0	0	0	3	0	2	35
Ginger Wasabi Slathering & Cooking	40	4	0	0	1	0	0	35
Ginger Wasabi Dressing & Dipping................	40	4	0	0	1	0	1	35
Neera's Tamarind Dipping Sauce & Glaze, 1 tsp	15	0	0	0	3	0	5	98
Prairie Thyme Blackberry Jalapeno Ambrosia .	35	0	0	0	9	0	8	5
Raspberry Jalapeño Ambrosia, Spicy or Original	35	0	0	0	9	0	8	5
Peach Habanero Ambrosia	35	0	0	0	9	0	8	5
Robt Rothschild Farm								
Ginger Wasabi Sauce, 1 tsp	10	1	0	0	1	0	1	10
Lemon Wasabi Sauce, 1 tsp.........................	20	2	1	0	1	0	0	30
Hot Raspberry Thunder Sauce, 1 tbsp	25	0	0	0	7	0	7	75
Wild Thymes Thai Chili Roasted Garlic Dipping .	38	0	0	0	9	0	8	18
Indian Vindaloo Curry Dipping......................	12	1	0	0	1	0	0	51
Moroccan Spicy Pepper Dipping Sauce	23	2	0	0	2	0	1	60
Indonesian Peanut Sesame Dipping Sauce	32	2	1	0	2	0	1	74

SAUCES – GRAVY AND CREAM SAUCES

	Cal	Fat	Sat	Chol	Carb	Fib	Sug	Sod
Turkey gravy, mix, prep, 1/4 cup	27	1	0	2	4	0	1	274
Canned, 1/4 cup	30	1	0	1	3	0	0	343
Beef gravy, canned, 1/4 cup	31	1	1	2	3	0	0	326
Brown gravy, mix, prep, 1/4 cup	25	1	0	1	4	0	1	339
30% less sodium mix, prep, 1/4 cup.............	25	1	0	0	3	0	0	230
Mushroom gravy, canned, 1/4 cup	30	2	0	0	3	0	0	339
Au jus, ready-to-use, 1/4 cup	20	1	0	0	3	0	0	340
Mix, 1 tsp...	9	0	0	0	1	0	0	348
Chicken gravy, canned, 1/4 cup.....................	47	3	1	1	3	0	0	343

Brands . . . *(1/4 cup unless noted)*

MIXES

	Cal	Fat	Sat	Chol	Carb	Fib	Sug	Sod
Med-Diet Premium Mushroom, Chicken or Brown	15	0	0	0	3	0	0	40
RC Fine Foods LS Instant Turkey or Chicken....	30	2	0	0	4	0	0	115
LS Instant Brown Gravy	25	1	0	0	5	0	0	130
Tony Chachere's Cream of Mushroom Mix	25	0	0	0	5	0	0	5

REDUCED SODIUM (LESS THAN GENERIC):

	Cal	Fat	Sat	Chol	Carb	Fib	Sug	Sod
Tony Chachere's Brown Gravy Mix	10	0	0	0	2	0	0	150
White Gravy Mix	20	0	0	0	4	0	0	170

GRAVY THICKENER

	Cal	Fat	Sat	Chol	Carb	Fib	Sug	Sod
Savoie's Instant Roux/Gravy Thickener, 2 tsp ...	30	0	0	0	6	3	0	5
Tony Chachere's Instant Roux Mix................	10	0	0	0	2	0	0	80

	Cal	Fat	Sat	Chol	Carb	Fib	Sug	Sod

SAUCES – HARD SAUCE

	Cal	Fat	Sat	Chol	Carb	Fib	Sug	Sod
Plum pudding hard sauce, 1 tbsp	180	8	5	15	26	0	25	65

Brands . . . *Most brands within generic average.*

SAUCES – HOLLANDAISE AND BEARNAISE SAUCE

	Cal	Fat	Sat	Chol	Carb	Fib	Sug	Sod
Hollandaise sauce, mix, 2 tsp	15	0	0	0	15	0	0	110
Bearnaise sauce, mix, 1 tsp	10	0	0	0	1	0	0	130

Brands . . .

	Cal	Fat	Sat	Chol	Carb	Fib	Sug	Sod
Blessac Hollandaise or Bernaise, 2 tsp mix	21	2	1	0	0	0	0	29
Knorr Hollandaise Mix	10	0	0	0	2	0	0	80
Bearnaise Mix	10	0	0	0	2	0	0	110
Mayacamus Hollandaise Sauce Mix	10	1	0	5	2	1	1	80
Simply Organic Hollandaise Mix	10	0	0	0	2	0	0	100
Wagner's Hollandaise Sauce Mix	15	1	0	10	2	0	0	75

SAUCES – HOT PEPPER SAUCE

(also see Hispanic/Latino Sauces, pg 164)

	Cal	Fat	Sat	Chol	Carb	Fib	Sug	Sod
Hot sauce, 1 tsp	1	0	0	0	0	0	0	124

Brands . . . *(1 tsp unless noted)*

	Cal	Fat	Sat	Chol	Carb	Fib	Sug	Sod
Arriba! Mango Pepper Sauce	5	0	0	0	1	0	0	10
Chipotle Pepper Sauce	5	0	0	0	0	0	0	15
Garlic Pepper Sauce	5	0	0	0	0	0	0	40
Chef Allen Orange-Chipotle Blasting Sauce	5	0	0	0	1	0	0	20
Dave's Gourmet Total Insanity	10	0	0	0	0	0	0	0
Ginger Peach or Ultimate Insanity	0	1	0	0	0	0	0	0
Temporary Insanity	10	0	0	0	0	0	0	10
Hurtin' Habanero or Cool Cayenne Pepper	10	0	0	0	0	0	0	15
Crazy Caribbean or Hurtin' Jalapeno	0	0	0	0	0	0	0	15
Jammin' Jerk Sauce	5	0	0	0	1	0	0	15
Hot Sauce & Garden Spray	0	0	0	0	0	0	0	15
Roasted Red Pepper/Chipotle	0	0	0	0	0	0	0	55
Scotch Bonnet Hot Sauce	0	0	0	0	0	0	0	60
Delicae Gourmet Key Lime Ginger Mango, 1 tbsp	15	0	0	0	4	0	3	0
Frontera Chipotle Hot Sauce	5	0	0	0	1	0	1	20
Red Pepper Hot Sauce	5	0	0	0	1	0	0	35
Habanero or Jalapeno Hot Sauce	5	0	0	0	1	0	0	35
Garlic Survival Co Roasted Garlic Hot Pepper	0	0	0	0	0	0	0	10
Glory Foods Hickory Smoked Hot Sauce	5	0	0	0	2	0	1	35
Island Grove Jamaican	10	0	0	0	0	0	1	25
West Indies Peppa Sauce	3	0	0	0	1	0	8	30
Bo Bo's Bajan Hot Sauce	10	0	0	0	0	0	0	40
Jump Up & Kiss Me Hot Sauce w/Passion	10	0	0	0	2	0	1	0
Spicy Passion Fruit Sauce, 1 tbsp	10	0	0	0	2	0	2	0
Chipotle Sauce, 1 tbsp	5	0	0	0	1	0	0	15
Marie Sharp's Belizean Heat Hot Sauce	24	0	0	0	5	0	2	12
McIlhenny Tabasco (original)	0	0	0	0	0	0	0	30
Mr. Spice Organic SF Tangy Bang	5	0	0	0	1	0	1	0
Phamous Phloyd's Hot Sauce	15	0	0	0	4	1	0	2
Pickapeppa	5	0	0	0	1	0	1	40
SOB Habanero Hot Sauce	6	0	0	0	0	0	0	48
Walkerswood Hot Jamaican Scotch Bonnet	0	0	0	0	0	0	0	45
Seriously Hot Jonkanoo Pepper Sauce	0	0	0	0	0	0	0	60
The Wizard's Hot Stuff	0	0	0	0	0	0	0	65

	Cal	Fat	Sat	Chol	Carb	Fib	Sug	Sod

SAUCES – LIQUID SMOKE

	Cal	Fat	Sat	Chol	Carb	Fib	Sug	Sod
Liquid smoke, 1 tsp	0	0	0	0	0	0	0	10

Brands . . . *Most brands within generic average.*

SAUCES – MINT SAUCE

	Cal	Fat	Sat	Chol	Carb	Fib	Sug	Sod
Mint sauce, 1 tsp	5	0	0	0	1	0	1	0

Brands . . . *Most brands within generic average.*

SAUCES – PASTA AND PIZZA SAUCE

(see Pasta Sauce, pg 205; Pizza Sauce, pg 150)

SAUCES – SEAFOOD SAUCES

	Cal	Fat	Sat	Chol	Carb	Fib	Sug	Sod
Cocktail sauce, 1/4 cup	80	2	0	0	16	1	14	680

Brands . . . *(1/4 cup unless noted)*

MIXES

	Cal	Fat	Sat	Chol	Carb	Fib	Sug	Sod
Blue Crab Bay Cocktail Sauce Seasoning Blend	0	0	0	0	0	0	0	0

READY-TO-USE

	Cal	Fat	Sat	Chol	Carb	Fib	Sug	Sod
Chef Allen Hot Mango Cocktail Sauce, 1 tbsp	10	0	0	0	3	0	2	30
Crosse & Blackwell Lemon Dill Sauce	130	0	0	0	33	0	29	15
Robert Rothschild Farm								
Peach Coconut Mango Habanero Seafood, 1 tbsp	25	0	0	0	6	0	6	5
Lemon Dill & Capers Sauce, 2 tbsp	70	6	0	5	1	0	1	130
Steel's Cocktail Sauce w/Dill & Lemon	35	0	0	0	9	2	6	85

SAUCES – SLOPPY JOE SAUCE

	Cal	Fat	Sat	Chol	Carb	Fib	Sug	Sod
Sloppy joe sauce, canned, 1/4 cup	30	0	0	0	6	1	5	370
Mix, 1/8 pkg	15	0	0	0	3	0	1	360

Brands . . .

	Cal	Fat	Sat	Chol	Carb	Fib	Sug	Sod
Dixie Diner Homestyle Sloppy Joe Mix, 7 oz	83	1	0	0	9	5	2	117

SAUCES – STEAK SAUCE

	Cal	Fat	Sat	Chol	Carb	Fib	Sug	Sod
Steak sauce, 1 tbsp	14	0	0	0	4	0	2	280

Brands . . . *(1 tbsp unless noted)*

	Cal	Fat	Sat	Chol	Carb	Fib	Sug	Sod
Braswell's Merlot Wine Sauce	15	0	0	0	3	0	2	75
Busha Browne's Planters Steak Sauce	5	0	0	0	2	0	1	10
Chef Allen Orange Chipotle Blasting	5	0	0	0	10	0	0	20
Crosse & Blackwell Mint Meat Sauce, 1 tsp	5	0	0	0	2	0	2	0
Delicae Gourmet Key Lime Steak & Grilling	15	0	0	0	4	0	3	40
Earp's Western Steak & Dinner	30	0	0	0	7	0	10	55
Mr. Spice	15	0	0	0	4	0	2	0
Newman's Own Steak Sauce	20	1	0	0	4	0	1	85
Robt Rothschild Farm Chop House Steak Sauce	50	4	0	0	4	0	3	65
Hot Raspberry Thunder Sauce	25	0	0	0	7	0	7	75
Southern Comfort	15	0	0	0	3	0	3	60
Stonewall Kitchen Mesquite Steak Sauce	50	0	0	0	12	0	10	95
World Harbors Steakhouse Sauce, 2 tbsp	35	0	0	0	7	0	5	135

SAUCES – TARTAR SAUCE

	Cal	Fat	Sat	Chol	Carb	Fib	Sug	Sod
Tartar sauce, 2 tbsp	190	20	3	15	1	0	0	250

Brands . . . *(2 tbsp unless noted)*

	Cal	Fat	Sat	Chol	Carb	Fib	Sug	Sod
Naturally Fresh Tartar Sauce (refrigerated)	130	14	2	10	2	0	2	85

	Cal	Fat	Sat	Chol	Carb	Fib	Sug	Sod

SAUCES – WORCESTERSHIRE SAUCE

	Cal	Fat	Sat	Chol	Carb	Fib	Sug	Sod
Worcestershire sauce, 1 tsp	4	0	0	0	1	0	1	55

Brands . . . *(1 tsp unless noted)*

	Cal	Fat	Sat	Chol	Carb	Fib	Sug	Sod
America's Choice (A&P) Worcestershire	0	0	0	0	0	0	0	30
Robbie's Worcestershire	5	0	0	0	1	0	1	20

VEGETABLE SPREADS

(also see Chutneys/Relishes–Vegetable, pg 76; Sandwich Spreads, pg 78; Cream Cheese/Spreads, pg 104; Dips/Spreads, pg 220)

	Cal	Fat	Sat	Chol	Carb	Fib	Sug	Sod
Bruschetta, 1 oz	20	2	0	0	2	1	1	240
Olive tapenade, 1 oz	60	4	0	0	2	0	0	320

Brands . . . *(1 oz unless noted)*

FROZEN/REFRIGERATED

	Cal	Fat	Sat	Chol	Carb	Fib	Sug	Sod
Sabra Caponata	55	5	1	0	2	1	0	65
Vegetarian Liver	70	6	0	30	2	0	1	70
Ratatouille	35	3	0	0	2	0	1	80

READY-TO-USE

	Cal	Fat	Sat	Chol	Carb	Fib	Sug	Sod
Bellino Bruschetta Tomato Topping	20	2	0	0	1	0	1	140
Bonavita								
Vegetarian Paté, Mushroom or Herb, 1 tbsp	30	2	0	0	1	0	0	80
Cantare Olive Tapenade French Black Olive	35	3	0	0	1	0	0	100
Classico Bruschetta								
Basil & Tomato or Extra Garlic, 1 tbsp	15	1	0	0	1	0	0	55
Delicae Gourmet								
Artichoke & Red Pepper Tapenade, 1 tbsp	15	1	0	0	1	0	0	20
Artichoke Lèmon Tapenade, 1 tbsp	25	2	0	0	1	0	0	35
Artichoke Parmesan Tapenade, 1 tbsp	25	2	0	0	1	0	0	50
Red Pepper Parmesan Tapenade, 1 tbsp	20	1	0	0	1	0	1	50
Truffled Artichoke Tapenade, 1 tbsp	25	2	0	0	1	0	0	55
Artichoke/Sun-Dried Tomato Tapenade, 1 tbsp	10	0	0	0	2	0	1	60
Artichoke & Green Olive Tapenade, 1 tbsp	20	2	0	0	3	0	0	115
Bruschetta Topping:								
Sun-Dried Tomato, 1 tbsp	70	6	1	0	3	1	1	70
Sun-Dried Tomato & Basil, 1 tbsp	40	3	0	0	3	1	2	85
Sun-Dried Tomato & Feta or Olive, 1 tbsp	70	7	2	5	1	0	1	120
Sun-Dried Tomato/Red Pepper, 1 tbsp	40	3	0	0	3	0	1	125
Bread Topper:								
Sun-Dried Tomato Merlot, 1 tbsp	30	3	0	0	1	0	1	55
Roasted Pepper Beaujolais, 1 tbsp	10	0	0	0	1	0	0	60
Olive Medley Chardonnay, 1 tbsp	15	1	0	0	1	0	0	80
Artichoke in Zinfandel, 1 tbsp	15	1	0	0	1	0	0	85
Dickinson's								
Hot or Mild Pepper Spread, 1 tbsp	50	0	0	0	12	0	8	5
Fischer & Wieser								
Sicilian Tomato Pesto, 1 tbsp	20	2	0	0	2	0	1	90
Cilantro Pepito Pesto Spread, 1 tbsp	50	4	1	0	1	0	0	120
Gaea Sundried Tomatoes Tapenade, 1 tbsp	26	2	0	1	1	1	1	70
Sweet Pepper/Goat Cheese Tapenade, 1 tbsp	17	1	0	1	1	0	1	95
Smoked Eggplant Tapenade, 1 tbsp	17	1	0	0	2	0	1	102
Gia Russa Mushroom Bruschetta	60	6	1	0	0	0	0	120
Artichoke Bruschetta	60	6	1	0	2	1	1	135
Marco Polo Bruschetta, 1 tbsp	20	1	0	0	2	1	1	45
Meditalia Sundried Tomato Tapenade	30	2	0	0	3	0	2	65

CONDIMENTS AND SAUCES
Vegetables – Pickled and Specialty Vegetables

	Cal	Fat	Sat	Chol	Carb	Fib	Sug	Sod
Roasted Red Pepper Tapenade	16	1	0	0	1	0	0	137
Eggplant & Tomato Tapenade	24	2	0	0	2	0	0	143
Robert Rothschild Farm								
Caramelized Onion Balsamic Spread	60	1	0	0	14	0	12	0
Roland								
Red Pepper Spread	30	1	0	0	5	0	2	100
Bruschetta	25	2	0	0	2	0	1	135
Sonoma Dried Tomato Tapenade, 1 tbsp	70	6	1	0	4	1	1	5
Stonewall Kitchen Eggplant Spread, 1 tbsp	25	1	0	0	4	0	4	90
Tartex Vegetarian Paté, all varieties	50	4	3	0	2	1	0	130
Tassos Bruschetta, all varieties, 1 tbsp	42	4	1	0	1	0	0	132
Wegmans *Italian Classics*								
Roasted Red Pepper Bruschetta	30	2	0	0	3	1	1	105
World Table Tomato-Basil Bruschetta	25	2	0	0	1	0	0	75

VEGETABLES – PICKLED AND SPECIALTY VEGETABLES

(also see Vegetable Spreads, pg 95; Asian–Pickled Foods, pg 159; Chili Peppers, pg 168)

	Cal	Fat	Sat	Chol	Carb	Fib	Sug	Sod
Sun-dried tomatoes, 0.3 oz	20	0	0	0	4	1	2	45
Sun-dried tomatoes in oil, 1/4 cup	59	4	1	0	6	2	0	73
Pickled beets, 1 oz	25	0	0	0	6	0	5	100
Giardiniera, 1/4 cup	5	0	0	0	0	0	1	170
Cocktail onions, 0.5 oz	5	0	0	0	1	0	0	250
Hot banana peppers, 1 oz	5	0	0	0	1	1	0	378
Jalapeños, 1 oz	18	0	0	0	4	0	0	441
Pepperoncini, 1 oz	8	0	0	0	2	1	0	453
Red peppers, 1 oz	10	0	0	0	2	1	0	480

Brands . . . *(1 oz or 2 tbsp unless noted)*

PICKLED AND MARINATED VEGETABLES

	Cal	Fat	Sat	Chol	Carb	Fib	Sug	Sod
Aunt Nellie's Sliced Pickled Beets, 4 slices	15	0	0	0	4	0	4	55
Whole Pickled Beets, 2	20	0	0	0	4	1	4	65
America's Choice Tiny Whole Pickled Beets, 2	20	0	0	0	5	1	4	65
B&G Salad Peppers w/Oregano & Garlic	20	0	0	0	5	0	3	75
Sweet Pepper Strips or Sweet Bell Pepper	20	0	0	0	5	0	3	75
Boscoli Family Spicy Pickled Asparagus, 1 spear	6	0	0	0	0	3	0	60
Cento Marinated Mushrooms, 1 oz	10	0	0	0	2	0	0	45
Forrest Floor Foods Pickled Mushrooms	15	0	0	0	4	0	4	105
Garden Fresh Marinated Garlic	24	0	0	0	6	0	2	3
Haddon House Hot Pickled Red Chili Peppers	15	1	0	0	3	2	0	60
London Pub Pickled Onions	10	0	0	0	2	0	1	50
Mother Teresa's Mediterranean, Giardiniera	15	1	0	0	2	0	0	45
Mediterranean Caponata, 1 tbsp	4	0	0	0	1	0	0	60
Mediterranean Garlic	35	0	0	0	8	1	0	75
Mushrooms	15	1	0	0	2	0	0	130
Mrs Renfro's Green Tomato Pickles	25	0	0	0	6	0	5	75
Napoleon Pickled White Asparagus, 3 spears	10	0	0	0	1	0	0	75
Pickled Mushrooms	10	0	0	0	2	1	1	100
Pickled Asparagus, 3 spears	15	0	0	0	2	0	1	100
Roland Pickled Baby Corn	10	0	0	0	2	0	2	65
Safies Sweet Pickled Beets, 1/3 cup	80	0	0	0	19	1	18	40
Square Pickled Sweet Red Peppers	38	0	0	0	8	0	1	50
Tillen Farms								
Pickled Sweet Bell Peppers, 1/4 cup	25	0	0	0	6	0	5	0
Sunnyside Tomatoes	40	3	1	0	4	1	3	5

	Cal	Fat	Sat	Chol	Carb	Fib	Sug	Sod
Pickled Crispy Carrots	30	0	0	0	7	1	6	5
Crispy Pickled Asparagus	10	0	0	0	1	0	0	75
Crispy Pickled Asparagus, Hot & Spicy	10	0	0	0	1	0	0	75
Vigo Cocktail Onions, 1 pc	0	0	0	0	0	0	0	30
Marinated Asparagus, 3 spears	10	0	0	0	1	0	0	75
Marinated Mushrooms, 3 pcs	15	1	0	0	1	0	0	135

SUN-DRIED TOMATOES AND ROASTED PEPPERS

Sun-dried tomatoes – *Most brands within generic average (45–73mg).*

	Cal	Fat	Sat	Chol	Carb	Fib	Sug	Sod
Alessi Fire Roasted Italian Style Peppers	10	0	0	0	1	0	1	83
Fire Roasted Red & Yellow Peppers	10	0	0	0	1	0	1	83
B&G Roasted Peppers w/Balsamic Vinegar	0	0	0	0	2	0	2	70
Roasted Peppers w/Oregano & Garlic	15	2	0	0	1	0	1	75
Hot Chopped Roasted Peppers, 1 tsp	5	0	0	0	1	0	0	120
Cento Roasted Peppers	5	0	0	0	1	0	1	85
Marinated Roasted Peppers	15	1	0	0	1	0	1	100
Delallo Sun-Dried Tomatoes in Oil	70	5	1	0	6	1	3	10
Dunbar's Sweet Roasted Peppers	5	0	0	0	1	0	1	85
Gaea Roasted Red Peppers, 1/2 cup	10	0	0	0	2	0	1	120
Haddon House Roasted Red Peppers, 5 oz	0	0	0	0	5	0	1	20
La Squisita Roasted Peppers, 1/2 cup	25	0	0	0	4	1	2	140
Mezzetta Roasted California Bell Peppers	10	0	0	0	1	0	1	110
Napoleon Roasted Piquillo Peppers, 3 oz	20	0	0	0	4	1	1	135
Vigo Flame Roasted Peppers	10	0	0	0	1	0	1	50

VINEGAR

	Cal	Fat	Sat	Chol	Carb	Fib	Sug	Sod
Vinegar, 1 tbsp	2	0	0	0	1	0	0	0
Balsamic vinegar, 1 tbsp	5	0	0	0	2	0	2	0
Rice vinegar, unseasoned, 1 tbsp	0	0	0	0	0	0	0	0
Seasoned, 1 tbsp	20	0	0	0	5	0	5	240

Brands . . . *Most brands within generic average.*

DAIRY AND NON-DAIRY ALTERNATIVES

See RESOURCES, *page 305, for a partial list of manufacturers and retailers offering low-salt products online or visit* **LowSaltFoods.com** *for additional sources.*

DAIRY AND NON-DAIRY ALTERNATIVES

BUTTER, MARGARINE AND BUTTER-LIKE SPREADS

	Cal	Fat	Sat	Chol	Carb	Fib	Sug	Sod
Butter spray, 2 sprays	0	0	0	0	0	0	0	5
Butter, whipped, 1 tbsp	60	6	4	15	0	0	0	55
Unsalted whipped butter, 1 tbsp	60	6	4	15	0	0	0	0
Butter, stick, 1 tbsp	102	12	7	31	0	0	0	82
Unsalted butter, stick, 1 tbsp	102	12	7	31	0	0	0	0
Butter-flavored granules, 1 tsp	5	0	0	0	2	0	0	120
Margarine, stick, 1 tbsp	100	11	2	0	0	0	0	132
Unsalted margarine, stick, 1 tbsp	100	11	2	0	0	0	0	0
Whipped margarine, 1 tbsp	101	11	2	0	0	0	0	93

Brands . . . *(1 tbsp unless noted)*

BUTTER AND BUTTER BLENDS

	Cal	Fat	Sat	Chol	Carb	Fib	Sug	Sod
Unsalted butter (stick/whipped) – Most brands within generic average (0mg).								
Downey's Honey or Cinnamon Honey Butter	60	1	1	5	11	0	11	10
Land O Lakes Honey Butter	90	8	4	15	4	0	3	40
Organic Valley Whipped	50	6	4	15	0	0	0	40
Pasture Butter Salted Cultured Butter	110	12	7	30	0	0	0	40
Smart Balance 50/50 Butter Blend, Unsalted	100	11	5	15	0	0	0	0
Vermont Butter & Cheese								
Cultured Butter, Lightly Salted	110	12	7	30	0	0	0	30

MARGARINE AND SPREADS – *The following have 80mg or less sodium:*

	Cal	Fat	Sat	Chol	Carb	Fib	Sug	Sod
Unsalted margarine – Most brands within generic average (0mg).								
Butter-flavored granules – Most brands within generic average of 120mg.								
Canola Harvest all varieties, 2 tsp	70	8	1	0	0	0	0	70
Earth Balance Natural Buttery Spread w/Olive Oil	80	9	3	0	0	0	0	70
Fleischmann's Original Light Spread	60	7	1	0	0	0	0	60
Great Value Cardio Choice Buttery Spread	80	9	2	0	0	0	0	70
Land O Lakes Fresh Buttery Taste Spread, soft	70	8	2	0	0	0	0	80
Country Morning Blend Spread, soft	100	11	3	0	0	0	0	80
Move Over Butter Whipped Spread	50	6	1	0	0	0	0	70
Parkay Whipped Spread	70	7	2	0	0	0	0	80
Smart Balance Whipped, Lightly Salted	65	7	2	0	0	0	0	30
Extra Virgin Olive Oil	60	7	2	0	0	0	0	70
Light Extra Virgin Olive Oil	50	5	2	0	0	0	0	70
Heart Right Light or *Light* Omega-3 (avg)	50	5	2	0	0	0	0	80
Spectrum Spread	80	10	1	0	0	0	0	55

CHEESE – BLOCK/WEDGE

(also see Cheese–Grated/Shredded, pg 102; Cheese–Sliced/Packaged, pg 102)

	Cal	Fat	Sat	Chol	Carb	Fib	Sug	Sod
Swiss, 1 oz	108	8	5	26	2	0	0	60
Mozzarella, fresh, 1 oz	70	5	3	10	0	0	0	85
Part-skim, low moisture, 1 oz	86	6	4	15	1	0	0	150
Whole milk mozzarella, 1 oz	85	6	4	22	1	0	0	178
Gruyere, 1 oz	117	9	5	31	0	0	0	95
Goat cheese, hard, 1 oz	128	10	7	30	1	0	1	98
Soft, 1 oz	76	6	4	13	0	0	0	104
Semisoft, 1 oz	103	8	6	22	1	0	1	146
Jack (monterey), 1 oz	106	9	5	25	0	0	0	152
Brick, 1 oz	105	8	5	27	1	0	0	159
Queso, Chihuahua, 1 oz	106	8	5	30	2	0	0	175
Asadero, 1 oz	101	8	5	30	1	0	0	186

	Cal	Fat	Sat	Chol	Carb	Fib	Sug	Sod
Anejo, 1 oz	106	8	5	30	1	0	0	321
Muenster, 1 oz	104	9	5	27	0	0	0	178
Brie, 1 oz	95	8	5	28	0	0	0	178
Colby/cheddar, 1 oz	113	9	6	28	1	0	0	180
Smoked cheddar, 1 oz	110	9	6	25	0	0	0	400
Havarti/tilsit, 1 oz	96	7	5	29	1	0	0	213
Stilton, 1 oz	110	9	5	30	0	0	0	220
Limburger, 1 oz	93	8	5	26	0	0	0	227
Fontina, 1 oz	110	9	5	33	0	0	0	227
Gouda, 1 oz	101	8	5	32	1	0	0	232
Camembert, 1 oz	85	7	4	20	0	0	0	239
Provolone, 1 oz	100	8	5	20	1	0	0	248
Edam, 1 oz	101	8	5	25	0	0	0	274
Feta, 1 oz	75	6	4	25	1	0	0	316
Romano, 1 oz	110	8	5	30	1	0	0	340
American (processed), 1 oz	100	9	6	25	1	0	0	380
Blue or gorgonzola, 1 oz	100	8	5	21	1	0	0	390
Asiago, 1 oz	110	9	5	0	1	0	1	400
Parmesan, 1 oz	111	7	5	19	1	0	0	454
Roquefort, 1 oz	105	9	6	26	1	0	0	513

Brands . . . *(1 oz unless noted)*

BLUE-VEIN CHEESES

	Cal	Fat	Sat	Chol	Carb	Fib	Sug	Sod
Clawson Lemon Zest White Stilton	100	7	4	20	6	1	4	120
White Stilton w/Blueberries or Apricot (avg)	100	8	5	28	4	1	3	130
REDUCED SODIUM (LESS THAN GENERIC):								
Clawson White Stilton w/Pear & Apple	100	7	5	20	5	1	3	150
White Stilton w/Mango & Ginger	100	6	4	20	7	1	6	150
White Stilton	100	9	6	30	1	0	1	180
White Stilton w/Cranberries or Blue Vinney	90	7	5	22	2	1	1	180
Saga Baby Blue	120	12	8	40	0	0	0	180

BRIE AND CAMEMBERT

	Cal	Fat	Sat	Chol	Carb	Fib	Sug	Sod
Cantare Baked Brie en Crioche Mushroom & Chive	80	5	3	25	5	0	1	115
Apple, Cinnamon, Raisin & Brandy	90	5	3	20	7	1	2	115
Cranberries, Apricots, Almonds & Brandy	80	4	2	16	7	0	2	120
Pesto, Pine Nuts & Roasted Vine Tomatoes	100	7	3	20	6	1	1	135
Original Recipe or Spinach Florentine	90	6	4	25	4	0	0	135
Meza Baked Brie in Pastry w/Mushrooms	100	7	4	25	6	0	1	120
Baked Brie in Pastry	100	7	5	30	5	0	0	135
Old Chatham Sheepherding Co								
Hudson Valley Camembert	100	10	6	32	0	0	0	95
President Brie Wedge/Log or Brie w/Herbs	100	9	4	20	0	0	0	120
REDUCED SODIUM (LESS THAN GENERIC):								
Joan of Arc Brie, wedge	100	8	6	20	0	0	0	150
President Brie, soft	80	7	3	15	0	0	0	150
Saint-Louis Brie	100	8	6	20	0	0	0	150
Wegmans Rich & Buttery Triple Cream Brie	110	11	8	35	0	0	0	145

CHEDDAR AND COLBY

	Cal	Fat	Sat	Chol	Carb	Fib	Sug	Sod
American Heritage LS Cheddar	110	9	6	30	1	0	0	5
Heluva Good Reduced Sodium Cheddar	110	9	6	30	1	0	0	25
Laughing Cow Mini Babybel Cheddar, 0.8 oz	70	5	3	20	0	0	0	140
Organic Valley Reduced Fat/Sodium Cheddar	90	6	4	15	1	0	0	125
REDUCED SODIUM (LESS THAN GENERIC):								
Clawson Innkeeper's Choice or Windsor Red	100	8	6	25	1	0	1	160
Crystal Farms Cheddar Jack	110	9	6	30	1	0	0	160
Hannaford 2% Colby Jack	90	6	4	20	0	0	0	160

	Cal	Fat	Sat	Chol	Carb	Fib	Sug	Sod
Sartori Reserve BellaVitano, all flavors	120	10	-	30	0	0	0	165

EDAM, FONTINA, GOUDA AND HAVARTI

	Cal	Fat	Sat	Chol	Carb	Fib	Sug	Sod
King's Choice Danish Fontina	120	9	6	30	0	0	0	140
Denmark's Finest Havarti w/Herbs & Spices	110	9	7	20	1	0	0	140
Dofino Havarti w/Caraway	120	10	7	25	0	0	0	140
REDUCED SODIUM (LESS THAN GENERIC):								
Denmark's Finest Havarti Creamy	120	10	7	25	0	0	0	150
Havarti w/Jalapeno	110	9	6	20	0	0	0	150
King's Choice Light Havarti	80	5	3	10	0	0	0	160
Kronenost Fontina	110	9	6	25	1	0	0	150

FETA AND GOAT *(also see Cheese Spreads/Balls/Logs pg 108)*

	Cal	Fat	Sat	Chol	Carb	Fib	Sug	Sod
Coach Farm Black Pepper Goat Cheese Buttons	65	5	4	25	1	0	1	70
Herb Goat Cheese Buttons	65	5	4	25	1	0	1	70
Fage Feta in Oil & Oregano	170	17	9	6	0	0	0	130
Firefly Farms Mt Top Blue Goat	90	7	5	15	1	0	0	30
Merry Goat Round	80	6	4	15	1	0	0	50
Allegheny Chevre	70	6	4	10	0	0	0	60
Le Chevrot Goat	70	6	0	13	1	0	0	50
Jacquin Le Chevrot	70	6	0	13	1	0	0	50
Mozzarella Co. – offers several no salt and lightly salted goat cheeses.								
Sainte-Maure Goat Cheese	70	6	0	13	1	0	0	50
Swissrose Dutch Goat	100	9	6	25	0	0	0	55
Vermont Butter/Cheese Chevre or Pepper Chevre	80	6	4	20	1	0	1	45
Creamy Goat	50	5	3	20	1	0	1	70
Woolrich Dairy Elite Lemon Poppyseed	60	3	2	15	7	0	5	55
Elite Cranberry w/Port or Blueberry Pomegranate	60	3	2	10	6	0	3	60

JACK, BRICK AND MUENSTER

	Cal	Fat	Sat	Chol	Carb	Fib	Sug	Sod
Alpine Lace Reduced Sodium Muenster	100	9	5	25	1	0	0	85
Tillamook Reduced Fat Monterey Jack	80	6	4	15	0	0	0	130

MISCELLANEOUS/SPECIALTY CHEESES

	Cal	Fat	Sat	Chol	Carb	Fib	Sug	Sod
Clawson Whirl Herb & Garlic	110	9	6	30	1	0	1	130
Heini's Yogurt Cultured Semi-soft, Original	100	8	5	20	0	0	0	140
Mozzarella Co. – offers a lightly salted queso blanco and queso fresco.								
Ski Queen Gjetost	130	9	6	30	7	0	7	90
St Marcellin Au Lait Pasteurise	70	6	4	20	0	0	0	55
Wegmans Brillo Pecorino Divino	116	9	6	27	1	0	0	130
Woolrich Dairy Tre Fratello	80	6	5	25	1	0	0	135

MOZZARELLA AND PROVOLONE

	Cal	Fat	Sat	Chol	Carb	Fib	Sug	Sod
Apple Smoked Cheese Smoked Provolone	100	8	5	23	1	0	0	84
Smoked Mozzarella	94	7	5	22	0	0	0	87
Bel Gioioso Fresh Mozzarella in Water	80	6	4	22	1	0	0	40
Fresh Ciliengini Mozzarella Balls, 3 pc	90	63	3	15	0	0	0	45
Boar's Head Lower Sodium Provolone	100	7	5	20	0	0	0	140
Cantare Fresh Mozzarella, all varieties	80	6	4	25	0	0	0	20
Burrata (Fresh w/Mascarpone Filling)	60	4	3	15	1	0	1	50
Cappiello Marinated Irish Fresh Mozzarella, 1.3 oz	120	9	6	25	1	1	0	10
Fresh Mozzarella Log	90	6	4	30	0	0	0	130
Sun-Dried Tomato or Basil or Pesto Italiano Marinated Mozzarella Braid, 1.3 oz	90	7	5	20	1	0	0	140
Jalapeno/Cilantro Marinated Mozzarella, 1.3 oz.	90	7	5	20	1	0	0	140
Cucina Andolina Fresh Mozzarella	70	6	4	10	0	0	0	10
Formaggio Fresh, Unsalted	80	6	4	20	1	0	0	60
Fresh & Healthy Dried Tomato/Basil Mozzarella	80	6	4	20	1	0	0	140
Miceli's Fresh Mozzarella Cheese	70	5	3	15	1	0	0	5

DAIRY AND NON-DAIRY ALTERNATIVES
Cheese – Grated and Shredded

	Cal	Fat	Sat	Chol	Carb	Fib	Sug	Sod
Mozzarella (pear shape)	90	7	5	20	0	0	0	95

Mozzarella Co. *– offers several unsalted and lightly salted mozzarellas.*

Mozzarella Fresca

	Cal	Fat	Sat	Chol	Carb	Fib	Sug	Sod
Fresh mozzarella, all non-marinated	60	5	3	15	0	0	0	25
Fresh mozzarella, all marinated varieties	100	14	4	15	0	0	0	65
Polly-O Fresh Mozzarella	80	7	4	20	0	0	0	15
Precious Fresh Mozzarella (Cilengini)	70	5	4	30	1	0	0	60
Primo Taglio Fresh Mozzarella Bocconcini	80	6	4	20	0	0	0	40
Sorrento Fresh Mozzarella (Cilengini)	70	5	4	30	1	0	0	60
Woolrich Dairy Mozzarella	100	8	5	25	1	0	0	100

PARMESAN/ROMANO/ASIAGO *– Most brands within generic average (340mg–454mg).*

SWISS, JARLSBERG AND GRUYERE

Most swiss brands within generic average (60mg), the following have less:

	Cal	Fat	Sat	Chol	Carb	Fib	Sug	Sod
Boar's Head Natural Swiss, NSA	110	8	5	25	1	0	0	10
Lacey Swiss, Reduced Fat/Sodium	90	6	4	15	0	0	0	35
Dietz & Watson Lacey Swiss	80	6	4	15	0	0	0	35
Hillandale Farms Swiss, NSA	100	8	5	25	1	0	0	10
Swissrose Swiss Cheese	100	8	6	25	0	0	0	15
Swiss Valley Farms NSA Swiss	100	8	5	25	1	0	0	5
Wegmans No Salt Swiss	100	8	5	25	1	0	0	10

YOGURT CHEESE

	Cal	Fat	Sat	Chol	Carb	Fib	Sug	Sod
The Cultured Way Jalapeno or Classic Original	100	9	6	20	0	0	0	120

CHEESE – GRATED AND SHREDDED

	Cal	Fat	Sat	Chol	Carb	Fib	Sug	Sod
Asiago, shredded, 1 tbsp	20	2	1	5	0	0	0	55
Swiss, shredded, 1/4 cup	103	8	5	25	0	0	0	60
Romano, grated, 1 tbsp	19	2	1	5	0	0	0	70
Parmesan, grated, 1 tbsp	22	2	1	5	0	0	0	90
Soy-based, parmesan, grated, 2 tsp	15	1	0	0	1	0	0	85
Mozzarella, whole milk, shredded, 1/4 cup	84	6	4	22	0	0	0	176
Part skim, shredded, 1/4 cup	85	6	3	15	0	0	0	149
Cheddar, shredded, 1/4 cup	114	9	6	30	0	0	0	180

Brands . . . *(1/4 cup or 1 oz unless noted)*

PARMESAN/ROMANO/ASIAGO – REFRIGERATED *(1 tbsp unless noted)*

	Cal	Fat	Sat	Chol	Carb	Fib	Sug	Sod
BelGioioso Freshly Shaved Parmesan	20	1	1	5	0	0	0	45
Buitoni Fresh Shredded Romano or Parmesan (avg)	20	2	1	5	0	0	0	55
Cucina Andolina Asiago	20	2	1	5	0	0	0	40
Parmesan	20	2	1	5	0	0	0	70
Crystal Farms Parmesan or Parmesan/Romano	25	2	1	5	0	0	0	70
Haolam Parmesan	19	2	1	4	0	0	0	62
Maggio Shredded Parmesan	20	1	1	0	0	0	0	35
Miller's Parmesan	19	2	1	4	0	0	0	62
Parma! Parmesan seasoning (non-dairy)	25	2	0	0	2	0	0	25
Sartori Signature Blends Tuscan	20	2	0	5	0	0	0	40
Signature Blends Sicilian or Caesar	20	2	0	5	0	0	0	45

PARMESAN/ROMANO/ASIAGO – SHELF-STABLE

	Cal	Fat	Sat	Chol	Carb	Fib	Sug	Sod
4C Homestyle Parmesan	20	2	1	5	0	0	0	70
Kraft Romano/Parmesan, Reduced Fat	20	1	0	1	2	0	0	75

OTHER GRATED/SHREDDED CHEESE

	Cal	Fat	Sat	Chol	Carb	Fib	Sug	Sod
Sargento Reduced Sodium Mild Cheddar	110	9	5	25	1	0	0	135
Reduced Sodium Mozzarella	80	6	4	15	1	0	0	140

CHEESE – SLICED/PACKAGED

	Cal	Fat	Sat	Chol	Carb	Fib	Sug	Sod
Swiss, 0.8 oz	85	6	4	21	1	0	0	43

Cheese – Sliced/Packaged

	Cal	Fat	Sat	Chol	Carb	Fib	Sug	Sod
Monterey jack, 0.8 oz	84	7	4	20	0	0	0	120
Mozzarella, 0.8 oz	60	5	3	10	1	0	0	130
Cheddar, 0.8 oz	90	7	5	24	0	0	0	139
Muenster, 0.8 oz	82	7	4	22	0	0	0	141
Provolone, 0.8 oz	79	6	4	15	0	0	0	196
Soy-based, mozzarella or american, 1 slice	20	0	0	0	3	0	1	220
American/Processed, 0.8 oz	40	2	1	6	2	0	1	226

Brands . . . *(0.8 oz slice unless noted)*

SWISS – *Most brands within generic average (43mg), the following have less:*

	Cal	Fat	Sat	Chol	Carb	Fib	Sug	Sod
Kraft *Deli Fresh* Swiss	80	7	4	20	0	0	0	35
Lorraine Cheese *Deli Sliced* Swiss	110	9	5	25	1	0	1	15
Deli Sliced Reduced Fat Swiss	110	6	4	20	1	0	1	35
Sargento Reduced Fat Swiss	60	4	2	15	1	0	0	30

JACK/CHEDDAR/MOZZARELLA/MUENSTER – *the following have 110mg or less:*

	Cal	Fat	Sat	Chol	Carb	Fib	Sug	Sod
Alpine Lace Muenster, Reduced Sodium	80	7	5	15	0	0	0	105
Andrew & Everett Mild Cheddar	60	5	3	15	0	0	0	100
Sargento *Reduced Sodium* Colby or Pepper Jack	70	6	4	15	0	0	0	90

OTHER SLICED CHEESE

	Cal	Fat	Sat	Chol	Carb	Fib	Sug	Sod
Alpine Lace Provolone, 25% Reduced Fat	60	5	3	10	0	0	0	130
Andrew & Everett Provolone	60	4	3	11	0	0	0	140
Bel Gioioso Mild Provolone	100	8	5	25	0	0	0	120
Haolam Havarti	120	10	3	25	0	0	0	130
Horizon Provolone	70	6	4	15	0	0	0	140
Jarlsberg Light	50	3	2	10	0	0	0	100
Sargento *Reduced Sodium* Provolone, 0.7 oz	70	5	4	15	0	0	0	100
Natural Jarlsberg, 0.9 oz	80	6	4	15	1	0	0	110
Natural Havarti, 0.7 oz	80	6	4	15	0	0	0	120
Natural Provolone, 0.8 oz	70	5	3	15	0	0	0	135
Reduced Fat Provolone, 0.7 oz	50	4	2	10	0	0	0	140

CHEESE ALTERNATIVES

	Cal	Fat	Sat	Chol	Carb	Fib	Sug	Sod
Follow Your Heart Vegan Mozzarella, 1 oz	70	8	1	0	1	1	0	120
Galaxy Nutritional *Rice Vegan* all flavors, 0.7 oz	40	2	1	0	5	0	0	120
Vegan American Flavor Soy Slices, 0.7 oz	40	2	0	0	5	0	0	120

CHEESE – SHELF-STABLE

	Cal	Fat	Sat	Chol	Carb	Fib	Sug	Sod
Processed, boxed, 1 oz	60	6	4	25	3	0	2	410
Processed spread, jar, 2 tbsp	90	7	3	10	4	0	2	440

Brands . . . *(2 tbsp unless noted)*

	Cal	Fat	Sat	Chol	Carb	Fib	Sug	Sod
Kraft Pineapple Spread	70	5	4	15	4	0	4	120

CHEESE – STRING/SNACK

	Cal	Fat	Sat	Chol	Carb	Fib	Sug	Sod
String cheese, 1 oz	90	6	4	20	1	0	0	200

Brands . . . *(1 oz unless noted)*

	Cal	Fat	Sat	Chol	Carb	Fib	Sug	Sod
Les Petites Fermieres Part Skim Mozarella	60	4	2	10	0	0	0	110
Micelo's String Cheese	90	7	5	20	0	0	0	95
Sargento *Reduced Sodium* Pepper Jack Sticks	70	6	4	15	0	0	0	90
Reduced Sodium Colby-Jack Sticks, 0.8 oz	80	7	5	20	1	0	0	105
Reduced Sodium Mild Cheddar Sticks, 0.8 oz	90	7	4	20	1	0	0	105
Reduced Sodium String Cheese, 0.8 oz	60	4	3	10	1	0	0	110

CHEESE SAUCE

(see Cheese Sauce, pg 91)

	Cal	Fat	Sat	Chol	Carb	Fib	Sug	Sod

CHEESE SPREADS, CHEESE BALLS AND LOGS

(see Cream Cheese/Cheese Spreads, Balls/Logs, pg 104)

COFFEE CREAMERS AND FLAVORINGS

(see Coffee Creamers/Flavorings, pg 38)

COTTAGE CHEESE AND RICOTTA

	Cal	Fat	Sat	Chol	Carb	Fib	Sug	Sod
Hoop cheese (dry curd cottage cheese), FF, 1 oz	24	0	0	4	1	0	1	4
Ricotta cheese, 1/4 cup	108	8	5	32	2	0	0	52
Part skim, 1/4 cup	86	5	3	19	3	0	0	78
Farmer cheese (dry curd cottage cheese), 1 oz..	40	3	2	10	0	0	0	120
Cottage cheese, small curd, 1/2 cup	110	5	2	19	4	0	3	410
LF, 2% milkfat, 1/2 cup	97	3	1	11	4	0	3	373
LF with fruit, 1/2 cup	110	4	3	15	5	0	3	389
Large curd, 1/2 cup	103	5	2	18	4	0	3	390

Brands . . .

COTTAGE CHEESE *(1/2 cup unless noted)*

	Cal	Fat	Sat	Chol	Carb	Fib	Sug	Sod
Crowley LF Cottage Cheese, NSA	100	2	1	15	6	0	4	75
Friendship LF Cottage Cheese, NSA	90	1	1	5	4	0	3	50
Hood LF Cottage Cheese, NSA	90	1	1	15	6	0	5	55
Lucerne NSA Cottage Cheese	80	2	1	10	4	0	3	45

RICOTTA *(1/4 cup unless noted)*

	Cal	Fat	Sat	Chol	Carb	Fib	Sug	Sod
Calabro FF Ricotta	25	0	0	0	1	0	1	30
Great Value Part Skim Ricotta	80	5	3	30	4	0	1	60
Miceli's Lite Ricotta	60	3	2	15	3	0	3	55
Mozzarella Co. NSA Ricotta	74	5	2	15	2	0	0	36
Polly-O Part Skim Ricotta	90	6	4	20	2	0	2	65
Precious Part Skim Ricotta	100	7	4	25	4	1	3	60
Sargento Light Ricotta	60	3	2	15	3	0	3	55
FF Ricotta	50	0	0	10	5	0	2	65
Sorrento Part Skim Ricotta	100	7	4	25	4	1	3	60
Wegmans Part Skim Ricotta	100	7	4	25	4	1	3	60

CREAM

	Cal	Fat	Sat	Chol	Carb	Fib	Sug	Sod
Light whipping cream, 1 tbsp	44	5	3	17	0	0	0	5
Half and half, 1 tbsp	20	2	1	6	1	0	1	6
FF, 1 tbsp	9	0	0	0	1	0	1	22
Light cream, 1 tbsp	29	3	2	10	1	0	0	6
Heavy whipping cream, 1 tbsp	52	6	4	21	0	0	0	6

Brands . . . *Most brands within generic average.*

CREAM – SOUR

	Cal	Fat	Sat	Chol	Carb	Fib	Sug	Sod
Sour cream, 2 tbsp	58	6	3	16	1	0	1	24
Light/reduced fat sour cream, 2 tbsp	54	4	3	11	2	0	0	21
Fat free sour cream, 2 tbsp	22	0	0	3	5	0	0	42
Imitation sour cream, 2 tbsp	62	6	5	0	2	0	2	31

Brands . . . *Most brands within generic average.*

CREAM CHEESE/CHEESE SPREADS, BALLS AND LOGS

	Cal	Fat	Sat	Chol	Carb	Fib	Sug	Sod
Cream cheese, 1 oz	100	9	6	35	1	0	1	105
Whipped, 2 tbsp	60	6	4	20	1	0	1	90
Flavored, 1 oz	90	8	5	30	5	0	4	120
Light, 1 oz	70	5	3	20	2	0	2	140

	Cal	Fat	Sat	Chol	Carb	Fib	Sug	Sod
FF, 1 oz	30	0	0	5	2	0	1	210
Cream cheese alternatives:								
Mascarpone, 1 oz	124	13	7	6	1	0	0	16
Neufchatel, 1 oz	72	6	4	20	1	0	1	95
Cheese spread, cream cheese base, 1 oz	84	8	5	26	1	0	1	191
Cheese ball, sharp cheddar, 1 oz	90	6	3	15	4	1	3	230
Cheese spread, pasteurized process, american, 1 oz	82	6	4	16	2	0	0	461

Brands . . . *(1 oz or 2 tbsp unless noted)*

CREAM CHEESE AND NEUFCHATEL – PLAIN

Neufchatel – Most brands within generic average (95mg).

	Cal	Fat	Sat	Chol	Carb	Fib	Sug	Sod
All Seasons Kitchen Plain Cream Cheese	90	9	6	35	1	0	1	80
Alta Dena Whipped Plain Cream Cheese	80	7	5	20	1	0	1	75
Breakstone's *Temp Tee* Whipped Cream Cheese	80	8	5	25	1	0	1	65
Crystal Farms Whipped Plain Cream Cheese	70	7	5	20	1	0	1	75
J&J Whipped Cream Cheese	80	7	5	20	1	0	1	75
Reduced Fat Whipped Cream Cheese	50	5	3	15	1	0	1	75
Lucerne Whipped Plain Cream Cheese	70	7	5	20	1	0	1	65
Morning Select Whipped Cream Cheese	67	7	4	20	1	0	1	60
Mozzarella Co *– Offers an unsalted and lightly salted cream cheese.*								
Nancy's Cultured or Organic Cultured	95	9	6	35	2	0	2	35
Norman's 1/2% Creamy White Soft Cheese	15	0	0	0	1	0	0	15
5% Creamy White Soft Cheese	30	2	1	5	1	0	0	75
Richfood Whipped Plain Cream Cheese	70	7	5	0	1	0	1	65
Swiss Valley Farms Plain Cream Cheese	100	10	6	30	1	0	1	85
TempTee Whipped Cream Cheese	80	8	5	25	1	0	1	65
Tnuva 5% or 9% Creamy Soft Cheese (avg)	40	3	2	8	1	0	0	80
Weight Watchers Reduce Fat Cream Cheese	60	5	4	15	4	3	1	80

CREAM CHEESE – FLAVORED

	Cal	Fat	Sat	Chol	Carb	Fib	Sug	Sod
All Seasons Kitchen Spring Chive or Very Veggie	90	9	6	35	1	0	1	80
Honey Nut	110	8	5	25	5	0	2	85
Brummel & Brown Creamy Fruit Spread	100	8	2	0	6	0	6	90
Certified Kosher Gourmet Scallion	90	9	6	30	0	0	0	100
Lox Spread	80	8	5	25	0	0	0	105
Great Value Strawberry	90	7	5	20	5	0	5	70
J&J Whipped Vegetable Cream Cheese	80	7	5	20	1	0	1	75
Lucerne								
Whipped Mixed Berry Flavor	60	5	4	15	4	0	4	50
With Strawberries	100	8	6	25	5	0	5	80
Philadelphia *Whipped* Mixed Berry	70	5	3	15	3	0	3	55
Whipped Cinnamon 'n Brown Sugar	70	6	4	20	3	0	2	55
Whipped Garlic 'n Herb	60	6	4	20	1	0	1	100
Blueberry, Raspberry, or Strawberry	90	7	5	30	5	0	5	110
Cream Swirls Peaches 'n Cream	90	7	4	30	5	0	4	110
Honey Nut or Pineapple	90	8	5	30	4	0	4	110

CREAM CHEESE ALTERNATIVES

Hoop – Most brands within generic average (15mg).
Mascarpone – Most brands within generic average (16mg).

	Cal	Fat	Sat	Chol	Carb	Fib	Sug	Sod
Cascade Fresh Mediterranean Style Yogurt	60	6	4	15	2	0	2	20
Friendship Farmer, NSA	50	3	2	10	0	0	0	10
Lifeway Farmer or Organic Farmer Cheese	40	2	1	6	4	0	4	10
Farmer Cheese Lite or Fat Free (avg)	23	1	0	3	2	0	2	10
Premium White Cheese	50	3	0	11	2	0	1	11

CHEESE SPREADS, BALLS AND LOGS

	Cal	Fat	Sat	Chol	Carb	Fib	Sug	Sod
Alouette Berries & Cream	80	6	4	15	4	0	1	60

DAIRY AND NON-DAIRY ALTERNATIVES
Egg Nog

	Cal	Fat	Sat	Chol	Carb	Fib	Sug	Sod
Light Garlic & Herbs or *Light* Cucumber Dill....	50	4	3	15	2	0	1	60
Spinach Artichoke	70	6	4	15	1	0	1	70
Savory Vegetable	70	6	5	15	1	0	1	80
Sun-Dried Tomato & Basil................................	80	7	5	15	1	0	1	95
Creamy Onion/Shallot......................................	80	7	5	20	1	0	1	100
Garlic & Herbs or Peppercorn Parmesan..........	80	8	5	20	1	0	1	100
Elegante Roasted Sweet Peppers & Olive	100	9	6	30	2	0	1	120
Elegante Sun-Dried Tomato & Garlic	100	9	6	30	2	0	1	130
Elegante Roasted Garlic & Pesto	100	9	6	30	2	0	1	140
Boursin Garlic & Roasted Red Pepper	120	12	8	30	2	1	2	110
Cibo Naturals Basil Walnut Cheese Spread.....	120	13	7	30	1	0	0	85
Garlic Sundried Tomato Cheese Spread	120	12	7	35	1	0	1	105
Smoked Jalapeño Cheese Spread	110	12	7	35	1	0	1	120
Coach Farm Honey Lemon Goat Cheese.........	45	3	2	10	4	0	3	50
Herbes de Provence or Traditional Chevre......	40	3	2	10	2	0	1	65
Garden Tomato & Garlic Goat Cheese Spread .	50	3	2	10	2	0	1	80
Kaukauna Swiss Almond...............................	90	7	4	20	3	0	3	140
Lifeway *Sweet Kiss* Sweet Cheese w/Raisins ...	45	1	1	5	6	0	6	10
Sweet Kiss Plain, Apple or Peach Sweet Cheese	50	2	1	5	6	0	6	10
Sweet Kiss Choc Choc Chip Cheese...............	100	7	5	8	8	0	7	50
Opaa! Sun-Dried Tomato Feta Spread.............	50	4	2	5	2	0	1	120
Private Harvest Asiago Cheese Bread Spread.	100	11	2	10	0	0	0	35
Rising Sun Farms								
Cranberry Orange Cheese Tortas	100	7	5	20	10	1	9	55
Marionberry Cheese Tortas............................	120	11	6	20	5	1	4	60
Key Lime w/Cranberries or Curry (avg)	110	9	6	25	8	0	6	65
Cheese DipnSpread Northwest Strawberry.....	90	7	5	20	7	0	7	70
Roasted Garlic or Chili Lime Cilantro (avg).....	100	9	6	25	4	1	3	100
Pesto Dried Tomato Cheese Tortas..................	100	9	6	25	5	1	3	105
Gorgonzola Cheese Tortas............................	110	9	6	25	5	0	4	110
Cheese DipnSpread Roasted Garlic & Chive....	110	11	5	20	3	0	2	110
Mediterranean Cheese Tortas........................	100	8	5	25	5	1	3	115
Sweet Pepper & Chipotle Cheese Tortas	110	10	6	25	5	1	2	140
Cheese DipnSpread Chili Lime......................	120	11	5	20	2	0	2	140
Robt Rothschild Farm Red Pepper Cheese.....	80	7	4	20	5	0	5	85
Rondele Garden Veg Spreadable Cheese	70	5	0	25	1	0	1	135
Artichoke & Garlic Spreadable Cheese...........	70	5	0	25	1	0	1	135
Chipotle & Tomato Spreadable Cheese	70	6	4	20	2	0	1	140
Wegmans Garlic & Herb Cheese Spread	140	13	3	20	1	0	1	115
Artichoke Asiago Cheese Spread	120	12	3	20	1	0	0	120

CHEESE LOG/SPREAD SEASONINGS *(see Cheese Ball Seasonings, pg 223)*

EGG NOG

	Cal	Fat	Sat	Chol	Carb	Fib	Sug	Sod
Egg nog, ready-to-drink, 1/2 cup.....................	280	18	11	105	26	0	23	110
Mix, prep w/whole milk, 1 cup	258	8	5	30	39	0	34	150

Brands . . . *(1/2 cup unless noted)*
MIXES

	Cal	Fat	Sat	Chol	Carb	Fib	Sug	Sod
Aspen Mulling Co Egg Nog Mix, 2 tsp............	80	0	0	0	20	0	20	40
Calorie Control Egg Nog Mix	80	2	1	0	12	1	7	70

READY-TO-DRINK

	Cal	Fat	Sat	Chol	Carb	Fib	Sug	Sod
Borden EggNog (shelf-stable)	160	9	5	75	17	0	13	80
Hood Golden or Vanilla EggNog	180	9	5	65	22	0	21	95
Light EggNog...	140	4	3	45	22	0	22	95
Organic Valley Organic Eggnog	180	10	6	90	18	0	17	85

	Cal	Fat	Sat	Chol	Carb	Fib	Sug	Sod
Promised Land 2% Egg Nog	139	3	2	42	23	0	21	56
Holiday Nog	160	7	4	43	23	0	21	58
Egg Nog	200	11	7	45	23	0	21	60
Swiss Valley Farms Egg Nog	190	9	5	60	24	0	23	90
Turkey Hill Egg Nog, 1 cup	190	9	5	65	23	0	23	90

NON-DAIRY EGG NOG

	Cal	Fat	Sat	Chol	Carb	Fib	Sug	Sod
Silk Soy Egg Nog (seasonal)	90	2	0	0	15	0	12	75

EGGS AND EGG SUBSTITUTES

	Cal	Fat	Sat	Chol	Carb	Fib	Sug	Sod
Egg yolk, large, 1	55	5	2	212	0	0	0	8
Egg, whole, small, 1	54	4	1	157	0	0	0	52
Medium, 1	65	4	1	186	1	0	0	62
Large, 1	74	5	2	212	0	0	0	70
Egg white, large, 1	17	0	0	0	0	0	0	55
Egg substitute, 1/4 cup (1 egg)	53	2	0	0	0	0	0	111

Brands . . .

EGGS – *Most brands within generic average (52-70mg).*

EGG SUBSTITUTES

	Cal	Fat	Sat	Chol	Carb	Fib	Sug	Sod
Great Value Liquid Egg Whites	25	0	0	0	1	0	0	75
Kineret Light 'n Tasty, 1/4 cup	30	0	0	0	1	0	1	80

MILK PRODUCTS

(also see Milk/Milk Substitutes–Canned/Powdered, pg 28)

	Cal	Fat	Sat	Chol	Carb	Fib	Sug	Sod
Milk, whole, 1 cup	146	8	5	24	11	0	11	98
2%, 1 cup	122	5	3	20	11	0	11	100
1%, 1 cup	102	2	2	12	12	0	12	107
NF, 1 cup	90	0	0	5	13	0	12	125
Goat milk, 1 cup	168	10	7	27	11	0	11	122
Choc milk, ready-to-drink, 1 cup	208	8	5	30	26	2	24	150
LF, 1 cup	158	3	2	8	26	1	25	153
Buttermilk, LF, 1 cup	98	2	1	10	12	0	12	257

Brands . . . *(1 cup unless noted)*

BUTTERMILK

	Cal	Fat	Sat	Chol	Carb	Fib	Sug	Sod
Alta Dena Culture LF	120	3	2	15	14	0	14	140
Friendship Buttermilk, LF	120	4	3	15	12	0	12	125

KEFIR *(also see Yogurt/Non-Dairy Drinks, pg 111)*

	Cal	Fat	Sat	Chol	Carb	Fib	Sug	Sod
Helios Kefir Strawberry or Raspberry	160	4	3	15	26	2	23	85
Kefir Plain	120	5	3	18	12	2	10	90
Kefir Peach, Vanilla, or Blueberry	160	2	2	10	25	3	21	125
Lifeway Organic LF Plain Kefir	110	3	2	10	12	3	8	125
Whole Milk Plain Kefir	160	8	5	30	12	3	8	125
Whole Milk Wildberries or Strawberries n' Creme	212	8	5	30	25	3	21	125
Nancy's Organic Kefir Strawberry	180	3	2	14	34	1	32	80
Peach, Blackberry, or Raspberry (avg)	180	3	2	15	34	2	32	80
Blueberry	200	3	2	15	38	2	35	85
Plain	110	3	3	15	14	1	13	105
Redwood Hill Farm Blueberry Pomegranate Kefir	220	6	4	15	32	1	26	75
Plain Kefir	140	7	5	20	9	0	5	90

FLAVORED MILK

	Cal	Fat	Sat	Chol	Carb	Fib	Sug	Sod
Hood LF Coffee Milk	170	3	2	15	28	0	26	125
Land O Lakes Strawberry Milk	190	8	5	30	22	0	22	125
Promised Land Very Berry Strawberry Milk	250	9	6	35	35	0	34	125
Swiss Valley Farms 1% Strawberry Milk	180	2	0	10	31	0	29	115

	Cal	Fat	Sat	Chol	Carb	Fib	Sug	Sod

NON-DAIRY MILK ALTERNATIVES

(also see Yogurt/Non-Dairy Drinks, pg 111)

	Cal	Fat	Sat	Chol	Carb	Fib	Sug	Sod
Rice milk, refrigerated, plain, 8 fl oz	120	3	0	0	23	0	10	80
Shelf-stable, chocolate, 8 fl oz	160	3	0	0	34	1	28	90
Shelf-stable, plain, 8 fl oz	120	3	0	0	24	0	11	100
Soy milk, refrigerated, vanilla, 8 fl oz	100	4	1	0	10	1	7	95
Refrigerated, chocolate, 8 fl oz	140	4	1	0	23	2	19	100
Refrigerated, plain, 8 fl oz	100	4	1	0	8	1	6	120
Shelf-stable, plain, 8 fl oz	132	4	1	0	15	1	10	125
Shelf-stable, chocolate, 8 fl oz	154	4	1	0	24	1	19	130
Almond milk, plain, 8 fl oz	60	3	0	0	8	1	7	150

Brands . . . *(8 fl oz unless noted)*

RICE MILK

Many brands are low-sodium, the following have 75mg sodium or less.

SHELF-STABLE

	Cal	Fat	Sat	Chol	Carb	Fib	Sug	Sod
Pacific Natural Foods Rice LF Plain	130	2	0	0	27	0	14	60
Rice LF Vanilla	130	2	0	0	27	0	14	75
Rice Dream Horchata	160	3	0	0	32	0	18	5
Supreme Vanilla Hazelnut	140	3	0	0	29	0	17	65
Supreme Choc Chai	160	3	0	0	35	1	21	75

SOY MILK

REFRIGERATED

	Cal	Fat	Sat	Chol	Carb	Fib	Sug	Sod
8th Continent Complete	80	3	0	0	8	3	6	95
Power Dream, Java Jolt, 11 fl oz	240	5	1	0	26	2	24	70
Silk Unsweetened or *Organic* Unsweetened	80	4	1	0	4	1	1	85
Vanilla or *Organic* Vanilla	100	4	1	0	10	1	7	95
Light Vanilla or *Heart Health* Vanilla	80	2	0	0	10	1	7	95
Westsoy Soy Drink, Plain, Unsweetened	90	5	0	0	5	4	0	30
Vanilla, Unsweetened	100	5	1	0	5	4	0	30
Wild Wood Organics Unsweetened Soymilk	70	4	1	0	3	1	2	70
Plain or Vanilla Soymilk (avg)	90	4	1	0	8	1	7	70
ZenSoy Plain or Vanilla (avg)	100	4	1	0	12	1	8	80

SHELF-STABLE

The following shelf-stable brands have 100mg sodium or less.

	Cal	Fat	Sat	Chol	Carb	Fib	Sug	Sod
Edensoy Unsweetened	120	6	1	0	5	1	2	5
Light Original	100	2	0	0	15	0	10	90
Extra Vanilla	150	3	0	0	23	1	15	90
Carob	170	4	1	0	28	1	13	95
Extra Original	130	4	1	0	13	1	7	100
Kikkoman Pearl Soymilk Creamy Vanilla	110	4	1	0	11	0	10	90
Green Tea Organic Soymilk	110	4	1	0	13	1	10	95
Pacific Soy Unsweetened Original	90	5	1	0	4	2	2	15
Silk Soymilk Unsweetened	80	4	1	0	4	1	1	85
Soymilk Vanilla	100	4	1	0	10	1	7	95
Soymilk Chocolate	150	3	1	0	25	2	21	100
Westsoy Unsweetened, Choc	100	5	1	0	6	5	1	30
Unsweetened, Vanilla or Almond	100	5	1	0	5	4	1	30
Organic, Unsweetened, Original	90	5	1	0	5	4	1	30
Lite, Vanilla Soy Milk	70	2	0	0	8	1	6	75
Lite, Plain Soy Milk	60	2	0	0	6	1	5	85
Low Fat, Vanilla Soy Milk	120	2	0	0	21	2	10	90
Low Fat, Plain Soy Milk	90	2	0	0	14	2	7	90

	Cal	Fat	Sat	Chol	Carb	Fib	Sug	Sod
OTHER NON-DAIRY PRODUCTS – SHELF-STABLE								
Almond Dream Original	50	3	0	0	6	1	5	100
Unsweetened	30	3	0	0	1	1	0	100
EdenBlend	120	3	1	0	18	1	8	90
Hemp Dream Original or Vanilla (avg)	105	6	1	0	10	1	8	5
Kidz Dream *Smoothie* Orange Cream	120	2	0	0	21	1	17	30
Smoothie Berry Blast	100	2	0	0	17	1	13	35
Oat Dream Original or Maple Brown Sugar	120	3	0	0	20	3	16	20

(SOUR CREAM)

(see Cream–Sour, pg 104)

(WHIPPED TOPPINGS)

(see Sauces/Toppings/Fruit Dips, pg 133)

(YOGURT)

	Cal	Fat	Sat	Chol	Carb	Fib	Sug	Sod
Yogurt, vanilla, LF, 6 oz	140	2	1	10	23	0	23	105
Yogurt, plain, 6 oz	170	8	5	25	12	0	12	125
LF, 6 oz	107	3	2	10	12	0	12	115
FF, 6 oz	80	0	0	0	13	0	13	120
Yogurt, fruit, LF, 6 oz	170	2	1	5	26	0	24	125
LF w/artificial sweetener, 6 oz	80	2	1	5	16	0	11	99

Brands . . . *(6 oz unless noted)*
Most yogurt is low sodium, the following have 85mg or less per 6-oz serving, 60mg or less per 4-oz serving, or 110mg or less per 8-oz serving.

	Cal	Fat	Sat	Chol	Carb	Fib	Sug	Sod
Breyers Smooth & Creamy all, 4 oz (avg)	115	1	1	10	24	0	19	50
Inspirations Vanilla Bean, 4 oz	110	1	1	5	21	0	17	60
Fruit on the Bottom all but Black Cherry (avg)	170	1	1	10	34	1	27	75
Light Vanilla Bean	80	0	0	5	11	0	7	80
Light – Strawberry Cheesecake or Mixed Berry	80	0	0	5	12	1	7	85
Brown Cow Greek Yogurt, Vanilla, 5.3 oz	110	0	0	0	12	0	12	55
Greek Yogurt, Plain, 5.3 oz	80	0	0	0	6	0	6	60
Greek Yogurt, Strawberry, 5.3 oz	130	0	0	0	18	0	17	65
Cream Top Blueberry, Raspberry, or Peach	180	6	4	20	27	0	24	75
Cream Top Cherry Vanilla or Strawberry (avg)	180	6	4	20	28	1	26	75
Cream Top Apricot Mango	170	6	4	20	23	0	20	80
Cream Top – Creamy Coffee, Maple, or Vanilla	160	7	4	25	19	0	18	85
Cabot Cabot Greek 2% Vanilla Bean, 8 oz	220	4	3	25	33	0	32	100
Cabot Greek Plain, 8 oz	290	23	15	75	12	0	7	105
Cabot Greek 2% Strawberry, 8 oz	220	4	3	25	33	0	32	105
Chobani Champions Veryberry, 4 oz	100	2	1	5	12	0	11	40
Champions Honeynana, 4 oz	100	2	1	5	14	0	13	40
2%, all flavors (avg)	160	3	2	5	21	0	20	65
0% Blueberry, Strawberry, or Raspberry (avg)	140	0	0	0	20	1	20	65
0% Peach	140	0	0	0	20	1	19	65
2% Plain	130	4	2	10	7	0	7	70
0% Black Cherry	150	0	0	0	22	0	21	70
0% Vanilla	120	0	0	0	13	0	13	75
0% Pomegranate or Honey (avg)	145	0	0	0	20	1	20	75
0% Lemon	140	0	0	0	20	0	18	80
0% Plain Greek Yogurt	100	0	0	0	7	0	7	80
Dannon Activa Fiber, all flavors, 4 oz	110	2	1	5	20	3	16	60
Greek Honey, 5.3 oz	140	0	0	10	23	0	21	50
Greek Plain, 5.3 oz	80	0	0	10	6	0	6	50

DAIRY AND NON-DAIRY ALTERNATIVES
Yogurt

	Cal	Fat	Sat	Chol	Carb	Fib	Sug	Sod
Greek Blueberry or Vanilla, 5.3 oz	120	0	0	10	17	0	16	50
Greek Strawberry, 5.3 oz (avg)	115	0	0	10	17	0	16	55
Light & Fit:								
Blackberry, Raspberry, or Blueberry............	80	0	0	5	16	0	11	75
Pineapple Coconut or Pomegranate Berry	80	0	0	5	16	0	11	75
Vanilla, Strawberry Banana, or Banana	80	0	0	5	16	0	11	75
Strawberry Kiwi or White Choc Raspberry....	80	0	0	5	16	0	11	75
Peach, Cherry, or Orange Bliss (avg)	80	0	0	5	16	0	10	75
Lemon Chiffon, Cherry Vanilla, or Strawberry .	80	0	0	5	16	0	11	80
Mixed Berry	80	0	0	5	15	0	10	85
Fage *Total* all varieties, 5.3 oz (avg)	250	12	9	20	28	0	28	35
Total 2% all varieties, 5.3 oz (avg)...............	180	3	2	5	29	0	29	40
Total 0% Blueberry Acai or Mango Guanabana..	120	0	0	0	18	0	16	45
Total 0% Cherry Pomegrante, 5.3 oz	120	0	0	0	19	0	20	50
Total 0% Honey, 5.3 oz.................................	160	0	0	0	30	0	29	50
Total 0% Strawberry Goji, 5.3 oz	110	0	0	0	17	0	16	50
Total Plain, 7 oz	260	20	16	35	6	0	6	65
Total 2% Plain, 7 oz	130	4	3	10	8	0	8	65
Total 0% Plain, 6 oz	90	0	0	0	7	0	7	65
Fiber One, all flavors, 4 oz	50	0	0	5	13	5	4	55
Great Value *Light* FF Yogurt								
Peach, Strawberry, or Strawberry Banana	100	0	0	5	19	0	14	85
Blueberry, Mixed Berry, or Raspberry	100	0	0	5	19	0	14	85
Lala Strawberry, 8 oz	210	3	2	15	27	0	23	80
Apple, Mango, or Peach, 8 oz (avg)	150	3	2	15	27	0	23	80
Strawberry Banana, 8 oz................................	160	3	2	15	29	0	25	80
Nancy's *Fruit on Top* Raspberry, 8 oz	240	5	3	20	43	3	43	110
Peach, Cherry, or Blackberry, 8 oz (avg)........	220	6	3	20	37	1	35	110
Norman's NF Blueberry Creamy, 6 oz	90	0	0	0	15	0	8	50
NF Black Cherry Creamy, 6 oz......................	90	0	0	0	16	0	10	55
Low Carb, all or NF Plain, 6 oz	60	0	0	0	8	0	3	80
NF Strawberry or NF Vanilla, 6 oz (avg).........	85	0	0	0	15	0	9	80
Redwood Hill Farm Goat Yogurt								
Strawberry or Blueberry (avg)	145	4	3	25	24	1	20	65
Vanilla or Cranberry-Orange (avg)................	145	5	4	23	20	0	18	75
Plain	100	5	3	30	7	0	7	80
Stonyfield Farm *Oikos* Greek Yogurt								
Honey, 5.3 oz	120	0	0	0	18	0	17	50
Vanilla or Strawberry, 5.3 oz.......................	110	0	0	0	12	0	11	60
Plain, 5.3 oz	80	0	0	0	6	0	6	60
Blueberry, 5.3 oz.......................................	120	0	0	0	16	0	15	70
Wallaby Organic *Downunder* Dark Choc	170	5	3	10	28	1	25	75
Low Fat, all flavors (avg)............................	140	3	2	15	23	0	19	75
Downunder Mango Tangerine	140	2	2	10	26	0	24	75
Nonfat, all flavors (avg)	130	0	0	10	25	0	20	80
Downunder Peach Passion or Strawberries/Cream.	140	2	2	10	25	0	23	80
Downunder Berries & Cream	140	2	2	10	25	0	23	85
Downunder Pink Grapefruit..........................	140	2	1	10	24	0	22	90
Wild Harvest Organic Peach, 8 oz	140	2	2	10	26	0	21	90
Strawberry, 8 oz	120	2	1	10	22	0	21	90
Plain, 8 oz...	100	2	1	10	14	0	9	105
Yoplait *Original,* fruit flavors......................	170	2	1	10	33	0	27	80
Original, Coconut Cream Pie	170	3	2	10	34	0	27	85
Light, most varieties (avg)	100	0	0	5	19	0	14	85

	Cal	Fat	Sat	Chol	Carb	Fib	Sug	Sod
NON-DAIRY YOGURT ALTERNATIVES								
Nancy's Cultured Soy Plain	150	3	0	0	25	2	15	20
Cultured Soy all flavors (avg)	140	4	0	0	22	3	12	20
Silk Live! Soy Yogurt, all flavors (avg)	150	2	0	0	29	1	21	25
Live! Soy Yogurt, Plain	150	4	1	30	22	1	12	30
Stonyfield Farm O'Soy Smooth/Creamy Choc..	160	3	0	0	26	0	22	30
Fruit at the Bottom Blueberry	170	3	0	0	26	2	26	30
O'Soy Smooth/Creamy Vanilla	150	3	0	0	24	1	21	40
O'Soy Fruit at the Bottom Peach	170	3	0	0	30	2	28	45
O'Soy Fruit at the Bottom Strawberry	170	3	0	0	29	2	27	55
WholeSoy & Co Lemon	160	4	0	0	29	2	18	15
Peach, Strawberry, or Cherry (avg)	165	4	0	0	30	2	20	20
Strawberry/Banana	180	4	0	0	35	2	22	20
Plain or Vanilla (avg)	150	4	0	0	28	2	12	25
Raspberry, Apple Mango, or Blueberry (avg) ..	160	4	0	0	30	2	19	25
Wild Wood Organics Soyogurt Probiotic								
Blueberry or Strawberry (avg)	150	3	0	0	26	5	16	40
Vanilla, Peach, or Raspberry (avg)	160	3	0	0	30	5	21	40
Plain	110	4	1	0	14	5	4	45

YOGURT – FROZEN

(see Frozen Yogurt, pg 123)

YOGURT AND NON-DAIRY DRINKS

(also see Kefir, pg 107)

	Cal	Fat	Sat	Chol	Carb	Fib	Sug	Sod
Fruit flavored yogurt drink, 10 oz	240	0	0	0	48	0	44	150
Brands . . . *(8 oz unless noted)*								
Bolthouse Farms Fruit Smoothies								
Blue Goodness	170	0	0	0	41	8	28	5
Strawberry Banana	120	0	0	0	29	1	27	10
C-Boost or Amazing Mango (avg)	151	0	0	0	37	1	32	15
Berry Boost	120	1	0	0	30	4	21	20
Green Goodness	140	0	0	0	33	1	27	25
Protein Plus Chocolate	190	3	1	5	26	1	23	110
Dannon Light 'n Fit Smoothie Strawberry, 7 oz	60	3	2	15	4	0	3	35
DanActive Immunity, all flavors, 3.1 oz	80	2	1	5	13	0	13	40
Activa Mixed Berry, Strawberry, or Vanilla, 6 oz	160	3	2	10	27	1	25	60
Activa Peach, 6 oz	160	3	2	10	27	1	25	65
0% Plus Smoothie Strawberry or Blueberry, 7 oz	70	0	0	5	13	0	12	70
0% Plus Smoothie Mixed Berry, 7 oz	70	0	0	5	14	0	12	70
0% Plus Smoothie Strawberry Banana, 7 oz	70	0	0	5	14	0	12	75
0% Plus Smoothie Peach, 7 oz	70	0	0	5	13	0	12	90
Kemps Yo-J, all, 8 oz	150	0	0	0	34	0	32	55
Lifeway Kefir Smoothie, FF, all	180	0	0	5	33	3	30	125
Kefir Smoothie, LF or Organic LF, all	160	2	1	10	25	3	21	125
Lassi Mango or Strawberry	160	2	2	10	25	3	21	125
Slim6 LF Kefir Plain or flavored, all	110	2	2	10	8	2	6	125
Stonyfield Smoothie Peach, 10 oz	230	3	2	10	41	1	40	140
Smoothie Vanilla, 10 oz	240	3	2	10	40	1	37	140
Yoplait Smoothie, all (frozen)	110	2	1	5	14	2	10	20

DESSERTS AND SWEETS

See RESOURCES, page 305, for a partial list of manufacturers and retailers offering low-salt products online or visit **LowSaltFoods.com** *for additional sources.*

DESSERTS AND SWEETS

BISCOTTI

(also see Cookies, pg 119)

	Cal	Fat	Sat	Chol	Carb	Fib	Sug	Sod
Biscotti, 1 oz	110	0	0	0	24	0	15	95

Brands . . . *(1 oz unless noted)*
Most biscotti are low sodium, the following have 75mg or less.

MIXES

	Cal	Fat	Sat	Chol	Carb	Fib	Sug	Sod
King Arthur Flour Traditional Almond	80	0	0	0	18	1	8	75

SHELF-STABLE

	Cal	Fat	Sat	Chol	Carb	Fib	Sug	Sod
Alessi Cantuccini Crisp Almond Cookies, 5	115	3	1	12	19	0	8	60
Aunt Gussie's Almond Biscotti, 0.8 oz	110	6	0	15	13	1	5	10
Choc Chip Almond Biscotti, 0.8 oz	110	6	1	15	13	1	6	10
Sugar Free Biscotti, all, 0.8 oz (avg)	110	6	1	15	14	1	0	10
Italian Biscotti w/Olive Oil, 1.2 oz	160	5	1	25	25	1	13	30
Breadsmith Choc Hazelnut Biscotti, 1.1 oz	110	4	1	20	19	1	10	70
Almond Biscotti, 1.1 oz	110	3	0	25	20	1	10	75
Catanzaro's Anisette Biscotti, 1	104	5	1	34	13	0	4	26
Eating Right Cranberry & Pistachio Mini	130	4	2	26	20	2	13	55
Foods by George Biscotti, 0.8 oz	90	5	0	0	11	1	6	25
Golden Star Bakery Biscotti, all, 2 oz	85	0	0	0	14	0	6	30
Nonni's Triple Milk Choc Biscotti	110	5	3	20	17	1	10	50
Original or Decadence Biscotti (avg)	100	4	2	20	16	1	8	65
Choc or Toffee Almond Biscotti (avg)	120	6	3	23	18	1	10	70
Limone or Turtle Pecan Biscotti (avg)	110	5	2	20	17	0	10	75
Almond Dark Choc Biscotti Bites	120	6	3	20	16	1	8	75
Sahale Biscotti Crisps Almond Vanilla Latte	130	4	2	30	22	1	11	50
Shabtai Gourmet Choc Chip Biscotti, 0.8 oz	100	6	2	15	11	1	4	40
Stella D'oro Choc Chunk, 0.7 oz	90	4	2	5	14	0	8	35
Choc Almond, 0.7 oz	90	4	1	5	13	1	7	40
Almond, 0.7 oz	100	5	1	5	13	1	6	45
French Vanilla, 0.7 oz	90	4	1	10	15	0	7	55
Tre Sorella Italian Vanilla Biscotti Mix	60	2	1	0	10	1	2	55

BLINTZES AND CREPES

(see Blintzes/Crepes, pg 138)

BROWNIES AND DESSERT BARS

	Cal	Fat	Sat	Chol	Carb	Fib	Sug	Sod
Lemon bar, mix, 1/16 pkg	150	4	1	0	29	0	24	80
Brownie, ready-to-eat, 2 oz square	227	9	2	10	36	1	21	175
Brownie, mix, 1/16 pkg	165	6	1	0	29	0	22	115

Brands . . . *(1 brownie)*
There are many low-sodium brownies, the following have 90mg or less.

FROZEN/REFRIGERATED

Duncan Hines Oven Ready! Brownies

	Cal	Fat	Sat	Chol	Carb	Fib	Sug	Sod
Choc Chip, Choc Fudge, or Milk Choc (avg)	170	8	2	18	24	1	15	85
Gillian's Foods Brownies, 1	60	0	0	0	14	1	10	35

MIXES – *Some mixes require added ingredients that may increase sodium content.*
Lemon bar mix – *Most brands within generic average (80mg).*

	Cal	Fat	Sat	Chol	Carb	Fib	Sug	Sod
1-2-3 Gluten Free Divinely Decadent Brownies	70	1	0	0	18	1	13	60
Devlishly Decadent Choc Chunk Brownies	100	2	1	0	21	1	15	65
Arrowhead Mills Gluten Free Brownie	110	2	2	0	21	1	13	40
Bake With Me Organic Brownie Mix	90	2	1	0	21	1	14	45

113

	Cal	Fat	Sat	Chol	Carb	Fib	Sug	Sod
Brownie Mix	90	2	1	0	21	1	14	65
Barefoot Contessa Lemon Bar Mix	340	0	0	0	83	1	60	30
Brownie Mix	150	6	4	0	28	2	22	60
Bernard Butterscotch or Choc Brownie	70	0	0	0	20	0	7	10
Betty Crocker Gluten Free Brownie, 1/16	110	2	1	0	24	1	18	60
Walnut Choc Chunk, 1/16	130	3	1	0	25	1	17	90
Fudge Brownies, 1/16	100	1	0	0	23	1	15	90
Big Train Choc Chip Brownie Mix	60	2	1	0	15	4	4	45
Canterbury Naturals Choc Brownie	130	3	1	0	27	1	19	80
Cause Your Special Choc Fudge Brownie	125	1	0	0	29	1	19	82
The Cravings Place Ooey Gooey								
Chocolatey Chewy Brownie Mix	113	3	2	0	23	1	15	22
Dixie Carb Counters One Carb Brownie	20	1	0	2	1	0	1	31
Homemade Rich & Think LF Mix	46	1	1	34	11	1	7	32
Caramel Overload Brownie	26	1	1	2	2	1	1	38
Duncan Hines Family Style Milk Choc Brownie	110	3	1	0	22	1	15	65
Decadent Milk Choc Chunk Brownie Mix	130	4	2	0	25	1	18	75
Eagle Brand Turtle Temptations	140	6	3	5	19	2	13	15
Magic Cookie Bars	110	5	3	5	15	1	9	50
Toffee Dream Bars	110	4	3	0	20	0	10	65
Peanut Butter Passion, 1/20	170	8	3	5	20	1	15	90
Firenza Triple Choc Brownie	110	2	2	0	25	1	16	70
Oatmeal Cranberry Bar	80	1	1	0	17	1	10	75
Gluten-Free Pantry Choc Truffle Brownie	150	3	2	15	31	1	23	65
Hodgson Mill Brownie Mix	120	1	1	0	28	2	19	80
Hol-grain Choc Brownie Mix	90	0	0	0	22	1	17	70
Krusteaz Raspberry or Pecan Bars (avg)	130	3	0	0	24	1	13	70
Miss Roben's Chewy Brownie Mix, 1/12	110	0	0	0	27	1	20	50
Naturally Nora Fantastic Fudgy Brownie, 1/20	120	0	0	0	27	1	21	60
Doubly Fudgy Brownie, 1/20	130	0	0	0	28	1	22	60
Rabbit Creek Gourmet all varieites (avg)	95	1	1	0	25	0	20	4
Really Great Food Co Aunt Tootsie's Brownie	80	1	0	0	22	1	16	70
SHELF-STABLE (READY-TO-EAT)								
Ener-G Brownies, 1.4 oz	150	6	2	15	22	2	15	70
Foods by George Brownies, 1.6 oz	180	9	1	40	24	1	16	45
Golden Star FF Cinnamon, 2 oz	107	0	0	0	24	0	16	30
FF Brownie, 2 oz	145	0	0	0	29	3	22	35
Isabella's Sugar Free Black Tie Brownie, 1.2 oz	100	5	2	20	19	1	0	75
Pillsbury *Sweet Moments Bite-Size Brownies*								
Choc Caramel or Choc Fudge, 1.5 oz (3)	180	9	4	15	25	1	20	85
Shabtai Gourmet Gluten Free Brownie	120	6	2	25	16	1	13	25
Gluten Free Brownie Bites, 0.8 oz	90	5	2	20	13	1	9	25

CAKE

(also see Cheesecake, pg 118, Snack Cakes/Pies/Other Sweet Snacks, pg 134)

	Cal	Fat	Sat	Chol	Carb	Fib	Sug	Sod
Fruitcake, 1/12	92	3	0	1	17	1	8	77
Sponge cake, 1/12	110	1	0	39	23	0	14	93
Ice cream cake, 4 oz	190	11	7	25	23	1	16	100
Pound cake, 1/12	109	6	3	62	14	0	13	111
Choc cake w/frosting, ready-to-eat, 1/12	154	7	2	18	51	1	42	140
Chocolate cake, mix, 1/12	186	7	1	0	32	1	17	359
Yellow cake w/frosting, ready-to-eat, 1/12	157	6	1	23	38	0	29	144
Yellow cake, mix, 1/12	188	5	1	1	34	1	19	286
Angel food cake, ready-to-eat, 1/12	72	0	0	0	16	0	13	210

	Cal	Fat	Sat	Chol	Carb	Fib	Sug	Sod
Angel food cake, mix, 1/12	127	0	0	0	29	0	15	251
Marble cake, pudding-type, mix, 1/12	179	5	1	0	34	1	25	223
Gingerbread, mix, 1/12	140	4	1	0	25	1	16	224
Carrot cake, pudding-type, mix, 1/12	176	4	1	0	34	2	24	240
German choc, pudding-type, mix, 1/12	172	4	1	0	34	2	21	276
White cake, mix, 1/12	185	5	1	0	34	0	24	289

Brands . . . *(1/12 serving unless noted)*

FROZEN/REFRIGERATED

	Cal	Fat	Sat	Chol	Carb	Fib	Sug	Sod
Pepperidge Farm 3 Layer Cakes								
Coconut or Vanilla Bean, 1/8 (avg)	230	10	3	20	35	1	25	120
Choc Fudge, Lemon, or Golden, 1/8 (avg)	235	10	3	20	33	1	23	130
Peppermint (seasonal), 1/8	230	11	3	25	31	2	21	135
Roland Torta Della Nonna Custard Cake, 1/14	340	14	0	40	47	2	24	100
Mixed Berry & Chantilly Cream Cake	290	14	0	20	36	2	19	115
Choc Cream Pear or Apple Cream Crostata (avg)	290	9	0	20	50	2	30	115
Black Forest Cake	290	10	0	65	45	2	27	140
Sara Lee Fudge Golden Layer Cake, 1/10	260	14	10	20	31	1	21	105
Weight Watchers Lemon Creme Cake, 1	80	3	1	20	17	5	8	65
Carrot Cake, 1	90	4	2	10	17	4	10	70
Choc Creme Cake, 1	80	4	2	20	16	4	9	95
Wholly Wholesome Golden Butter Pound, 1/4	330	18	12	150	36	0	19	130

REDUCED SODIUM (LESS THAN GENERIC):

	Cal	Fat	Sat	Chol	Carb	Fib	Sug	Sod
Sara Lee Vanilla Layer Cake, 1/10	250	14	10	25	29	0	20	150

MIXES – *Some mixes require additional ingredients that may raise sodium content.*

	Cal	Fat	Sat	Chol	Carb	Fib	Sug	Sod
Arrowhead Mills Organic Vanilla Cake	160	0	0	0	37	1	20	140
Authentic Foods Lemon Cake Mix	110	1	0	0	24	1	14	45
Choc Cake Mix	100	1	0	0	23	1	14	105
Barefoot Contessa Choc Ganache, 1/16	110	3	2	0	22	1	15	0
Lemon Angel Food, 1/16	140	0	0	0	33	0	26	70
Old Fashioned Gingerbread Mix, 1/9	250	0	0	0	60	1	29	75
Decadent Molten Choc Cake Mix, 1/6	220	12	6	0	34	2	28	90
Orange Pound Cake Mix, 1/16	150	0	0	0	36	0	26	115
Lemon Pound Cake & Glaze, 1/16	150	0	0	0	36	0	26	120
Bob's Red Mill Gluten Free, Choc, 1/16	110	1	0	0	24	2	12	85
'Cause You're Special Golden Pound, 1/10	207	0	0	0	50	1	27	120
Cravings Place Raisin Spice Cookie & Cake	140	0	0	0	24	2	12	120
Dixie Carb Counters								
Choc Snackin Cake & Frosting, 1/9	35	1	0	0	4	2	1	60
Molten Choc Royale Cake Mix, 1/6	84	5	2	5	5	1	3	76
Lemon Pound Cake Mix, 1/16	23	0	0	0	5	2	2	126
Classic Pound Cake Mix, 1/16	22	0	0	0	5	2	1	136
Almond Cream Coffee Cake Mix	46	1	0	0	5	1	3	140
Dr. Oetker *Lava* Caramel, 1/4	240	2	1	0	56	0	36	50
Lava Choc or *Lava* Choc Raspberry, 1/4 (avg)	255	2	1	0	55	2	41	50
Black Forest Cake Mix, 1/16	110	1	1	0	25	0	16	70
Ener-G Pound Cake, 1/6	140	7	1	40	19	1	9	115
Gefen Honey Cake, 1/9	190	8	2	35	26	0	18	40
Choc or Marble Cake, 1/9 (avg)	215	10	4	40	29	0	18	55
Choc Chip Cake, 1/9	230	11	4	40	31	0	18	55
Gluten-Free Pantry Choc Chip Cookie/Cake	120	2	1	0	25	1	14	135
King Arthur Flour Buttermilk Lemon, 1/14	190	0	0	0	43	1	25	100
Complete Fruit Cake, 1/15	320	1	0	0	77	2	48	110
Choc Indulgence Cake, 1/14	190	9	6	0	26	3	23	140
Honey Lemon, 1/18	160	0	0	0	36	1	19	140
Kinnikinnick Angel Food, 1/4	430	0	0	0	107	1	67	75

DESSERTS AND SWEETS
Cake

	Cal	Fat	Sat	Chol	Carb	Fib	Sug	Sod
Miss Roben's Angel Food Cake Mix, 1/10	120	0	0	0	30	0	20	120
Namaste Vanilla Cake Mix, 1/16	170	0	0	0	41	1	17	50
Naturally Nora Alota Dots, 1/12	180	1	0	0	41	1	19	140
Cookie Cookie or Surprising Stars, 1/12	190	2	0	0	42	1	22	140
Pantry Shelf *Classic Desserts Collection*								
Pineapple Upside Down Cake, 1/6	150	0	0	0	35	1	27	75
Rabbit Creek Gourmet Hot Caramel Pudding Cake	106	0	0	0	28	0	25	33
Coca Cola Cake w/Frosting, 1/16	130	0	0	0	31	0	28	40
Sugar Free Yummy!! Choc, 1/16	25	1	1	0	6	2	0	60
Hot Fudge Pudding Cake Dessert Mix	1240	0	0	0	30	0	22	126
Stonewall Kitchen Choc Molten Lava Cake, 1/6	310	7	5	0	62	2	50	60
Eggnog Pound Cake Mix, 1/15	130	0	0	0	29	0	16	85
Sweet 'N Low Snack Cake Mix, all, 1/5	160	3	1	0	36	1	1	30
REDUCED SODIUM (LESS THAN GENERIC):								
Barefoot Contessa Coconut Layer, 1/16	260	5	4	0	54	1	39	150
Cherrybrook Kitchen Yellow	140	5	4	0	34	0	21	150
Dixie Carb Counters Classic Devil's Food	35	0	0	0	5	1	3	146
Naturally Nora Sunny Yellow, 1/12	170	1	0	0	39	1	23	150
Cherry Chocolate, 1/12	170	1	0	0	37	1	21	150
SHELF-STABLE								
Entenmann's Ultimate Madeline's Petite								
Butter Cakes, 2 (2 oz)	240	14	9	80	26	0	16	80
Foods by George Crumb Cake, 1/9	280	14	9	40	36	1	12	80
Hill & Valley Sugar Free Yellow Square, 1.4 oz	140	8	4	10	17	0	0	75
Sugar Free White or Choc Square Cake (avg)	140	8	4	8	18	0	0	85
Sugar Free 8" Yellow Cake, 2.2 oz	220	13	7	15	27	0	0	110
Sugar Free 8" White Cake, 2.2 oz	220	12	6	10	28	0	0	120
Sugar Free Pound Cake, 1 oz	110	5	3	30	13	0	0	120
Sugar Free 8" Choc Cake, 2.2 oz	210	12	6	15	26	2	0	125
Sugar Free Pumpkin Spice Creme Cake, 1.1 oz	80	3	1	15	11	0	0	130
Sugar Free Blueberry Creme Cake, 1.1 oz	90	3	1	20	11	0	1	135
Choc Creme or Marble Creme Cake, 1.1 oz	90	4	1	20	12	1	0	140
Sugar Free Angel Food Bar, 0.9 oz	35	0	0	0	11	1	0	140
Kuchen Meister Rum Stollen, 1.8 oz	190	8	5	0	28	1	15	65
Marzipan or Black Forest Stollen, 1.8 oz (avg)	203	9	4	3	29	2	16	60
Shabtai Gourmet Swiss Choc Roll, 1/6	290	20	9	35	26	1	23	30
Sponge or Marble Cake, 1/8	120	5	2	90	17	1	9	55
Raspberry or Apricot Roll, 1/8	180	6	3	65	29	1	22	55
Devil's Food or White 7-Layer Cake, 1/8	220	13	5	75	25	1	16	60
Honey Loaf Cake, 2.9 oz	140	9	4	40	13	0	8	65

CHEESECAKE *(see Cheesecake, pg 118)*

COFFEE CAKE *(see Pastries/Other Breakfast Sweets, pg 72)*

CUPCAKES

	Cal	Fat	Sat	Chol	Carb	Fib	Sug	Sod
MIXES								
Arrowhead Mills Bake w/Me Organic or Vanilla	120	0	0	0	27	1	10	110
Gluten Free Choc	120	1	0	0	27	2	11	120
Barefoot Contessa Vanilla w/Milk Choc Frosting	300	6	4	5	66	1	51	135
Vanilla & Cream Cheese Frosting	240	2	1	5	58	1	43	140
Duncan Hines Snack Size Confetti Cupcakes	90	2	1	0	17	0	10	135
Snack Size Classic Yellow Cupcakes	90	2	1	0	17	0	9	135
Iveta Gourmet Choc Coconut	200	4	3	0	40	1	7	120
Robt Rothschild Farm Red Velvet (w/o frosting)	230	1	0	0	46	1	35	88
White Cupcake Mix (w/o frosting)	100	0	0	0	22	0	13	100
SHELF-STABLE								
Hill & Valley Sugar Free White Mini, 0.9 oz	80	5	3	5	11	0	0	30

	Cal	Fat	Sat	Chol	Carb	Fib	Sug	Sod
Sugar Free Choc Mini Cupcakes, 0.9 oz	80	5	3	5	11	1	0	35
Sugar Free White Cupcakes, 2 oz	200	11	6	10	25	0	0	105
Sugar Free Choc Cupcakes, 2 oz	190	11	6	10	24	2	0	110
Shabtai Gourmet Gluten Free Ring Ting	220	13	5	60	24	1	17	40

ICE CREAM CAKES

	Cal	Fat	Sat	Chol	Carb	Fib	Sug	Sod
Carvel Celebration Ice Cream Cake, 1/15	190	10	7	20	21	0	17	75
Lil' Love Ice Cream Cake, 1/7	210	12	8	25	24	0	20	90
Snickers Ice Cream Cake, 1/10	250	15	8	35	27	1	21	125
Celebrate Confetti Fudge Ice Cream Cake, 1/9	190	11	7	25	23	1	16	100
Jon Donaire Caramel Brownie, 1/10	250	13	8	20	32	1	24	110
Strawberry Cheesecake Ice Cream Cake, 1/8	220	10	6	25	29	1	20	125

CAKE FROSTING, ICING AND DECORATIONS

	Cal	Fat	Sat	Chol	Carb	Fib	Sug	Sod
Sprinkles, 1 tsp	20	1	1	0	3	0	3	0
Icing, decorating, 1 tsp	30	1	0	0	5	0	4	10
Frosting, mix, fluffy white, 1/12 pkg	61	0	0	0	16	0	15	38
Ready-to-spread, cream cheese, 2 tbsp	137	6	2	0	22	0	21	63
Ready-to-spread, vanilla, 2 tbsp	153	6	1	0	25	0	23	67
Ready-to-spread, choc, 2 tbsp	140	5	2	0	23	1	20	100
Mix, choc, 1/12 pkg	121	2	0	0	29	1	24	130

Brands . . . *(2 tbsp or 1/12 unless noted)*
There are many low-sodium frostings, the following have 65mg or less.

MIXES

	Cal	Fat	Sat	Chol	Carb	Fib	Sug	Sod
Calorie Control Lemon	140	5	2	0	12	0	2	40
Vanilla, Choc, or Cream Cheese	100	5	2	0	12	0	2	40
Cherrybrook Kitchen Choc or Vanilla (avg)	80	0	0	0	20	1	19	20
Dixie Carb Counters White or Choc Butter	15	0	0	0	6	5	0	20
Dr Oetker Organics Choc or Vanilla (avg)	110	0	0	0	26	0	25	65
Duncan Hines *Whipped* Fluffy White or Vanilla	150	7	2	0	22	0	20	60
King Arthur Flour Vanilla Glaze	35	0	0	0	9	0	8	0
Vanilla Buttercream	90	0	0	5	22	1	21	30
Choc Fudge	80	1	0	10	19	1	16	60
Miss Roben's Milk Choc Buttercream	260	1	1	0	60	1	50	0
Vanilla Buttercream	386	0	0	0	64	0	54	5
Namaste Toffee Vanilla Frosting Mix, 1/16	150	5	3	10	29	0	27	65
Naturally Nora Extraordinary Vanilla	100	0	0	0	25	0	23	5
Cheerful Choc	100	0	0	0	24	0	21	15
Alot'a Dots or Surprising Stars (avg)	110	0	0	0	26	0	23	15
Pillsbury *Home Style* Fluffy White	100	0	0	0	24	0	23	55
Sweet N'Low White Frosting, 1/16	60	2	2	0	9	0	0	10
Chocolate Frosting, 1/16	45	2	2	0	6	1	0	50

READY-TO-SPREAD

	Cal	Fat	Sat	Chol	Carb	Fib	Sug	Sod
Betty Crocker *Whipped* Whipped Cream	100	5	2	0	15	0	13	25
Whipped Fluffy White or Strawberry Mist	100	5	2	0	15	0	14	25
Whipped Vanilla or Butter Cream	100	5	2	0	15	0	14	25
Whipped Cream Cheese	100	5	2	0	15	0	13	45
Whipped Milk Choc	100	5	2	0	14	1	12	55
Rich & Creamy Coconut Pecan	140	7	3	0	19	1	16	55
Home Style Fluffy White	100	0	0	0	24	0	23	55
Whipped Choc	90	5	2	0	14	1	12	60
Cherrybrook Kitchen Vanilla	120	6	3	0	18	0	17	25
Duncan Hines *Whipped* Fluffy White or Vanilla	150	7	2	0	22	0	20	60
Pillsbury *Whip Supreme* Fluffy White or Cr Cheese	100	5	2	0	14	0	13	20
Strawberry, Vanilla, or Vanilla Funfetti	100	5	2	0	15	0	14	20

117

	Cal	Fat	Sat	Chol	Carb	Fib	Sug	Sod
Whipped Supreme Milk Choc	100	5	1	0	14	0	13	50
Reduced Sugar Milk Choc	100	6	2	0	17	2	9	50
Sugar Free Vanilla	100	6	2	0	17	3	0	55
Reduced Sugar Vanilla	120	7	2	0	18	3	10	60
Creamy Supreme Coconut Pecan	160	10	4	0	17	1	16	60
Creamy Supreme Pink Vanilla Funfetti	140	5	2	0	23	0	22	65

ICING AND DECORATIONS – *Most brands within generic average (0–10mg).*

CANDY AND CHEWING GUM

	Cal	Fat	Sat	Chol	Carb	Fib	Sug	Sod
Chewing gum, 1 stick	5	0	0	0	1	0	1	0
Candy:								
Breath savers, 1 pc	10	0	0	0	2	0	0	0
Sweet choc candy, 1 oz	143	10	6	0	15	2	12	0
Gumdrops, 1 oz	34	0	0	0	9	0	21	4
Jelly beans, 1 oz	104	0	0	0	26	0	18	7
Choc coated fondant, 1 oz	102	3	2	0	22	0	21	7
Choc coated raisins, 1 oz	109	4	2	1	19	1	17	10
Lollipop, 0.6 oz (1)	60	0	0	0	16	0	12	10
Hard candy, 1 oz	106	0	0	0	28	0	20	11
Butterscotch, 1 oz	112	1	0	3	2	0	24	12
Choc coated peanuts, 1 oz	145	9	4	3	14	1	11	12
Caramels, choc-flavored roll, 1 oz	103	2	0	0	22	0	19	24
Caramel, 1 oz	108	2	2	2	22	0	24	70
Candy bars:								
Sweet choc bar, 1.5 oz	207	14	8	0	24	2	21	7
Milk choc bar w/almonds, 1.5 oz	216	14	7	8	22	3	18	30
Milk choc bar, 1.6 oz	235	13	6	10	26	2	23	35
Milk choc w/rice cereal, 1.5 oz	223	12	7	9	29	2	25	65
Crisped rice bar, choc chip, 1 oz	113	4	3	1	20	1	9	78

Brands . . . *Most brands within generic average.*

CHEESECAKE

	Cal	Fat	Sat	Chol	Carb	Fib	Sug	Sod
Cheesecake, ready-to-eat, 1/6 of 17 oz	401	28	12	69	32	1	27	259
Mix, 1/6	271	13	7	29	35	2	27	376

Brands . . . *(1/6 unless noted)*

FROZEN/REFRIGERATED

	Cal	Fat	Sat	Chol	Carb	Fib	Sug	Sod
Chatila's Bakery Mini Dbl Choc, 3 oz	120	3	1	25	8	0	4	135
Lean on Me Choc Dipped Cheesecake, 2 oz	140	10	6	35	13	0	2	105
Blueberry Cheesecake, 2 oz	120	9	5	35	7	0	2	120
Original or Marble Cheesecake, 2 oz	130	10	6	45	7	0	2	140
Sara Lee Simple Singles								
Creamy Cheesecake w/Strawberry Sauce, 1	250	10	7	0	37	0	26	85
Wholly Wholesome Cheesecake Bites, 1.9 oz	190	12	7	60	18	0	13	110

MIXES – *Some mixes require additional ingredients which may raise sodium content.*

	Cal	Fat	Sat	Chol	Carb	Fib	Sug	Sod
Calorie Control Cheesecake	60	2	1	5	7	0	4	80
Choc or Choc Chip Cheesecake	60	2	1	5	7	0	4	80
Dixie Carb Counters Classic, 1/9	11	0	0	0	2	1	0	23
Strawberry-Daiquiri Cheese Cake, 1/9	25	0	0	0	3	1	2	23
Pecan Praline Cheese Cake, 1/9	40	3	0	0	4	2	1	23
Almond Cream Coffee	46	1	0	0	5	1	3	140
Expert Foods Wise Choice Cheesecake	23	0	0	0	4	4	0	44
King Arthur Flour Key Lime Cheesecake Bars	130	1	1	0	28	0	18	55
Rabbit Creek Gourmet No Bake Cheesecakes								
Key Lime or Peaches & Cream, 1/8 (avg)	25	0	0	0	5	0	5	0

	Cal	Fat	Sat	Chol	Carb	Fib	Sug	Sod
Pumpkin Pie, 1/8	30	1	1	0	5	1	4	0
Three Berry or Wild Raspberry, 1/8	25	0	0	0	6	1	6	10
Sugar Free Raspberry or Strawberry, 1/8	5	0	0	0	1	1	0	10
Sans Sucre Cheesecake Mousse, 1/8	60	2	1	5	8	0	4	80
Choc Cheesecake Mousse, 1/8	60	2	1	5	8	0	4	80

COFFEE CAKES

(see Pastries/Other Breakfast Sweets, pg 72)

COOKIES

	Cal	Fat	Sat	Chol	Carb	Fib	Sug	Sod
Sugar wafers w/creme filling, 1 oz	145	7	1	0	20	0	10	42
Ladyfingers, 1 oz	103	3	1	83	17	0	11	42
Marshmallow, choc coated, 1 oz	119	5	1	0	19	1	13	48
Coconut macaroons, 1 oz	115	4	3	0	20	1	20	70
Choc chip cookies, soft, 1 oz	127	6	3	0	18	1	11	76
Refrg dough, 1 oz	126	6	2	7	17	0	10	59
Mix, 1 oz	141	7	2	0	19	0	14	82
Graham crackers, choc covered, 1 oz	137	7	4	0	19	1	12	82
Wafers, vanilla, 1 oz	134	6	1	0	20	1	11	88
Choc, 1 oz	123	4	1	1	21	1	8	164
Fig Bar, 1 oz	99	2	0	0	20	1	13	99
Sandwich, vanilla w/creme filling, 1 oz	137	6	1	0	20	0	11	99
Choc w/creme filling, 1 oz	131	6	2	0	20	1	11	141
Butter cookies, 1 oz	132	5	3	33	20	0	6	100
Sugar cookies, 1 oz	136	6	2	15	19	0	13	101
Refrg dough, 1 oz	124	6	1	8	17	0	7	120
Oatmeal cookies, 1 oz	128	5	1	0	19	1	7	109
Mix, 1 oz	131	5	1	0	19	1	11	134
Animal crackers, 1 oz	126	4	1	0	21	0	4	111
Peanut butter, 1 oz	135	7	1	0	17	1	9	118
Refrigerated dough, 1 oz	130	7	2	8	15	0	9	113
Mix, 1 oz	120	4	1	0	20	0	12	140
Shortbread, 1 oz	142	7	2	6	18	1	4	129
Molasses, 1 oz	122	4	1	0	21	0	5	130
Gingersnaps, 1 oz	118	3	1	2	22	1	10	185

Brands . . . *(1 oz unless noted)*
There are many low-sodium cookies, the following have 50mg or less sodium.

FROZEN/REFRIGERATED

	Cal	Fat	Sat	Chol	Carb	Fib	Sug	Sod
Wholly Wholesome Oatmeal Cranberry Dough	110	5	3	15	15	1	8	50

MIXES

	Cal	Fat	Sat	Chol	Carb	Fib	Sug	Sod
Arrowhead Mills Bake with Me Organic Sugar	90	1	0	0	20	1	9	45
Canterbury Organics Coconut Macaroon, 1	50	3	3	0	7	1	5	15
Cherrybrook Kitchen Sugar	70	0	0	0	16	0	9	50
Cravings Place Peanut Butter	50	0	0	0	10	0	3	15
Choc Chunk	80	2	1	0	12	1	5	30
Double Choc Chunk Cookie & Muffin	70	2	1	0	11	1	4	30
Dixie Carb Counters Beanit Butter, 1	23	1	0	0	2	1	0	24
Gluten Free Essentials Choc Chip, 1	38	1	0	0	8	1	8	45
King Arthur Flour Coconut Macaroon	100	6	5	0	12	1	8	10
Traditional Shortbread	50	0	0	0	11	1	4	20
Vanilla Sugar Cookie	60	0	0	0	12	1	6	30
Rabbit Creek Gourmet White Choc Cranberry Drop	40	1	1	0	9	1	6	20
Oatmeal Raisin Or Choc Chip Drop (avg)	30	0	0	0	7	3	3	40
Peanut Butter Drop Cookie	36	1	1	0	6	0	3	45

	Cal	Fat	Sat	Chol	Carb	Fib	Sug	Sod
Sugar Free Sugar Cookie	24	0	0	0	3	0	0	45
Gluten Free Choc Chip Cookie	38	1	0	0	8	1	0	45
Really Great Food Co Coconut Macaroon	80	5	4	0	9	1	7	5
Stonewall Kitchen Choc Macaroon Cookie	110	6	5	0	14	2	11	10
Peppermint Snowball Cookie Mix	70	0	0	0	16	0	7	25
Vanilla Sandwich Cookie Mix	100	0	0	0	23	1	16	35
Peanut Butter Cookie	80	3	1	0	14	0	8	45
Sweet 'N Low Choc Chip Cookie	100	3	1	0	22	1	0	30
SHELF-STABLE								
Alessi Biscotti Savoiardi Lady Fingers, 4	120	1	0	35	25	1	14	50
Almondina Anniversary or Original (avg)	134	4	0	0	22	1	10	8
Pumpkin Spice	121	5	1	0	15	1	7	8
Cinnaroma	130	4	0	0	21	1	12	10
Gingerspice or Sesame (avg)	137	4	0	0	22	1	8	10
BranTreats or Coconut (avg)	130	4	0	0	22	2	10	12
Chocolate Dipped	130	5	2	0	16	4	13	15
AlmonDuo	135	5	1	0	20	1	8	44
Andre's Carbo-Save Mini Cookies, all	130	9	5	15	3	1	1	5
Aunt Gussie's Sugar Free Latte	110	6	3	15	18	0	0	40
Pecan Meltaways	150	10	5	20	14	1	3	40
Pecan Meltaways, Dark Choc Drizzled	180	12	6	25	16	1	4	45
Sugar Free Choc Chip	120	8	5	15	16	1	0	45
Mexican Wedding Cakes	180	10	5	20	19	1	8	45
Sugar Free Pecan Meltaways	150	10	5	20	14	1	0	45
Choc Chip	140	8	5	15	16	1	9	50
Bahlsen Afrika Dark Choc Wafers, 1.1 oz	170	10	6	5	12	1	9	20
Choco Leibniz Dark Choc	140	7	4	5	18	1	10	50
Barbara's Bakery Fig Bars Blueberry, 1.4 oz	120	1	0	0	27	1	16	45
Fig Bars Multigrain, 1.4 oz	110	1	0	0	26	2	15	50
Fig Bars Wheat Free Raspberry, 1.4 oz	120	0	0	0	27	2	16	50
Fig Bars Whole Wheat, 1.4 oz	110	1	0	0	25	2	8	50
Barry's Bakery French Twists, all, 0.5 oz	60	2	1	0	9	0	4	25
Barry's Bakery/Parisian Sweets Meringues	100	0	0	0	24	0	24	45
Bear Naked Fruit & Nut Granola Cookies	130	6	2	0	18	2	9	40
Catanzaro's Egg Biscuit	100	4	1	15	14	0	5	45
Chatila's Bakery Choc Choc Chip, 1	50	1	0	15	9	2	0	20
Vanilla Chip or Vanilla Walnut, 1 (avg)	45	1	0	15	10	2	0	20
Pistachio, 1	45	0	0	20	9	2	0	25
Peanut, 1	60	4	0	15	8	2	0	30
Macaroon, 1	80	5	5	0	12	3	1	30
Dipped Macaroons, 1	130	8	7	0	20	4	1	40
Lemon	45	1	0	20	10	2	0	40
Cherrybrook Kitchen Snickerdoodle Mini	110	4	2	0	18	0	8	15
Choc Chip or Gluten Free Choc Chip Mini (avg)	120	5	3	0	21	1	10	30
Dare Pure Choc Whippet, Original, 1.2 oz (avg)	155	5	3	0	26	1	18	50
DeBenkelaer Pirouline, Choc Hazelnut, 3	150	7	5	0	20	0	9	25
Ener-G Cinnamon	160	9	5	0	21	0	9	10
White Choc Chip, 0.6 oz	80	4	1	15	10	0	6	20
Choc, 0.6 oz	60	3	2	10	9	0	4	25
Ginger, 0.5 oz	50	2	1	0	9	0	4	30
Choc Chip Potato, 0.6 oz	70	3	2	10	11	0	6	35
Vanilla, 0.6 oz	90	4	0	10	11	0	5	45
Choc Chip Potato or Sunflower, 0.6 oz	80	5	1	0	7	1	4	50
Fifty/50 Creme Filled Wafers, all, 1.2 oz (avg)	160	9	4	0	22	0	0	30

	Cal	Fat	Sat	Chol	Carb	Fib	Sug	Sod
Choc Chip, 1.3 oz	170	9	3	0	22	1	7	35
Coconut	170	8	2	0	23	1	8	45
Choc Wafers, 1.2 oz	160	9	2	0	21	1	0	45
Butter, 1.4 oz	190	9	6	30	24	1	9	50
Franz Choc Striped Shortbread, 3	150	7	5	0	20	1	10	45
Vanilla Wafers, 4	120	5	3	10	17	0	9	45
Ginger Snaps, 4	130	6	3	0	19	0	9	50
Gefen Almond Cookies	125	6	1	21	17	1	8	10
Glutino Wafers, all	160	8	5	5	19	0	14	25
Golden Star Bakery FF Cookies, all, 2 oz	115	0	0	0	25	0	12	35
Great Value FF Devil's Food Choc Cookie Cakes	50	0	0	0	12	0	7	25
Fudge Marshmallow Cookies	120	5	4	0	19	1	13	45
Health Valley Oatmeal Raisin, 0.8 oz	90	4	0	0	14	1	8	50
Jennie's Coconut Macaroons	130	7	6	0	17	3	15	10
Keebler Fudge Shoppe Fudge Sticks, 3	150	8	5	0	20	1	15	40
Fudge Shoppe Peanut Butter Fudge Sticks, 3	160	9	5	0	17	1	12	40
E L Fudge Original, 1 (0.6 oz)	90	4	1	5	13	1	6	50
Kinnikinnick K-Kritters Animal Cookies, 8	90	2	1	0	17	1	2	25
Ginger Snaps, 1	40	1	1	0	7	0	2	50
KinniToos Fudge Sandwich Creme, 1	60	3	1	0	9	1	4	50
KinniToos Choc Vanilla Sandwich, 1	60	3	1	0	9	1	4	50
Lu Le Chocolatier	150	9	7	0	17	1	12	5
Pim's Raspberry, 2	100	3	2	10	16	1	13	30
Pim's Orange, 2	100	3	2	10	17	0	14	35
Petit Ecolier, Extra Dark Choc, 2	130	7	5	5	15	2	7	50
Petit Ecolier, Dark Choc, 2	130	6	4	5	17	1	9	50
Cinnamon Sugar Spice, 2	120	5	3	0	18	0	10	50
Luv U Almond Cookies, 0.6 oz	70	3	1	4	10	1	3	1
Miss Meringue Meringues, all (avg)	110	0	0	0	27	0	26	20
Traditional Madeleines, 1.2 oz	160	9	5	55	19	0	11	20
Choc Madeleines or Chocolettes Meringues	160	9	6	55	18	1	11	25
Murray Sugar Free Vanilla Creme Wafers, 4	130	8	3	0	19	4	0	20
Sugar Free Fudge Dipped Vanilla Wafers, 4	150	10	7	0	19	4	0	20
Nabisco Snackwell's Devil's Food, 0.6 oz	50	0	0	0	12	0	7	25
Snackwell's Choc Mint, 0.6 oz	50	1	0	0	12	0	7	40
Cookie Cakes Black Forest, 0.6 oz	50	1	0	0	12	0	7	40
Mallomars	120	5	3	0	18	1	2	40
Pinwheels	120	5	3	0	20	0	14	45
Pamela's Lemon Shortbread, 0.8 oz	120	6	4	15	15	1	5	50
Papadopoulos Caprice Creme-Filled Wafers (avg)	150	7	3	0	20	1	15	40
Pepperidge Farm Pirouette, Choc Fudge (2)	120	4	2	0	18	1	12	30
Tahiti Coconut, 2	170	10	6	5	17	2	8	40
Milano Raspberry or Strawberry, 2	130	7	5	5	16	1	8	40
Pirouette Choc Hazelnut, 2	120	5	2	5	19	1	13	40
Pirouette French Vanilla or Mint Choc, 2 (avg)	120	5	3	5	18	0	12	40
Reko Pizzelle Anise, Lemon, Maple, or Vanilla	150	6	1	15	20	0	8	20
Ritter Sport Neapolitan Wafers, 1.4 oz	210	13	7	5	18	2	17	35
Roland Amaretti Cookies	130	2	0	0	25	1	24	15
Gallettes	180	8	0	20	23	0	10	35
Sables	180	8	0	15	23	1	10	40
Schar Hazelnut Wafers, 1.8 oz	250	12	7	0	33	2	14	15
Shortbread Cookies	130	5	2	10	20	1	5	20
Choc Hazelnut Bars, 1.3 oz	200	12	6	5	22	1	14	30
Ladyfingers	110	2	1	40	22	1	10	40
Shabtai Gourmet Gluten Free Bon Bons	110	12	6	0	15	1	13	10

DESSERTS AND SWEETS
Dessert Mixes

	Cal	Fat	Sat	Chol	Carb	Fib	Sug	Sod
Gluten Free Florentine Lace Cookies	150	9	2	5	15	1	11	15
Gluten Free Rainbow Cookie Squares	120	8	1	20	11	1	8	20
Gluten Free Mini Black & White, 1.5 oz	200	12	3	15	23	1	15	25
Gluten Free Lady Fingers, 0.5 oz	45	1	0	40	7	0	4	25
Gluten Free Choc Chip	120	6	2	10	15	1	6	30
Gluten Free Pecan Meltaway Cookies	140	7	3	5	17	1	9	35
Susanna's Shortbread, Strawberry	110	2	0	5	20	1	5	10
Shortbread, Lemon or Key Lime	110	2	0	5	20	1	5	10
Shortbread, Butterscotch	140	6	0	20	19	1	4	55
Voortman Coconut, 0.7 oz	90	5	3	0	10	1	5	30
Mocha Cappuccino, Sugar Free	80	9	4	0	19	1	0	25
Vanilla, Choc, or Strawberry Wafers, 1.1 oz	140	6	2	0	20	0	12	25
Fudge Vanilla Wafers, No Sugar Added, 1.1 oz	150	9	4	0	20	0	0	25
Chunky Chip, 0.7 oz	100	5	2	0	14	1	7	40
Fudge Choc Chip, Sugar Free, 0.8 oz	90	5	1	0	13	1	0	40
Shortbread Swirl, Sugar Free, 0.8 oz	100	6	1	0	12	0	0	40
Apple or Strawberry Turnover	110	4	1	0	18	0	9	50
Wafer Cookies, Sugar Free, all	130	8	2	0	17	0	0	40
Choc Chip, Sugar Free, 0.8 oz	80	5	2	0	13	0	0	50
Oatmeal, Sugar Free, 0.8 oz	70	4	1	0	10	1	0	50
Peanut d'arachide, No Sugar Added, 1.1 oz	140	8	4	0	20	0	0	50
Wegmans Swiss Crepes, 8	160	8	5	0	19	0	4	35
Italian Classics Choc Swirl, 0.9 oz	160	6	3	5	30	1	12	40

DESSERT MIXES

(also see Pudding/Mousse, pg 131)

Brands . . .

	Cal	Fat	Sat	Chol	Carb	Fib	Sug	Sod
Barefoot Contessa Brownie Pudding Mix	340	2	1	0	86	4	70	0
Concord Foods Apple Crisp Mix	100	0	0	0	25	0	18	0
Fran Gare Choc Bake Mix, 1 oz	90	1	1	5	9	2	0	55
Almond Bake Mix, 1 oz	100	4	0	5	7	2	0	80

DESSERTS – FROZEN

(also see Pastries/Other Breakfast Sweets, pg 72; Ice Cream/Ices/Frozen Yogurt, pg 123)

Brands . . .

	Cal	Fat	Sat	Chol	Carb	Fib	Sug	Sod
Market Day Brownie Fudge Sunday Cup	360	17	9	55	49	1	32	120
Roland Plain Cream Puffs, Mini, 6	270	21	0	110	16	0	9	45
Choc Topped Cream Puffs, Mini, 6	250	17	0	70	23	1	16	60
Mini Eclairs, Plain, 6	220	14	0	90	19	0	12	70
Mini Eclairs, Choc Topped, 6	260	17	0	85	23	1	15	70
Belgian Crepes, Raspberry Filled, 1	180	7	0	15	27	1	12	120
Belgian Crepes, Blueberry Filled, 1	180	7	0	25	26	1	13	130
Belgian Crepes, Choc Filled, 1	290	16	0	50	33	2	17	130
Wegmans *Italian Classics* Mini Cannoli, 2	200	10	5	25	23	0	13	55
Italian Classics Tiramisu, 1/6	290	20	11	95	22	1	15	60
Weight Watchers *Smart Ones*								
Choc Fudge Brownie Sundae, 2.4 oz	140	3	2	5	26	1	14	70
Turtle Sundae, 2.2 oz	130	3	1	5	23	0	10	75
Mocha Fudge Sundae, 2.4 oz	160	4	2	5	27	1	15	85
Peanut Butter Cup Sundae, 2.3 oz	170	5	3	5	28	3	13	90
Choc Chip Cookie Dough Sundae, 2.7 oz	170	3	2	5	32	1	15	100
Mint Choc Chip Sundae, 2.5 oz	150	3	2	5	28	1	16	130

	Cal	Fat	Sat	Chol	Carb	Fib	Sug	Sod

DONUTS

(see Donuts, pg 68)

FUDGE

	Cal	Fat	Sat	Chol	Carb	Fib	Sug	Sod
Fudge, chocolate, 0.6 oz piece	70	2	1	2	13	0	12	8

Brands . . . *Most fudge within generic average.*

GELATIN

	Cal	Fat	Sat	Chol	Carb	Fib	Sug	Sod
Unflavored gelatin, 1 envl..............................	23	0	0	0	0	0	0	14
Regular gelatin, 1/2 cup	80	0	0	0	19	0	18	98
Sugar free, 1/2 cup	13	0	0	0	5	0	0	55

Brands . . . *Most gelatins within generic average.*

ICE CREAM, ICES AND FROZEN YOGURT

	Cal	Fat	Sat	Chol	Carb	Fib	Sug	Sod
Sherbet, orange, 1/2 cup	107	1	1	0	23	2	18	34
Ice cream, strawberry, 1/2 cup	127	6	3	19	18	1	15	40
Ice cream, choc, 1/2 cup..............................	143	7	4	22	19	1	17	50
Ice cream, vanilla, 1/2 cup	137	7	4	29	16	1	14	53
Sugar-free, light, 1/2 cup...........................	115	5	3	18	15	0	4	65
Fat-free, 1/2 cup	91	0	0	0	20	1	4	64
Frozen yogurt, choc, 1/2 cup	110	3	2	11	19	1	19	55

Brands . . . *(1/2 cup unless noted)*

SHERBET, SORBET AND ICES
Most brands are very low sodium, the following have less than 30mg per serving.

	Cal	Fat	Sat	Chol	Carb	Fib	Sug	Sod
Ben & Jerry's Berried Treasure Sorbet...........	110	0	0	0	29	1	24	5
Berry Berry Extraordinary or Lemonade (avg) ..	100	0	0	0	27	1	22	5
Jamaican Me Crazy Sorbet...........................	130	0	0	0	33	1	29	10
Mango Mango Sorbet.................................	100	0	0	0	27	1	23	10
Blue Bunny Pineapple or Rainbow Sherbet	110	0	0	0	26	0	20	25
Häagen-Dazs Raspberry or Strawberry Sorbet	120	0	0	0	31	2	27	0
Cranberry Blueberry Sortbet.......................	100	0	0	0	25	1	20	0
Orchard Peach Sorbet...............................	130	0	0	0	33	1	29	0
Mango Sorbet..	120	0	0	0	37	0	36	10
Zesty Lemon Sorbet	110	0	0	0	28	1	29	25
Hood *New England Creamery*								
Orange, Rainbow, or Wildberry Sherbet........	110	0	0	0	27	0	21	25
Venice Premium Ice Cherry Lemon	100	0	0	0	24	0	23	0
Venice Premium Ice Pomegranate Blueberry ..	110	0	0	0	28	0	23	5
Fruit Rainbow Sherbet	120	1	1	5	26	0	17	15
Orange Grove Sherbet	120	1	1	5	26	0	18	20

FROZEN YOGURT
Most brands are low sodium, the following have 50mg or less per serving.

	Cal	Fat	Sat	Chol	Carb	Fib	Sug	Sod
Blue Bunny Strawberry Banana	100	2	1	20	19	2	16	45
Bordeaux Cherry Choc or Dbl Raspberry (avg).	115	3	2	20	21	2	18	50
Dreyer's/Edy's *Slow Churned Yogurt Blends*								
Peach	100	2	2	10	17	0	14	30
Black Cherry Vanilla Swirl or Vanilla	100	3	2	10	17	0	13	35
Choc Vanilla Swirl	100	3	2	10	16	0	13	35
Slow Churned Yogurt Blends								
Cappucino Chip or Choc Fudge Brownie (avg)...	115	4	3	10	18	0	14	40
Caramel Praline Crunch.............................	120	4	2	10	19	0	16	45
Häagen-Dazs Vanilla Raspberry Swirl	170	3	2	25	32	0	24	35
Wildberry	180	2	1	35	34	0	27	40

DESSERTS AND SWEETS
Ice Cream, Ices and Frozen Yogurt

	Cal	Fat	Sat	Chol	Carb	Fib	Sug	Sod
Peach	170	2	1	40	31	0	23	40
Tart Natural	180	3	1	45	30	0	21	45
Coffee	200	5	3	65	31	0	20	50
Hood FF Strawberry-Banana	90	0	0	0	20	0	16	45
Frozen Tangy Strawberry or Blueberry	110	1	1	5	24	0	18	40
Frozen Tangy Mango Peach or Mixed Berry	110	1	1	5	24	0	19	40
Frozen Tangy Raspberry Vanilla	110	1	1	5	23	0	18	40
Frozen Tangy Pomegranate Blueberry	110	1	1	5	23	0	18	45
Frozen Tangy Vanilla	110	1	1	5	23	0	18	45
FF Strawberry	80	0	0	0	18	0	14	45
Frozen Tangy Cherry Vanilla	110	1	1	5	23	0	18	50
Stonyfield Organic Minty Choc Chip	140	3	2	5	25	1	21	50

ICE CREAM

Most ice cream is low sodium, the following have 50mg or less per serving.

	Cal	Fat	Sat	Chol	Carb	Fib	Sug	Sod
Ben & Jerry's Chocowlate Chip	230	13	9	55	25	0	22	30
Orange & Cream	152	6	4	31	23	1	20	30
Chunky Monkey	240	14	5	45	24	0	22	35
Strawberry Cheesecake	210	11	6	40	24	0	20	35
Strawberry	170	9	6	45	18	0	16	35
Coffee Coffee BuzzBuzzBuzz	120	14	10	50	23	1	21	40
No Sugar Added Vanilla Fudge Chip	180	13	10	45	20	3	3	40
Mint Choc Chunk	230	14	10	50	23	1	20	45
NY Super Fudge Chunk	250	17	9	25	24	2	21	45
Cherry Garcia	240	14	9	60	27	1	22	50
Chocolate	250	15	8	40	25	2	22	50
Coffee or Vanilla	190	11	8	60	18	0	16	50
Blue Bunny *Light* Vanilla	100	4	2	15	16	3	8	30
French Vanilla	130	7	5	50	15	0	12	40
Orange Dream or Strawberry (avg)	120	5	3	22	18	0	14	40
Strawberry Cheesecake	130	5	4	20	19	0	14	40
Premium Double Strawberry	140	6	4	25	20	0	18	40
Premium Bordeaux Cherry Choc	160	8	5	25	20	0	17	40
Hot Fudge Sundae	150	7	4	20	18	0	12	40
Premium Coffee Break	130	7	5	25	16	0	15	45
Premium Homemade Choc	150	7	5	35	16	0	16	45
Vanilla or Neapolitan (avg)	130	7	4	25	16	0	11	45
Light Butter Pecan	100	4	2	10	16	3	8	45
Premium Berry Me Please!	150	6	5	25	21	0	18	45
Choc Chip or Mint Chip	140	7	5	25	17	0	11	45
Premium Choc Lovers Triple Choc Cake	190	10	5	25	25	1	19	45
Premium Banana Split	170	8	4	25	22	0	18	50
Premium French Vanilla or Vanilla (avg)	140	8	5	40	16	0	14	50
Premium Pistachio Almond	150	8	4	25	15	1	13	50
Light Choc Raspberry Cheesecake	100	3	2	10	18	3	10	50
Light Super Fudge Brownie	120	3	2	10	22	3	12	50
Premium All Natural Vanilla	160	9	6	55	16	0	16	50
Hi Lite Mint Chip	110	4	3	10	18	0	14	50
Ozark Black Walnut	140	7	4	25	17	0	12	50
Breyer's *All Natural* Peach	120	5	3	15	17	0	16	30
All Natural Choc Crackle	160	10	7	15	15	0	15	35
All Natural Natural Vanilla	135	7	5	45	14	0	14	35
All Natural Lactose Free Vanilla	130	7	5	20	14	0	14	35
All Natural Vanilla, Choc, Strawberry	130	6	4	20	15	0	15	35
All Natural French Vanilla	140	7	5	45	14	0	14	40

	Cal	Fat	Sat	Chol	Carb	Fib	Sug	Sod
All Natural Strawberry	110	5	3	15	16	0	15	40
All Natural Rocky Road	160	7	5	15	21	1	17	40
Smooth & Dreamy FF Strawberry	90	0	0	0	21	3	13	40
All Natural Nascar Checkered Flag	140	8	5	20	16	0	14	45
All Natural Choc	140	7	5	20	17	1	16	45
All Natural Black Raspberry Choc	150	7	5	15	21	0	17	45
All Natural Mint Choc Chip or Choc Chip (avg)	150	8	6	15	18	1	17	45
Carb Smart Vanilla	90	6	4	15	13	4	4	45
Smooth & Dreamy FF Creamy Vanilla	90	0	0	5	21	3	13	45
Smooth & Dreamy No Sugar Added Vanilla	90	4	3	10	15	4	4	45
Smooth & Dreamy No Sugar Triple Choc	90	5	3	30	15	4	4	45
Smooth & Dreamy No Sugar French Vanilla	90	5	3	30	15	4	4	45
Smooth & Dreamy No Sugar Vanilla/Choc/Straw	90	5	3	30	15	4	4	45
All Natural Extra Creamy Vanilla	140	7	4	20	16	0	13	50
All Natural Coffee or Vanilla Caramel (avg)	130	7	4	20	16	0	14	50
Smooth & Dreamy LF Vanilla Bean	110	4	2	10	16	0	16	50
Smooth & Dreamy LF Creamy Vanilla	110	4	2	10	16	0	16	50
Smooth & Dreamy LF Vanilla/Choc/Strawberry	110	3	2	10	17	0	16	50
Overload! Very Choc Cherry	120	3	2	5	21	1	16	50
Deans Vanilla	150	8	5	30	17	0	16	40
Light Vanilla	100	3	2	15	17	0	13	50
Dreyer's/Edy's *Grand* Vanilla Choc	150	8	5	25	16	1	14	30
Grand Real Strawberry	130	6	4	20	16	0	15	30
Slow Churned Choc	100	4	2	20	15	0	13	30
Slow Churned Rocky Road	120	4	2	15	17	0	14	30
Grand Vanilla or Vanilla Bean (avg)	140	8	4	25	15	0	13	35
Grand Rocky Road	170	10	5	30	19	1	14	35
Grand Neapolitan or Choc (avg)	145	7	5	25	16	0	15	35
Grand French Vanilla	150	9	5	50	16	0	11	35
Grand Coffee	130	7	4	25	15	0	13	35
Slow Churned Neapolitan	100	3	2	20	15	0	12	35
Slow Churned Double Fudge Brownie	120	4	2	20	17	0	15	35
Slow Churned French Vanilla, No Sugar Added	100	3	2	30	15	2	3	35
Dreyer's/Edy's								
Slow Churned Strawberry	110	3	2	15	18	0	13	40
Slow Churned Neapolitan, No Sugar Added	90	3	2	10	14	2	3	40
Grand Double Vanilla	140	7	5	35	16	0	15	40
Slow Churned Coffee, Vanilla Bean, or Vanilla	105	4	2	20	15	0	11	45
Slow Churned Choc Chip	120	4	3	20	17	0	13	50
Slow Churned Fudge Tracks or Mint Choc Chip	120	5	3	20	18	0	13	50
Häagen-Dazs Java Chip	300	18	12	90	26	2	24	40
Five Strawberry	210	11	6	65	24	0	22	40
Five Passion Fruit	220	11	6	70	25	0	24	45
Chocolate	260	17	10	90	22	1	19	45
Green Tea	250	17	10	105	20	0	19	50
Mango	250	14	8	85	28	1	17	50
Vanilla Honey Bee	270	17	10	110	23	0	20	50
Five Mint or Coffee (avg)	220	12	7	70	24	0	22	50
Five Ginger or Vanilla Bean (avg)	230	12	7	70	25	0	22	50
Five Lemon	210	10	6	60	26	0	24	50
Hood Strawberry	130	7	5	25	17	0	12	45
Choc Chip	150	9	6	25	19	0	14	45
Maple Walnut or Natural Vanilla Bean	150	9	5	25	17	0	12	45
Fudge Twister	140	6	4	25	20	0	16	45
Chocolate	140	6	4	25	18	1	15	50

DESSERTS AND SWEETS
Ice Cream, Ices and Frozen Yogurt

	Cal	Fat	Sat	Chol	Carb	Fib	Sug	Sod
Creamy Coffee	140	7	5	30	16	0	12	50
Golden Vanilla, Patchwork, or Classic Trio (avg)	140	7	5	30	17	0	12	50
Birthday Party	150	8	5	25	19	0	13	50
Light Maine Blueberry & Sweet Cream	110	3	2	10	18	0	14	50
Light Choc Chip	120	5	3	10	18	0	14	50
New England Creamery:								
Maine Blueberry & Sweet Cream	110	3	2	10	18	0	14	45
New England Lighthouse Coffee	170	9	6	25	19	0	16	45
Martha's Vineyard Black Raspberry	150	7	4	25	20	0	16	50
Boston Vanilla Bean	140	7	5	30	17	0	13	50
Kemps Caribou Coffee *Light* Java Chunk	130	5	4	10	20	0	16	40
Orange Cream Dream	130	4	3	15	23	0	18	40
Old Fashioned Strawberries 'n Cream	130	6	4	25	17	0	14	45
Cotton Candy or Strawberry (avg)	125	7	4	28	16	0	13	45
Churned White Choc Raspberry Truffle	120	4	2	10	20	0	15	50
Vanilla, Vanilla Bean, or NY Vanilla	130	7	4	30	16	0	13	50
Homemade Vanilla or Pink Peppermint (avg)	140	7	5	33	17	0	15	50
Old Fashioned Vanilla Custard	150	8	5	50	19	0	12	50
Doubles, Choc Chip, or Mint Choc Chip (avg)	140	7	5	28	17	0	14	50
Neopolitan	130	6	4	30	16	0	13	50
Churned Dutch Choc or Vanilla	105	3	2	13	17	0	13	50
Churned Choc Chip or Mint Choc Chip	120	5	3	10	18	0	14	50
Black Jack Cherry	140	6	4	25	19	0	15	50
Lactaid Strawberry & Cream	140	7	5	30	18	0	14	30
Vanilla or Choc (avg)	155	8	5	33	17	0	12	35
Ruggles Cherry Cordial	150	8	5	25	19	0	13	50
Smith's Vanilla Orange Cream	130	5	3	15	21	0	15	50
Stonyfield Farm Vanilla Chai	240	16	10	60	21	0	20	45
Gotta Have Vanilla or Gotta Have Java	250	16	10	60	21	0	20	45
After Dark Choc	240	16	10	60	22	0	20	35
Tillamook Banana Split	160	9	5	20	19	1	13	50
Expresso Mocha or Oregon Strawberry (avg)	160	10	6	25	17	0	11	50
French Vanilla or Wild Mountain Blackberry	160	9	5	45	18	0	11	50
Old-Fashioned Vanilla or Vanilla Bean	160	9	6	25	17	0	10	50
Mint Choc Chip	180	11	7	20	19	1	12	50
Cinnamon Banana Bliss	170	8	5	20	22	0	15	50
Turkey Hill Premium Orange Cream Swirl	130	6	4	20	19	0	14	35
Premium Strawberries & Cream	120	6	4	20	16	1	12	35
Premium Black Cherry	130	6	4	25	18	0	13	40
Premium Black Raspberry	130	7	5	25	16	0	11	40
Premium Neapolitan	140	7	5	25	17	0	13	40
Premium Choco Mint Chip	160	9	6	25	17	1	13	45
Premium Vanilla & Choc	140	7	5	25	17	0	13	45
Premium Colombian Coffee	140	7	5	25	16	0	12	45
Premium Original Vanilla or Vanilla Bean	140	7	5	30	16	0	12	45
Premium Dutch Choc or Choc	150	7	5	25	19	1	14	45
Premium Fr Vanilla or Homemade Vanilla	140	7	5	50	16	0	12	45
All Natural Recipe Choc	150	8	5	30	18	0	17	45
All Natural Recipe Mint Choc Chip	160	9	5	25	18	0	18	45
All Natural Recipe Neapolitan	140	7	5	25	17	0	16	45
All Natural Recipe Coffee or Vanilla Bean	140	8	5	30	16	0	16	50
Premium Party Cake	160	8	5	25	20	0	15	50

NON-DAIRY ICE CREAM ALTERNATIVES
(also see Non-Dairy Alternatives–Bars, pg 129)

	Cal	Fat	Sat	Chol	Carb	Fib	Sug	Sod
Brands . . . *(1/2 cup unless noted)*								
Purely Decadent *Dairy Free* Belgian Choc	180	7	2	0	30	4	25	15
Dairy Free Pralines Pecan	210	10	1	0	33	5	15	20
Dairy Free Cherry Nirvana	190	6	2	0	26	5	18	30
Dairy Free Choc Obsession	210	7	3	0	27	5	20	30
Dairy Free Cookie Avalanche	180	7	1	0	27	5	19	30
Dairy Free Purely Vanilla	170	5	1	0	22	5	17	35
Dairy Free Pomegranate Chip	200	7	3	0	29	5	24	35
Dairy Free Mocha Almond Fudge	200	8	1	0	25	5	19	40
Dairy Free Peanut Butter Zig Zag	230	12	3	0	24	5	16	45
Dairy Free Mint Choc Chip	190	7	3	0	24	5	18	50
So Delicious *Coconut Milk* Coconut Almond Chip	180	12	8	0	20	6	12	5
Coconut Milk Coconut or Mint Chip (avg)	170	9	9	0	20	6	12	5
Coconut Milk Choc or Vanilla Bean (avg)	150	8	8	0	20	6	12	5
Coconut Milk Green Tea or Cookies/Cream (avg)	135	7	6	0	20	6	12	5
Coconut Milk Passionate Mango	150	7	6	0	19	5	13	10
Coconut Milk Pomegranate Chip	130	7	6	0	20	6	13	10
Coconut Milk Cherry Amaretto	130	6	5	0	22	6	10	10
Coconut Milk German Choc	180	12	9	0	22	6	14	15
Coconut Milk Mocha Almond Fudge	180	9	6	0	21	5	14	30
Coconut Milk Cookie Dough	190	9	8	0	24	5	15	30
Coconut Milk Turtle Trails	160	8	6	0	26	4	19	40
Coconut Milk Choc Peanut Butter Swirl	210	13	9	0	21	6	12	40
Dairy Free Choc Velvet	130	4	1	0	23	1	14	50
Coconut Milk Choc Brownie Almond	170	9	6	0	23	6	14	55
Dairy Free Creamy Vanilla	130	3	0	0	24	3	13	55
Dairy Free Mint Marble Fudge	140	3	1	0	27	2	17	55
Dairy Free Neapolitan or Strawberry (avg)	120	4	1	0	23	2	13	55
Dairy Free Choc Peanut Butter	140	5	1	0	23	2	13	60

ICE CREAM, ICES AND FROZEN YOGURT – NOVELTIES

	Cal	Fat	Sat	Chol	Carb	Fib	Sug	Sod
Bar, fruit and juice, 1 bar	87	0	0	0	20	1	17	4
Yogurt bar, choc, 1 bar	120	0	0	0	22	0	15	45
Bar, choc covered, 2.2 oz bar	220	15	11	15	18	0	15	55
Drumstick, 3.4 oz	340	20	11	20	34	1	23	85
Sandwich, 2.3 oz	180	7	4	20	26	0	12	160

Brands . . . *(1 bar or sandwich unless noted)*

FRUIT JUICE BARS – *Most brands within generic average (4mg).*

ICE CREAM AND YOGURT BARS
   Most bars are low sodium, the following have 50mg or less.

	Cal	Fat	Sat	Chol	Carb	Fib	Sug	Sod
Ben & Jerry's Cherry Garcia Bar	260	16	11	40	23	1	19	40
Vanilla Bar	300	20	13	50	25	1	22	40
Blue Bunny *FrozFruit* Chunky Pineapple	120	0	0	0	30	0	23	10
FrozFruit Bananas & Cream	160	6	4	25	27	1	19	15
FrozFruit Chunky Strawberry or Mango (avg)	135	0	0	0	34	1	26	15
FrozFruit Double Lime	120	0	0	0	32	0	22	15
FrozFruit Creamy Coconut	200	14	10	35	19	1	17	25
FrozFruit Strawberries & Banana	160	5	4	20	27	1	25	25
FrozFruit Creamy Pina Colada	190	4	3	5	37	1	31	25
Dream Bar Orange	70	1	1	5	15	0	12	25
Root Beer Float Bar	90	3	2	10	15	0	12	25
Sweet Freedom Black Raspberry Bar	100	7	5	5	11	2	2	25
Sweet Freedom Ice Cream Lites Bar	100	8	6	5	11	1	3	30
Sweet Freedom Caramel Lites or Krunch Lites	100	7	6	5	10	1	2	30

DESSERTS AND SWEETS
Ice Cream, Ices and Frozen Yogurt – Novelties

	Cal	Fat	Sat	Chol	Carb	Fib	Sug	Sod
Big Star Bar Vanilla	110	7	6	5	11	0	9	30
Star Bars	110	7	6	5	11	0	9	30
Naturally Vanilla Bean or Strawberry Bar	140	8	6	20	14	0	13	35
Big Star Bar Choc Choc	120	7	6	5	12	0	10	35
Homemade Vanilla	160	11	9	20	13	0	12	35
English Toffee Bar	130	9	7	15	12	0	9	40
Big Star Bar	130	8	7	5	13	0	11	40
Choc Raspberry Ice Cream Bar	270	18	12	35	25	1	20	45
Sweet Freedom Vanilla Fudge & Fudge Bar	60	0	0	0	15	4	4	45
Sweet Freedom Almond Bar	150	11	7	5	16	2	3	45
Aspen Frozen Yogurt Granola Bars	150	8	7	5	19	3	13	50
Milk Choc Ice Cream Bar	300	21	14	45	25	0	22	50
Crunch Caramel Bar	150	10	8	15	14	0	11	50
Sweet Freedom Vanilla Caramel Bar	190	14	9	5	20	2	3	50
Breyers Smooth & Dreamy								
No Sugar Added Creamy Vanilla Bar	150	9	8	5	18	3	6	35
CarbSmart Almond Bar	180	15	10	15	9	2	5	40
CarbSmart Ice Cream Bar	170	15	11	15	9	2	5	45
Smooth & Dreamy Triple Choc Chip Bar	130	6	4	5	17	1	13	45
Smooth & Dreamy Choc Covered Strawberry	120	5	4	5	17	0	13	45
CarbSmart Fudge Bar	100	7	5	20	9	1	3	50
Creamsicle No Sugar Added Bars	50	0	0	0	5	1	1	10
Low Fat Bars	70	1	0	5	13	0	8	20
100 Calorie Bars	100	2	1	5	20	0	12	30
Fruitful Cream-Based Fruit Bars								
Pina Colada or Raspberry Cream (avg)	100	3	2	10	17	1	13	20
Banana or Strawberry Cream (avg)	110	3	2	15	19	0	15	25
Coconut	130	5	4	15	18	0	13	25
Mango Cream	170	7	5	20	26	1	20	25
Lucuma (Mamay)	180	8	5	22	25	2	19	31
Cream-Based Bars Peaches 'n' Cream	150	5	4	25	24	2	21	50
Good Humor Strawberry Shortcake Bar	170	9	4	5	21	0	12	40
Toasted Almond Bar	240	12	4	10	30	1	23	40
The Original Bar	160	10	9	5	17	0	13	40
Häagen-Dazs Snack Size Vanilla & Almonds	190	14	8	35	14	1	12	25
Choc & Dark Choc Bar	290	20	12	65	24	2	20	30
Snack Size Coffee & Almond Crunch Bar	190	13	8	40	15	1	13	35
Vanilla & Almonds Bar	310	22	13	65	22	1	20	40
Vanilla & Dark Choc Bar	300	21	13	70	23	1	21	45
Happy Indulgence Decadent Dips								
Banana Cream	240	15	11	5	26	0	22	35
Banana Split	290	16	12	10	34	0	28	40
Cherry Cream	280	15	11	15	33	0	27	45
Coconut Cream	300	15	7	10	37	0	23	50
Strawberry Cream	270	16	12	10	29	0	29	50
Healthy Choice Sorbet & Ice Cream Bar	80	1	0	5	18	1	12	25
Mocha Swirl Bar	90	1	1	5	17	1	13	40
Hood Ice Cream Bars	150	11	9	15	12	1	9	30
Orange Cream Bar	90	2	1	5	19	0	13	40
Kemps 100 Calorie Minis Vanilla, 1	100	7	6	10	8	0	6	15
Caribou Coffee Nuggets, 1	120	7	5	10	13	0	11	25
Orange Cream Bar	80	3	2	10	13	0	9	25
Ice Cream Bar	150	10	8	15	13	0	10	30
Vanilla Ice Cream Cups	150	10	7	15	13	0	11	35

128

	Cal	Fat	Sat	Chol	Carb	Fib	Sug	Sod
Toffee Bar	160	12	9	15	14	0	10	40
Klondike 100 Calorie Vanilla Bar	100	6	5	5	11	2	8	25
100 Calorie French Vanilla Bar	100	6	5	10	12	2	8	30
100 Calorie English Toffee Bar	100	6	5	5	12	2	8	30
Ruggles Vanilla Orange Cream Bar	90	3	2	10	15	0	12	30
Vanilla Ice Cream Bar	140	9	7	15	12	0	10	35
Turkey Hill Vanilla Ice Cream Bar	320	23	16	25	26	2	20	40

DRUMSTICKS

	Cal	Fat	Sat	Chol	Carb	Fib	Sug	Sod
Blue Bunny Champ! Mini Swirls Choc Cone	140	8	6	10	17	1	12	40
Sweet Freedom Snack Size Vanilla Cone	120	6	3	5	17	2	2	50
Champ! Mini Swirls Vanilla Cone	140	8	6	10	16	1	11	50
Champ! Mini Swirls Birthday Party Cone	160	8	6	5	22	0	17	50
Durango Frozen Yogurt Granola Cones	180	5	4	5	30	4	17	55
Champ! Banana Split Cone	220	8	6	10	33	1	20	65
Sweet Freedom Choc Cone	170	8	3	5	28	3	4	75
Champ! Hot Fudge Brownie Cone	230	9	7	10	35	1	22	75
Good Humor Sundae Cone	260	15	9	15	29	1	18	80
Kemps 100 Calorie Minis Choc Cone	100	4	3	5	15	0	10	45
100 Calorie Minis Vanilla Cone	100	5	4	10	14	0	9	50

SANDWICHES

	Cal	Fat	Sat	Chol	Carb	Fib	Sug	Sod
Blue Bunny Birthday Party Sandwich	140	3	2	10	23	0	14	40
Mini Ice Cream Sandwich Variety Pack	100	2	1	5	18	0	8	70
Snack Size Vanilla & Choc Sandwich	80	2	1	5	18	2	2	70
Mint Grasshopper Sandwich	140	4	2	5	26	1	13	80
Peanut Butter Fudge Chip Sandwich	170	7	3	5	26	1	14	100
Naturally Vanilla Bean or Milk Choc Sandwich	160	4	2	25	26	1	16	105
Sweet Freedom Vanilla Sandwich	130	2	1	5	32	4	4	110
Breyers Smooth & Dreamy								
Choc Chip Cookie Dough Sandwich	160	4	2	5	30	1	15	115
Good Humor LF Vanilla Sandwich	130	2	1	5	26	2	12	80
Vanilla Sandwich	160	5	3	10	26	0	13	90
Hood Mini Ice Cream Sandwich	100	4	2	10	14	0	7	50
Kemps 100 Calorie Minis Vanilla Sandwich	100	4	2	10	14	0	7	50
100 Calorie Minis Choc Chip Sandwich	100	4	2	10	14	0	7	50
Mini Ice Cream Sandwiches Vanilla	100	4	2	10	14	0	7	80
Kempwich	350	18	9	20	45	0	34	95
Ice Cream Sandwiches Vanilla	160	5	3	20	26	0	14	110
Klondike No Sugar Added Vanilla Sandwich	100	2	1	5	20	2	3	90
100 Calorie Choc Sandwich	100	2	1	5	21	2	9	100
100 Calorie Vanilla Sandwich	100	2	1	0	21	2	10	105
Ruggles Mini Vanilla Sandwich	100	4	2	10	15	0	6	100
Turkey Hill Light Vanilla Bean Sandwich	160	3	2	10	32	3	15	95
Vanilla Bean Sandwich	190	7	4	20	29	1	15	95
Double Decker Sandwich	190	7	4	20	30	1	16	105

OTHER NOVELTIES

	Cal	Fat	Sat	Chol	Carb	Fib	Sug	Sod
Kemps IceeBits, all	30	0	0	0	7	0	3	15
IttiBitz Cotton Candy, Vanilla or Strawberry	160	11	7	40	12	0	8	45
IttiBitz Choc & Fudge, 1 cup	190	12	9	40	17	0	12	50

NON-DAIRY ALTERNATIVES – BARS

	Cal	Fat	Sat	Chol	Carb	Fib	Sug	Sod
So Delicious Coconut Milk Sugar Free Fudge	70	4	3	0	10	3	6	0
Coconut Milk Organic Minis Fudge Bar	70	4	3	0	10	3	6	0
Coconut Milk Coconut Almond Bar Minis	170	10	7	0	15	3	10	10
Coconut Milk Sugar Free Vanilla Bar	150	7	6	0	14	3	10	10
Dairy Free Creamy Orange Bar	80	2	0	0	18	2	12	30

	Cal	Fat	Sat	Chol	Carb	Fib	Sug	Sod
Dairy Free Creamy Fudge Bar	90	2	0	0	18	2	12	30
Almond Milk Vanilla Bar	140	7	3	0	18	3	8	40
Almond Milk Mocha Almond Fudge Bar	150	7	3	0	19	3	10	50
Coconut Milk Vanilla Minis	100	4	3	0	15	2	7	50
Sweet Nothings Non-Dairy Fudge Bars	100	0	0	0	23	0	12	5
Non-Dairy Mango Raspberry Bar	100	0	0	0	23	0	12	10

NON-DAIRY ALTERNATIVES – DRUMSTICKS AND SANDWICHES

	Cal	Fat	Sat	Chol	Carb	Fib	Sug	Sod
So Delicious *Dairy Free Minis*, all soy sandwich.	100	4	3	0	15	2	7	50
Dairy Free Minis Choc or Vanilla (avg)	90	2	1	0	18	2	8	70
Almond Milk Vanilla Sandwich	90	3	1	0	17	2	6	70
Dairy Free Minis Mint Sandwich	90	2	1	0	18	1	8	80
Dairy Free Choc, Mint or Vanilla Sandwich	150	3	1	0	28	2	13	105
Tofutti Cuties Choc Sandwich	130	6	1	0	16	0	9	110
Cuties Mint Choc Chip Sandwich	130	6	1	0	19	0	10	110

ICE CREAM CONES

	Cal	Fat	Sat	Chol	Carb	Fib	Sug	Sod
Cone, cake or wafer-type, 1	17	0	0	0	3	0	3	6
Sugar cone, 1	40	0	0	0	8	0	3	32
Ice cream cone, waffle, 1 oz cone	121	2	0	0	23	1	2	41

Brands . . . *Most brands are within the generic range.*

ICE CREAM TOPPINGS

(see Sauces/Toppings/Fruit Dips, pg 133)

MUFFINS AND SCONES

(see Muffins/Scones, pg 56)

PASTRIES

(see Pastries/Other Breakfast Sweets, pg 72)

PIES AND COBBLERS

(also see Snack Cakes, Pies/Other Sweet Snacks, pg 134)

	Cal	Fat	Sat	Chol	Carb	Fib	Sug	Sod
Choc creme pie, 1/6	344	22	6	6	38	2	-	154
Coconut creme pie, 1/6	191	11	4	0	24	1	23	163
Lemon meringue pie, 1/6	303	10	2	51	53	1	27	165
Cherry pie, 1/6	304	13	3	0	47	1	17	288
Apple pie, 1/6	277	13	4	0	40	2	18	311
Peach pie, 1/6	261	12	2	0	39	1	7	316
Pecan pie, 1/6	541	22	4	56	79	3	33	319
Banana creme pie, no-bake mix, prep, 1/6	309	16	9	36	39	1	-	357
Blueberry pie, 1/6	271	12	2	0	41	1	12	380
Pumpkin pie, 1/6	323	13	3	35	46	2	25	450

Brands . . . *(1/6 slice unless noted)*

FROZEN/REFRIGERATED

	Cal	Fat	Sat	Chol	Carb	Fib	Sug	Sod
Amy's Apple Pie, 4 oz	230	8	5	25	37	2	15	135
Weight Watchers Smart Ones Key Lime Pie	190	5	2	10	33	1	25	85
Wholly Wholesome Apple Pie, 1/6	310	14	7	0	42	3	27	40
Cherry Pie, 1/6	320	14	7	0	46	3	32	65
Blueberry Pie, 1/6	310	14	7	0	42	4	26	70
Wisconsin Door County Cherry Apple Crisp, 1/6	210	8	3	10	35	2	22	65
Rhubarb Apple Crisp, 1/6	160	8	3	7	37	2	19	76
Apple Crisp, 1/6	240	8	3	10	41	2	28	80

REDUCED SODIUM (LESS THAN GENERIC):

	Cal	Fat	Sat	Chol	Carb	Fib	Sug	Sod
Wholly Wholesome Dairy-Free Pumpkin, 1/5	310	13	7	0	45	4	29	160

	Cal	Fat	Sat	Chol	Carb	Fib	Sug	Sod
MIXES								
Calhoun Bend Mill Pecan Pie Mix, 1/8	110	0	0	0	28	0	16	10
Concord Foods Apple Crisp, 1/9	100	0	0	0	25	0	18	0
Chef Hans Apple Crisp, 1/2 cup	280	1	0	0	64	0	45	85
Dixie Carb Counters Key Lime Dessert, 1/9	76	4	0	3	8	5	1	112
Double Choc Torte Mix, 1/9	112	8	1	0	8	6	1	112
SHELF-STABLE								
Hill & Valley Sugar-Free Pecan Pie, 1/8	270	15	5	30	34	2	1	135
Oberweis Pumpkin Pie, 1/8	400	23	14	45	45	1	29	95
REDUCED SODIUM (LESS THAN GENERIC):								
Chatila's Bakery Blueberry Pie, 1/8	90	1	0	0	20	3	4	150
Hill & Valley Sugar-Free Choc Creme Pie, 1/8	210	9	6	0	34	1	0	150
Oberweis Peppermint Pie, 1/8	360	21	10	40	40	1	31	155

PUDDING AND MOUSSE

(also see Pastry/Pie Fillings, pg 28)

	Cal	Fat	Sat	Chol	Carb	Fib	Sug	Sod
Egg custard, mix for 1/2 cup serv	86	1	0	54	17	0	12	59
Choc, regular (cooked), mix for 1/2 cup serv	91	1	0	0	22	1	11	88
Ready-to-eat, 1/2 cup	153	5	1	1	25	0	19	164
Instant, mix for 1/2 cup serv	95	0	0	0	22	1	17	357
Flan, mix for 1/2 cup serv	73	0	0	0	19	0	11	91
Rice pudding, mix for 1/2 cup serv	102	0	0	0	25	0	15	99
Ready-to-eat, 1/2 cup	133	3	2	20	22	1	16	139
Tapioca, mix for 1/2 cup serv	85	0	0	0	22	0	15	110
Ready-to-eat, 1/2 cup	134	4	1	0	22	0	20	180
Vanilla, ready-to-eat, 1/2 cup	143	4	1	1	25	0	19	156
Regular (cooked), mix for 1/2 cup serv	83	0	0	0	21	0	17	166
Instant, mix for 1/2 cup serv	94	0	0	0	23	0	23	360
Brands . . . *(1/2 cup unless noted)*								
FROZEN/REFRIGERATED								
Echo Farm Royal's Rice Pudding, 3/4 cup	195	6	5	53	23	0	12	45
Misty's Indian Pudding, 1/2 cup	180	5	3	30	30	1	19	65
Miracle's Choc Pudding, 3/4 cup	255	6	4	23	44	2	33	98
Ticket's Tapioca, 3/4 cup	255	8	5	45	32	0	26	98
Lolly's Butterscotch Pudding, 3/4 cup	230	6	4	20	38	0	18	110
Candle's Coffee Caramel Tapioca, 3/4 cup	255	8	5	53	39	0	27	113
Kozy Shack Creme Caramel Flan, 1 cup	150	4	2	35	27	0	16	85
Bread Pudding, Peach, 1 cup	150	4	2	40	25	0	17	100
Bread Pudding, Apple Cinnamon, 1 cup	150	4	2	40	27	0	19	105
Bread Pudding, Apple Raisin, 1 cup	160	4	2	45	29	1	19	105
Pumpkin, 1 cup	120	5	3	20	10	1	13	105
CowRageous! Choc, 3.8 oz	100	1	1	5	21	3	14	105
Choc w/LF Milk, 1 cup	110	1	1	5	20	4	15	110
No Sugar Added Vanilla, 1 cup	90	3	2	10	10	4	5	115
Original Rice or Cinn Raisin Rice, 1 cup (avg)	135	3	2	15	24	0	15	120
Banana Cream, 1 cup	130	5	3	15	19	0	15	120
No Sugar Added Rice, 1 cup	70	1	0	10	11	3	5	120
Honey Lemon Tapioca, 1 cup	130	3	2	10	24	0	19	125
No Sugar Added Strawberry, 1 cup	80	1	1	5	10	3	5	125
CowRageous! Strawberry, 3.8 oz	100	1	0	5	18	3	14	125
Simply Well Green Tea Chai or Lemon Ginger	100	1	1	10	17	3	14	125
Simply Well Pear Mangosteen	100	1	0	10	17	3	14	125
Tapioca, 1 cup or Strawberry (avg)	130	3	2	13	22	0	17	130
CowRageous! Vanilla, 3.8 oz	100	1	0	10	21	3	15	130
No Sugar Added Choc, 1 cup	60	1	1	5	10	4	4	130

DESSERTS AND SWEETS
Pudding and Mousse

	Cal	Fat	Sat	Chol	Carb	Fib	Sug	Sod
Simply Well French Vanilla...............	100	1	1	10	18	3	15	130
European Style Rice, 1 cup...............	130	4	2	20	21	0	14	135
Restaurant-Style Flan, 1 cup............	190	6	3	50	28	0	23	135
No Sugar Added Tapioca, 1 cup.........	70	1	0	5	11	4	5	135
Choc, 1 cup..........................	140	4	2	15	24	1	19	140
No Sugar Added Choc Mint, 1 cup.......	70	1	1	5	10	3	5	140
Lean on Me Choc Mousse, 2 oz	150	11	5	15	17	1	0	70
MIXES – *Some mixes require additional ingredients which may raise sodium content.*								
Barefoot Contessa Brownie Pudding, 1/6 pkg .	340	2	1	0	86	4	70	0
Calorie Control Mousse, all flavors......	50	3	2	0	6	0	0	25
Vanilla Custard, No Bake, 2/3 cup........	70	1	0	0	10	0	9	100
Concord Foods								
Banana Pudding/Pie Filling, 1/8.........	100	2	2	0	21	0	14	60
Con-Gelli Caramel Custard Flan.........	80	0	0	0	19	0	15	45
Dixie Carb Counters Tapioca, 1/6 pkg...	20	0	0	0	3	1	0	37
Choc Mousse, 1/4 pkg	25	0	0	0	2	1	1	47
Raspberry or Vanilla Mousse, 1/4 pkg ...	16	0	0	0	1	0	1	47
Dr Oetker								
Mousse Supreme Pistachio, 1/4 pkg.....	100	2	2	0	19	0	15	25
Panna Cotta, 1/4 pkg..................	120	0	0	0	29	0	26	25
Pudding Choc or Almond, 1/4 pkg (avg)...	40	0	0	0	9	0	1	30
Pudding Raspberry, Creme, or Lemon, 1/4 pkg.	40	0	0	0	10	0	1	30
Pudding Vanilla, 1/4 pkg	40	0	0	0	10	0	4	45
Flan Creme Caramel, 1/4 pkg...........	100	0	0	15	23	0	21	45
Mousse Supreme Milk Choc, 1/4 pkg.....	100	4	3	0	15	0	13	45
Mousse Supreme Double Choc, 1/4 pkg...	130	4	3	0	21	1	17	45
Mousse Supreme Choc Irish Cream, 1/4...	130	4	4	0	21	1	17	45
Mousse Supreme Choc Raspberry, 1/4 ...	130	4	4	0	21	1	17	45
Mousse Supreme Light Strawberry, 1/5...	35	2	2	0	3	0	1	70
Mousse Supreme Mocha Choc, 1/4	70	3	2	0	13	0	11	80
Lemon Pie Filling & Dessert Mix, 1/8...	100	0	0	0	26	0	18	80
Key Lime Pie Filling & Dessert Mix, 1/8..	100	0	0	0	26	0	18	80
Mousse Supreme Light French Vanilla, 1/5...	35	2	2	0	3	0	2	85
Mousse Supreme Dark Choc Truffle, 1/4...	100	4	3	0	15	0	11	85
Classic Creme Brûlée, 1/4 pkg	110	2	1	10	23	0	18	90
Hannaford								
Choc Cook & Serve Pudding/Pie	100	1	0	0	23	0	17	120
Vanilla Cook & Serve Pudding/Pie Filling...	80	0	0	0	21	0	16	130
Harvest Direct *Soy Pudding*, all, 1/3 pkg...	150	3	0	0	26	2	14	105
Hy-Vee Cooked Pudding & Pie, Choc or Vanilla..	100	0	0	0	23	0	17	130
Inspired Cuisine *European* Creme Brulee, 1/4 pkg	90	0	0	0	21	0	19	15
Dark Choc Mousse, 1/4 pkg	80	4	3	0	13	2	9	70
Mocha Mousse, 1/4 pkg	80	2	2	0	16	1	14	70
Milk Choc or Milk Choc Raspberry Mousse, 1/4 pkg	80	3	2	0	14	1	11	75
Jell-O Cook & Serve Pudding, Lemon........	50	0	0	0	12	0	6	70
Cook & Serve Pudding, Choc...........	90	0	0	0	22	1	15	110
Cook & Serve Pudding, Choc Sugar Free...	30	0	0	0	7	1	0	110
Cook & Serve Pudding, Vanilla Sugar Free...	20	0	0	0	5	0	0	115
Cook & Serve Pudding, Butterscotch.....	100	0	0	0	24	0	19	130
Cook & Serve Pudding, Vanilla	80	0	0	0	20	0	16	135
Junket Custard Mix (avg)	45	0	0	0	10	0	10	0
Meijer Cook/Serve Pudding/Pie, Choc or Vanilla..	100	0	0	0	23	0	17	130
Mori-Nu *Mates* Choc or Vanilla, 1/4 pkg (avg)...	110	2	2	0	22	1	18	5
Lemon Creme, 1/4 pkg	120	3	2	0	22	0	18	5

132

	Cal	Fat	Sat	Chol	Carb	Fib	Sug	Sod
My*T*Fine Pudding & Pie, Sugar Free Choc....	50	0	0	0	12	1	0	85
Pudding & Pie Filling, Lemon	50	0	0	0	12	0	5	120
Pudding & Pie Filling, Vanilla	70	0	0	0	18	0	13	120
Pudding & Pie Filling, Chocolate Fudge	80	0	0	0	20	1	12	125
Pudding & Pie Filling, Chocolate	80	0	0	0	20	1	13	130
Noh Hawaiian Coconut, 1/8 pkg	100	4	3	0	16	1	9	15
RC *Bavarian* Sugar Free, Vanilla	40	2	2	0	8	5	0	15
Bavarian Sugar Free, Strawberry or Choc	40	2	2	0	8	5	0	20
Lemon *Bavarian*	90	4	4	0	13	0	12	30
Bavarian Vanilla or Unflavored	90	4	4	0	13	0	11	35
Choc *Bavarian*	110	6	5	0	14	1	10	45
No Bake Custard	50	0	0	0	13	0	11	45
Key Lime *Bavarian*	90	5	5	0	12	0	10	50
Raspberry *Bavarian*	110	5	5	0	15	0	13	55
Roland Spanish Flan	60	0	0	0	17	0	14	90
Royal Flan	70	0	0	0	18	0	18	30
Cook & Serve Choc Pudding	80	0	0	0	20	1	13	80
Sans Sucre French Vanilla or Lemon Mousse...	50	3	2	0	8	0	0	25
Strawberry, Choc, or Mocha Cappuccino Mousse	50	3	2	0	8	0	0	25
Key Lime Pie Filling & Mousse	50	3	2	0	8	0	0	25
Pumpkin Pie Filling & Pudding, 1/8	50	1	1	0	7	1	4	80
Uncle Ben's *Rice Pudding* French Vanilla	120	0	0	0	28	1	10	90
READY-TO-EAT (SHELF-STABLE)								
Ambrosia Devon Custard	130	4	2	5	21	0	15	50
Kraft *Handi-Snacks* Rice Pudding	140	6	1	0	19	0	11	130
Handi-Snacks Tapioca	100	1	1	0	21	0	14	140
Snack Pack Lemon Pudding	130	3	2	0	25	0	20	65
Sugar Free Vanilla	60	3	2	0	11	0	0	100
Sugar Free Caramel	60	3	2	0	11	0	0	105
Sugar Free Choc	70	4	2	0	15	1	0	110
Brownie Mix	130	4	2	0	23	1	18	125
Cinnamon Roll or Blueberry Muffin	110	4	2	0	20	0	15	125
Ice Cream Sandwich or Choc Fudge (avg)	120	4	2	0	21	1	16	130
Vanilla or Tapioca (avg)	120	4	2	0	21	1	14	135
Choc	130	3	2	0	23	1	16	140
FF Choc	80	0	0	0	20	1	15	140
ZenSoy Vanilla or Banana Pudding, 4 oz (avg)	105	1	0	0	22	1	15	75
Chocolate Pudding, 4 oz	130	1	0	0	29	2	21	75
Choc/Vanilla Swirl Pudding, 4 oz	120	1	0	0	26	1	20	75

SAUCES, TOPPINGS AND FRUIT DIPS

(also see Cream, pg 104)

	Cal	Fat	Sat	Chol	Carb	Fib	Sug	Sod
Whipped topping, ready-to-eat, 1 tbsp	13	1	1	0	1	0	1	1
Powdered mix, prep, 1 tbsp	8	0	0	0	1	0	1	2
Pressurized, 1 tbsp	8	0	0	2	0	0	0	4
Strawberry, 2 tbsp	107	0	0	0	28	0	12	9
Pineapple, 2 tbsp	106	0	0	0	28	0	9	18
Marshmallow cream, 2 tbsp	91	0	0	0	22	0	13	23
Fruit dip, choc, 2 tbsp	120	7	1	0	15	1	13	100
Choc fudge sauce, 2 tbsp	133	3	2	1	24	1	13	131
Butterscotch or caramel sauce, 2 tbsp	103	0	0	0	27	0	9	143

Brands . . . *(2 tbsp unless noted)*
FROZEN/REFRIGERATED

	Cal	Fat	Sat	Chol	Carb	Fib	Sug	Sod
Marie's Honey Vanilla Cream Dip	60	4	3	15	5	0	4	20

DESSERTS AND SWEETS
Snack Cakes, Pies and Other Sweet Snacks

	Cal	Fat	Sat	Chol	Carb	Fib	Sug	Sod
Marzetti Light French Vanilla Yogurt Fruit Dip......	45	0	0	0	9	0	9	45
Chocolate Cream Cheese Fruit Dip...............	110	2	1	0	23	1	16	85
Strawberry Cream Cheese Fruit Dip.............	70	4	2	15	9	0	8	90
100 Calorie Pack Cream Cheese Fruit Dip	100	5	3	20	14	0	12	120

MIXES

	Cal	Fat	Sat	Chol	Carb	Fib	Sug	Sod
RC Fine Foods Pineapple Coulis Mix...............	20	0	0	0	7	0	7	10
Kiwi or Lemon Coulis Mix...........................	30	0	0	0	7	0	6	15
Raspberry, Blackberry, Blueberry or Strawberry	30	0	0	0	7	0	7	20
Mango Coulis Mix	30	0	0	0	7	0	7	35

READY-TO-USE

Fruit toppings – *most brands within generic average (9-18mg sodium)*

	Cal	Fat	Sat	Chol	Carb	Fib	Sug	Sod
Ah!Laska Organic Choc Syrup......................	0	0	0	0	25	0	22	0
Delicae Gourmet Choc Raspberry Liqueur.......	45	1	0	0	10	0	7	0
Espresso Choc Liqueur Sauce, 1 tbsp...........	40	1	0	0	9	0	8	5
Black Forest Choc Liqueur Sauce, 1 tbsp	30	1	0	0	6	0	5	10
Port Wine Choc Liqueur Sauce, 1 tbsp...........	20	2	1	0	8	0	7	10
East Shore Dipping Sauces, all (avg).............	115	7	4	15	15	0	15	25
Mrs Richardson's Butterscotch Caramel	130	2	1	5	28	0	19	50
Hot Fudge	140	6	6	0	19	1	16	55
Naturally Fresh Caramel Dip.......................	100	4	3	5	16	0	12	20
Choc Dip	70	0	0	0	12	0	13	55
Robt Rothschild Farm Raspberry Choc Dip....	70	3	2	0	12	0	8	10
Cinnamon Bun Gourmet Sauce......................	90	2	1	5	18	0	8	30
Old-Fashioned Caramel Sauce......................	90	2	1	5	18	0	8	30
Old-Fashioned Hot Fudge Sauce	80	3	2	0	15	0	10	35
Choc S'mores Dip.......................................	90	4	2	5	13	0	12	40
Nutcracker Dip..	100	5	3	5	13	0	8	50
Gingerbread Dip..	110	6	4	15	15	0	6	65
Steel's All Natural Fudge Sauce	80	2	0	0	19	0	0	15
All Natural Caramel Sauce	90	6	5	12	7	1	6	15
Stonewall Kitchen Black Cherry Cognac........	60	0	0	0	16	0	16	0
Choc Peanut Butter Sauce	110	6	3	5	13	1	10	5
Choc Hazelnut Sauce	110	5	2	0	15	0	12	10
Coffee Caramel Sauce..................................	90	2	1	5	17	0	15	20
Bittersweet Choc or Mocha Espresso	90	3	0	0	16	0	14	25
Choc Peppermint Sauce	110	5	3	5	17	0	13	25
Dulce De Leche Sauce	90	2	1	5	17	0	14	30
Spiced Rum Butterscotch Sauce	110	4	2	10	18	0	15	30
Dark Choc Toffee	130	8	5	20	14	0	10	45
Walden Farms Caramel Dip	0	0	0	0	0	0	0	20
Choc Dip	0	0	0	0	0	0	0	35
Wax Orchards Fudge Sauces, all	90	0	0	0	20	4	18	40

SNACK CAKES, PIES AND OTHER SWEET SNACKS

(also see Pastries/Other Breakfast Sweets, pg 72; Cake, pg 114; Pies/Cobblers, pg 130)

	Cal	Fat	Sat	Chol	Carb	Fib	Sug	Sod
Cake, sponge, creme-filled, 1.7 oz.................	157	5	2	17	27	0	16	168
Cupcake, choc w/frosting, creme-filled, 1.8 oz......	200	8	1	9	30	2	19	195
Pie, fruit filled, fried, 4.6 oz	404	21	3	0	55	3	27	479

Brands . . . *(1 oz unless noted)*

FROZEN/REFRIGERATED

	Cal	Fat	Sat	Chol	Carb	Fib	Sug	Sod
Kraft Snack Bites Choc Covered Strawberry	130	7	3	10	15	0	10	55
Snack Bites Turtle	130	7	4	10	14	0	10	70
Snack Bars Strawberry Cheesecake, 1.5 oz....	180	9	3	10	22	0	13	80

	Cal	Fat	Sat	Chol	Carb	Flb	Sug	Sod
Snack Bars Classic Cheesecake, 1.5 oz..........	190	11	3	15	20	0	12	85
Snack Bars Marble Brownie, 1.5 oz..............	170	9	4	25	20	1	14	110
SHELF-STABLE								
Dolly Madison Raspberry Cream Filled *Zingers* ...	160	6	5	15	25	1	20	95
Iced Vanilla Cake w/Filling *Zingers*, 1.4 oz.........	160	5	2	10	27	0	21	120
Iced Devil's Food w/Filling *Zingers*, 1.4 oz.........	150	5	3	10	25	1	20	140
Drake's Devil Dogs, 1	170	7	3	0	27	1	20	125
Entenmann's Devil's Food Cookie Cake..........	60	1	0	0	13	0	8	40
100 Calorie Choc Chip Muffins, 0.8 oz	100	5	1	10	13	0	9	65
100 Calorie Blueberry Muffins, 0.8 oz...........	100	4	1	10	12	0	7	90
Little Bites Banana Choc Chip Muffins, 1.7 oz .	180	8	2	20	25	1	17	125
Little Bites Choc Chip Muffins, 1.7 oz	190	9	3	20	26	1	17	135
Hostess Brownie Bites, 1.3 oz (3)..................	170	9	2	30	22	1	17	80
MiniMuffins Banana Walnut, 2 oz	230	14	2	30	24	1	15	125
100 Calorie Cinnamon Coffee Cake, 3	100	3	1	10	21	5	7	135
100 Calorie Choc Cake w/Filling, 1 pkg.........	100	3	2	10	22	5	10	140
Little Debbie 100 Calorie Nutty Bar, 1...............	90	5	1	0	9	1	5	40
Petites Yellow Cakes	100	3	1	5	18	0	13	80
Caramel Cookie Bar, 1.2 oz..........................	160	8	2	0	22	0	16	85
Fudge Rounds, 1.2 oz	150	6	2	0	23	1	14	85
Petites Strawberry Cake.............................	100	3	1	5	18	0	13	95
Petites Red Velvet Cake	100	4	1	5	17	0	13	100
Petites Choc Cake	100	3	1	5	17	1	12	115
Nutty Bars, 2 oz..	320	20	8	0	33	1	22	125
Mrs Freshley's Buddy Bars	140	7	4	0	17	1	11	75
Iced Honey Buns..	250	13	7	0	31	1	17	130
Honey Buns..	210	10	5	0	27	1	13	140
Tastykake Hippity Hops, 1 pkg	170	9	7	0	22	2	15	45
Kandy Kakes Ghostly Goodies, 1 pkg	170	9	8	0	22	2	15	70
Kandy Kakes Peanut Butter, 1 pkg	180	10	5	10	20	1	15	85
Witchy Treats, 1.4 oz	150	6	2	30	24	1	16	90
Koffee Kake Cupcakes, most, 1 pkg (avg)......	220	7	2	35	36	3	21	130
Koffee Kake Cupcakes, Cream-Filled, 1 pkg ..	250	11	4	35	35	0	22	140

DINNERS, LIGHT MEALS AND ENTREES

See RESOURCES**,** *page 305, for a partial list of manufacturers and retailers offering low-salt products online or visit* **LowSaltFoods.com** *for additional sources.*

DINNERS, LIGHT MEALS AND ENTREES

APPETIZERS AND SNACKS – FROZEN

(also see Dips, pg 220; Egg Rolls/Spring Rolls, pg 157)

	Cal	Fat	Sat	Chol	Carb	Fib	Sug	Sod
Pizza snacks, cheese, 1 oz	70	3	1	3	8	0	1	140
Buffalo wings, 1 oz	45	3	1	33	1	0	0	275
Cheese nuggets, 1 oz	70	4	1	3	7	1	1	317
Brands . . . *(1 oz unless noted)*								
Alexia Mushroom Bites	55	2	0	0	8	1	1	140
Amy's Snacks, Cheese Pizza, 1.2 oz	38	1	1	2	4	0	1	78
Snacks, Spinach Pizza, 1.2 oz	40	1	1	3	5	0	0	84
Apollo Spanakopita	80	4	1	10	9	1	1	120
Artisanal Gougeres (Cheese Puffs), 1.2 oz	100	7	4	60	5	0	0	95
Athens Fillo Appetizers Spanakopita	80	4	1	10	9	1	1	120
Black Tie Mini Cheese Soufflé	127	10	6	173	4	0	1	107
Mushroom Turnovers	84	5	3	14	9	1	2	140
Dr. Praeger's Kids Sweet Potato Littles, 1.3 oz	60	2	0	0	9	1	2	85
California Veggieballs, 1	40	2	0	0	5	2	1	95
Kids Broccoli Littles, 1.3 oz	40	2	0	0	4	1	0	100
Kids Spinach Littles, 1.3 oz	45	3	0	0	5	1	0	100
Kids Potato Littles, 1.4 oz	60	3	0	15	7	1	0	115
Health is Wealth Spinach Munchies	60	2	0	0	8	1	0	107
Hot Tamale Munchies	53	1	0	0	9	1	0	110
Broccoli & Cheese Munchies	53	1	0	0	9	1	1	140
Ian's Chicken Nuggets, 1.2 oz	88	4	0	10	8	0	0	120
Lotus Restaurant Cream Cheese Wonton	120	8	2	10	9	0	0	110
Matlaw's Clams Organata, 2	80	5	0	6	6	0	0	125
Michael Angelo's Mini Calzones	80	4	2	10	8	0	0	135
Nate's Mini Burritos Bean/Rice/Cheese, 3 oz	230	2	2	5	44	1	1	115
Crispy Burritos Mini Jalapeno/Cr Cheese, 3 oz	290	10	6	30	41	0	1	115
Ore-Ida Hot Bites Stuffed Jalapeno Peppers, 1	70	5	2	5	7	0	1	130
Original Rangoon Mini Beef Wellington, 2	180	13	4	13	11	1	1	90
Deli Swirls Garden Vegetable	80	4	2	5	8	1	0	115
Crab Rangoons	80	3	2	15	9	0	1	135
Snapps Mushroom Bites	30	3	1	0	7	0	0	110
Snack Bites Cream Cheese Pepper Bites, 1.4 oz	110	6	2	5	12	1	0	140
Wegmans Hors D'Oeuvres								
Profiterole Puffs, 3	60	4	3	40	4	0	0	25
Bengal Shrimp Sugar Cane Skewer, 1 pc	30	1	1	20	3	0	1	65
Blue Cheese & Fig Lollipop, 1.2 oz	130	8	3	10	12	2	5	70
Classic Escargot Profiteroles, 1.1 oz	120	9	6	55	5	0	1	85
Mini Quiche Collection, 1 pc (avg)	70	5	4	30	4	0	0	90
Ratatouille & Artichoke Fillo Cup, 1 oz	25	1	0	0	3	0	0	90
Spinach & Artichoke Tortilla Crisps, 0.6 oz	50	3	2	10	3	0	0	95
Mini Mushroom Fillo Triangles, 1.1 o	70	5	3	10	6	0	0	110
Smoked Salmon Rye Profiteroles, 1.4 ozz	110	9	6	45	4	0	0	115
Potato Skins, 1.2 oz	80	6	2	8	6	1	1	125
New England Lobster Pot Pie, 1 pc	90	6	4	25	5	0	0	140
Portobello Mushroom/Herb Empanada, 1.2 oz	100	7	4	15	7	1	0	140
REDUCED SODIUM (LESS THAN GENERIC):								
Cohen's Potato Puffs, 2 oz	170	12	4	0	14	1	0	150
Health is Wealth Mexican Munchies	57	1	0	0	9	1	1	143

137

DINNERS, LIGHT MEALS AND ENTREES
Blintzes and Crepes

	Cal	Fat	Sat	Chol	Carb	Fib	Sug	Sod
Michelina's Lean Gourmet								
Pepperoni Pizza Rolls, 1.5 oz	100	4	1	5	12	1	1	145
Nancy's Mini Cheese Souffle, 1.5 oz	190	16	8	260	7	0	1	160
Original Rangoon Deli Swirls Pesto Chicken..	80	5	2	10	7	1	0	150

BLINTZES AND CREPES

	Cal	Fat	Sat	Chol	Carb	Fib	Sug	Sod
Crepes, 1	45	1	1	5	9	0	3	60
Fruit blintz, 2.2 oz	80	2	0	10	16	1	5	160
Cheese blintz, 2.2 oz	100	3	1	10	15	2	4	170
Potato blintz, 2.2 oz....................................	90	4	1	5	15	2	2	170

Brands . . . *(2.2 oz unless noted)*
FROZEN

	Cal	Fat	Sat	Chol	Carb	Fib	Sug	Sod
Empire Kosher Cheese Blintzes	80	2	1	15	13	2	5	135
Flaum Potato Blintzes, 3 oz..........................	110	5	1	50	14	1	1	125
Golden Blueberry Cheesecake Crepes, 2.3 oz ..	140	7	1	0	19	1	14	60
Strawberry Cheesecake Crepes, 2.3 oz..........	140	7	1	0	19	1	14	60
Cheese Blinzes	80	2	1	15	13	2	5	135
J&J Potato Blintzes, 2.3 oz..........................	90	5	1	14	13	1	1	130
Cheese Blintzes, 2.5 oz	132	4	1	7	10	1	4	132
Lupita's Apple Cinnamon Crepes, 2.5 oz........	110	3	1	0	20	1	12	60
Crepas de Mango, 2.5 oz.............................	110	3	1	0	20	1	12	60
Market Day Cherry & Cheese Blintz, 2.3 oz	110	4	2	25	16	1	11	135
Mendelsohn's Cheese Blintz........................	140	7	3	85	15	0	10	115
Mon Dairy Cheese Blintzes, 2.5 oz	180	7	3	90	24	0	8	125
Ratner's/King Kold Blueberry Blintzes, 2.1 oz..	80	1	0	25	17	1	7	105
Potato Blintzes, 2.1 oz	90	1	0	25	18	1	8	105
Cheese Blintzes, 2.1 oz	100	2	1	30	16	0	5	140
Tuv Taam Blueberry or Strawberry Blintz, 3 oz..	140	6	1	75	23	1	13	65
Apricot & Walnut, 3 oz	190	6	2	85	29	1	7	70
Apple Cinnamon, 3.9 oz...............................	160	5	1	85	27	1	14	75
Cheese/Blueberry or Cheese/Cherry, 3 oz (avg).	155	6	2	80	22	1	11	80
Cheese, 3 oz	160	7	3	100	18	0	15	95
Cheese Strawberry w/Custard Sauce, 5 oz........	260	11	5	100	34	0	21	105
Cheese w/Choc Sauce, 5 oz..........................	300	13	7	105	37	1	24	115
Cheese w/Strawberry Sauce, 5 oz	250	7	4	95	39	1	26	115
Unger's Cherry Blintzes, 3 oz........................	160	2	1	10	31	1	20	130
REDUCED SODIUM (LESS THAN GENERIC):								
Golden Apple Raisin Blinzes	80	2	0	10	16	1	5	150
Blueberry or Cherry Blinzes (avg)...............	95	1	0	8	18	2	7	150
MIXES								
Dixie Carb Counters French Crepe Mix, 1	12	0	0	0	2	2	0	46

BREAKFAST MEALS AND ENTREES

(see Breakfast Meals – Frozen, pg 63; Pancakes/Waffles/French Toast, pg 70)

DINNERS AND MEALS – FROZEN

(also see Dinners/Meals–Shelf-Stable, pg 143; Entrees/Light Meals, pg 143; Pizza, pg 147)

	Cal	Fat	Sat	Chol	Carb	Fib	Sug	Sod
Baked lemon pepper fish dinner, 9.1 oz	220	6	2	40	55	7	10	630
Beef and potatoes complete meal, 9.1 oz	270	10	4	71	19	4	12	742
Lasagna w/meat sauce, 10 oz........................	359	13	7	45	36	4	6	792
Spaghetti w/meat sauce, 10 oz	330	9	3	15	47	4	7	800
Grilled chicken and veg skillet, 12.5 oz...........	360	9	3	50	43	3	8	870
Fettuccine alfredo, 10 oz	653	39	16	64	58	2	4	902

	Cal	Fat	Sat	Chol	Carb	Fib	Sug	Sod
Veal parmigiana complete meal, 9.1 oz	362	19	6	26	35	7	15	964
Seafood scampi, 12 oz	410	12	5	75	56	5	5	1050
Turkey and stuffing complete meal, 9.4 oz	280	10	3	52	34	3	7	1060
Macaroni and cheese, 12 oz	370	15	8	0	38	48	26	1070
Salisbury steak complete meal, 9.6 oz	398	25	9	51	28	3	7	1140
Fried chicken complete meal, 8.1 oz	470	27	9	89	35	2	3	1500
Meatloaf and potatoes complete meal, 14 oz	460	34	10	80	39	9	7	1510

Brands . . . *(10 oz serving unless noted)*
The minimum serving size for the following dinners and meals is 8.1 ounces. Items that are 8 ounces or less are listed in Entree/Light Meals, pg 143.

	Cal	Fat	Sat	Chol	Carb	Fib	Sug	Sod
LaBriute Meatballs & Spaghetti, 12 oz	380	14	5	55	44	3	14	95
Vegetarian Pepper Steak, 12 oz	280	2	0	0	24	11	3	105
Pritikin Seared Tasmanian Trout, 10.4 oz	220	8	2	65	12	3	6	85
Roasted Bison, 8.4 oz	200	4	1	80	15	3	4	115
Bison Bolognaise w/Spaghetti, 9.5 oz	360	19	8	80	22	4	3	125
Vegetable Lasagna, 9.7 oz	120	1	0	0	24	6	6	130

REDUCED SODIUM (LESS THAN GENERIC):

	Cal	Fat	Sat	Chol	Carb	Fib	Sug	Sod
Amy's *Lite in Sodium Bowls* Brown Rice/Veg	260	9	1	0	36	5	7	270
Lite in Sodium Macaroni & Cheese, 9 oz	400	16	10	40	47	3	6	290
Lite in Sodium Shepherd's Pie, 8.1 oz	160	4	0	0	27	5	5	290
Lite in Sodium Veg Loaf/Potatoes/Veg	290	8	1	0	47	7	6	340
Lite in Sodium Veg Lasagna, 9.5 oz	290	8	4	15	41	4	8	340
Lite in Sodium Bowls Country Cheddar	430	21	6	20	45	4	3	345
Lite in Sodium Bowls Mexican Casserole	370	16	5	20	48	7	4	390
Lite in Sodium Indian Mattar Paneer	320	8	2	20	54	6	8	390
Thai Stir Fry, 9.5 oz	310	11	7	0	45	5	2	420
Bowls Brown Rice & Veg	260	9	1	0	36	5	7	550
Indian Paneer Tikka, 9.5 oz	320	7	0	20	36	5	6	550
Cedarlane Chicken Parmigiana	400	10	4	45	57	5	2	520
Burrito Grande w/Chili Verde	230	10	4	20	27	2	3	540
Eating Right (Safeway/Vons)								
5-Grain Chicken w/Plum Sauce, 9 oz	310	5	1	25	49	5	19	190
Butternut Squash Ravioli, 8.4 oz	280	10	3	30	42	5	7	330
Sesame Chicken, 9 oz	370	5	1	25	67	3	19	450
Cashew Chicken, 9.7 oz	290	4	1	30	44	3	6	460
Sweet & Sour Chicken	320	4	1	30	57	2	26	470
Chicken w/Basil Cream Sauce, 8.5 oz	280	7	2	35	34	2	5	480
Chicken Poblano, 9 oz	310	8	3	40	37	2	3	490
Mediterranean Style Chicken, 10.5 oz	230	6	1	30	30	5	4	500
Lemongrass Chicken, 9.3 oz	230	7	3	40	26	3	5	500
Santa Fe Style Rice & Beans, 9 oz	310	8	3	5	48	8	4	500
5-Grain Beef & Vegetable, 8.8 oz	280	5	1	25	43	4	6	500
Orange Glazed Chicken, 8.8 oz	300	5	1	30	33	3	24	500
Three Cheese Pasta, 8.8 oz	320	7	4	10	46	3	6	500
Chicken w/Peanut Sauce, 9 oz	280	10	1	25	33	7	6	500
Beef Portobello, 9 oz	260	6	2	25	36	3	5	550
Chicken Enchilada, 9 oz	300	6	3	30	43	3	3	550
Ethnic Gourmet Lemongrass/Basil Chicken	380	9	5	30	56	5	13	310
Shahi Paneer, 11 oz	560	30	13	60	49	7	7	400
Malay Chicken Curry	410	11	5	35	59	3	15	530
Healthy Choice Pineapple Chicken, 8.6 oz	380	7	1	10	70	4	29	190
Spicy Caribbean Chicken, 8.6 oz	290	3	1	30	52	5	20	260
Honey Ginger Chicken, 8.6 oz	320	5	1	30	53	5	18	280
Cafe Steamers Sesame Chicken, 10.4 oz	340	5	1	30	55	4	19	330

139

DINNERS, LIGHT MEALS AND ENTREES
Dinners and Meals – Frozen

	Cal	Fat	Sat	Chol	Carb	Fib	Sug	Sod
Honey Roasted Turkey, 10.9 oz	250	4	2	40	36	5	20	350
Herb Crusted Fish, 11.1 oz	270	5	2	25	40	5	8	370
Cafe Steamers Sweet/Spicy Orange Chicken	310	3	1	30	52	4	16	380
Cafe Steamers Pineapple Chicken, 10.6 oz	330	5	1	30	53	4	21	400
Roasted Chicken Marsala, 10.5 oz	240	5	2	40	29	4	6	420
Sundried Tomato & Chicken Alfredo, 10.5 oz	270	7	3	40	31	5	4	430
Roasted Sesame Chicken, 12 oz	410	10	2	20	63	8	21	460
Sweet & Tangy Chicken BBQ, 10.6 oz	320	4	1	30	56	4	29	470
Sweet & Sour Chicken, 12 oz	390	10	2	20	60	7	19	460
Chicken Romano Fresca, 8.1 oz	230	5	2	25	29	4	0	490
Lemon Herb Chicken, 8.8 oz	200	4	1	30	26	3	3	480
Tortellini Primavera Parmesan, 9 oz	230	5	2	20	37	5	7	490
Cafe Steamers Roasted Beef Merlot	220	6	2	35	25	5	5	500
Beef Pot Roast, 11 oz	250	6	2	40	32	5	14	500
Roasted Chicken Verde, 8.7 oz	230	4	1	30	35	3	5	500
Salisbury Steak, 8.1 oz	170	5	2	30	18	4	2	500
Rosemary Chicken & Sweet Potatoes, 8.8 oz	180	3	1	30	26	5	10	500
Garlic Herb Chicken, 12 oz	250	5	2	40	34	6	12	500
Cafe Steamers Grilled Basil Chicken, 10.7 oz	270	6	2	25	35	6	4	500
Portabella Marsala Pasta, 9.1 oz	260	6	3	10	38	5	4	500
Honey Balsamic Chicken, 8.8 oz	210	4	1	25	32	4	8	500
Cafe Steamers Gen'l Tso's Chicken, 10.9 oz	300	3	1	30	53	4	12	500
Cafe Steamers Thai-Style Chicken & Veg	260	5	1	35	36	4	10	500
Top Chef Chicken Linguini, 10.4 oz	260	6	3	40	28	5	3	510
Slow Roasted Turkey Medallions, 8.6 oz	210	5	2	30	28	4	14	520
Beef & Broccoli, 11.1 oz	280	6	2	45	37	4	4	520
Lobster Cheese Ravioli. 9.1 oz	260	5	3	15	41	4	9	520
Golden Roasted Turkey breast, 10.6 oz	270	4	1	30	38	7	13	520
Bacon & Smokey Cheddar Chicken, 8.7 oz	250	6	3	45	31	2	2	520
Cafe Steamers Lemongrass Chicken/Shrimp	280	4	1	45	42	6	11	530
Oven Roasted Chicken, 11.5 oz	240	5	2	35	37	5	10	540
Ravioli Florentine Marinara, 8.6 oz	250	5	3	25	37	6	11	540
Lemon Garlic Chicken, 10.6 oz	310	9	2	25	41	6	8	540
Cafe Steamers Balsamic Garlic Chicken, 10 oz	250	4	1	30	36	5	7	540
Classic Meatloaf, 12.1 oz	330	7	3	30	51	7	16	550
Portabella Spinach Parmesan, 9.5 oz	270	7	2	10	39	5	3	550
Top Chef Grilled Chicken Pesto w/Veg, 10.8 oz	310	9	3	40	34	3	2	550
Top Chef BBQ Steak w/Red Potatoes, 9.6 oz	330	6	2	45	47	4	15	550
Kashi Mayan Harvest Bake	340	9	2	0	58	8	19	380
Sweet & Sour Chicken	320	4	1	35	55	6	25	380
Black Bean Mango	340	8	1	0	58	7	11	380
Red Curry Chicken, 9.6 oz	300	8	3	20	42	6	9	420
Chicken Pasta Pomodoro	280	6	2	25	38	6	5	470
Chicken Florentine	290	9	5	45	31	5	1	550
Kid Cuisine KC's Kickin Ravioli, 8.2 oz	320	7	3	20	54	7	14	290
Spaghetti w/Mini Meatballs, 10.3 oz	450	13	4	25	63	9	21	470
LaBriute Vegetarian Stuffed Cabbage, 12 oz	335	7	0	0	50	7	11	364
Vegetarian Stuffed Shells in Sauce, 12 oz	310	4	1	0	61	9	10	450
Chicken Primavera w/Noodles, 8.6 oz	150	4	1	30	15	2	2	510
Cheese Ravioli in Tomato Sauce, 12 oz	320	4	2	10	61	4	7	520
Lean Cuisine Thai Chicken Spring Rolls, 8 oz	200	7	2	25	23	1	4	390
Spinach Artichoke Dip w/Pita Bread, 8 oz	200	6	3	20	29	2	5	410
Garlic Chicken Spring Rolls, 8 oz	200	8	2	20	24	2	4	420
Broccoli Cheddar Dip w/Pita Bread, 8 oz	200	6	2	10	29	2	4	420

	Cal	Fat	Sat	Chol	Carb	Fib	Sug	Sod
Garden Veg Dip w/Pita Bread, 8 oz	190	5	2	10	29	2	4	440
Glazed Chicken, 8.5 oz	240	5	1	45	26	2	6	450
Hunan Stir Fry w/Beef, 8.5 oz	280	8	2	20	36	5	12	460
Chicken w/Almonds, 8.5 oz	250	4	0	30	38	4	13	490
Tortilla Crusted Fish, 8 oz	300	9	2	30	41	2	7	490
Sweet & Sour Chicken, 10 oz	300	3	0	30	51	2	16	490
Grilled Chicken & Penne Pasta, 12 oz	340	5	2	30	55	4	24	500
Classic Macaroni & Beef, 9.5 oz	260	3	1	30	42	4	9	500
Chicken w/Basil Cream Sauce, 8.5 oz	230	6	3	35	28	2	5	510
Rosemary Chicken, 8 oz	210	4	2	30	27	5	5	510
Fajita-Style Chicken Spring Rolls	200	7	2	30	20	2	3	510
Lemon Pepper Fish, 9 oz	290	8	2	25	40	2	4	520
Apple Cranberry Chicken	320	5	2	30	55	6	23	520
Beef & Broccoli, 9 oz	270	5	2	20	43	2	9	520
Beef Chow Fun, 9 oz	320	5	2	20	54	3	18	520
Asian-Style Pot Stickers, 9 oz	260	4	1	10	49	2	9	530
Chicken Fried Rice, 9 oz	260	5	1	25	41	4	5	530
Chile Lime Chicken, 9 oz	240	2	0	25	38	2	8	530
Garlic Chicken Caesar, 8.5 oz	240	6	2	35	30	3	1	530
Herb Roasted Chicken, 8 oz	170	3	1	35	19	3	4	540
Salisbury Steak, 9.5 oz	260	8	3	40	23	3	3	540
Ranchero Braised Beef, 8.3 oz	240	4	2	30	34	3	23	540
Butternut Squash Ravioli, 9.9 oz	260	7	2	20	40	5	11	550
Beef Pot Roast, 9 oz	210	6	2	25	26	3	3	550
Beef Portabello, 9 oz	200	6	3	30	24	3	6	550
Lemongrass Chicken, 9 oz	260	6	1	25	33	5	7	550
Szechuan Style Stir Fry w/Shrimp, 9 oz	210	2	0	50	37	5	11	550
Chicken Chow Mein w/Rice, 9 oz	240	4	1	25	39	3	3	550
Chicken in Peanut Sauce, 9 oz	280	6	1	25	35	5	5	550
Lightlife Linguine Siciliano, 12.2 oz	280	7	3	10	44	10	9	280
Zesty Mexican, 11.5 oz	330	6	1	5	57	12	7	300
Indian Veggie Masala, 12.5 oz	390	9	4	20	65	11	15	320
Tuscan Portobello, 11.8 oz	250	5	1	0	40	10	4	400
Michael Angelos *Natural* Mediterranean Shrimp	310	7	1	85	43	6	5	460
Natural Chicken Alfredo w/Broccoli	360	11	6	60	40	3	2	510
Michelina's *Authentico* Spaghetti Marinara	250	2	0	0	47	3	5	430
Authentico Four Cheese Lasagna, 8.1 oz	280	6	3	15	43	3	4	500
Authentico Lasagna Mozzarella, 8.1 oz	260	7	4	20	39	3	5	540
Michelina's Budget Gourmet								
Angel Hair Pasta in Meat Sauce, 8.1 oz	290	5	2	10	48	4	5	410
Penne & Italian Sausage, 8.1 oz	280	7	2	10	41	3	4	410
Ziti Parmesano, 8.1 oz	250	7	3	10	37	3	3	500
Italian Veg & White Chicken, 8.1 oz	270	5	1	10	44	4	4	540
Macaroni & Cheese w/Cheddar, 8.1 oz	260	7	3	15	40	2	3	550
Michelinas Lean Gourmet Penne Primavera	280	6	3	15	43	3	3	470
Glazed Chicken, 8.1 oz	250	3	1	20	46	1	8	470
Macaroni & Cheese, 9.1 oz	280	5	2	10	48	2	3	490
Cheese Stuffed Rigtoni, 8.1 oz	220	6	3	30	33	3	7	510
Shrimp w/Pasta & Veg, 8.1 oz	280	6	3	45	41	2	4	540
Milano's Italian Grille Chicken Marsala, 9 oz	270	5	1	60	29	2	1	470
Mon Cuisine Vegan Meatless Italian Pasta	250	3	0	0	43	11	5	210
Vegetarian Stuffed Cabbage in Sauce	220	5	0	0	36	5	8	260
Braised Veal in Mushroom Gravy	610	15	3	180	72	9	17	400
Chicken Mediterranean	330	7	2	80	32	4	2	420

141

DINNERS, LIGHT MEALS AND ENTREES
Dinners and Meals – Frozen

	Cal	Fat	Sat	Chol	Carb	Fib	Sug	Sod
Vegetarian Salisbury Steak in Gravy	320	7	1	0	36	14	2	430
Vegetarian Spaghetti & Meatballs	360	4	0	0	54	9	8	440
Vegan Moroccan Couscous	280	4	1	0	46	10	10	440
Vegan Veal Style Schnitzel in Sauce............	300	8	1	0	38	7	2	440
Vegetarian Steak in Mushroom Gravy	250	6	1	0	29	12	3	470
Moosewood Pasta e Fagioli	260	5	1	0	47	6	8	340
Farfalle & Spinach Pasta Sauce	370	11	5	20	56	4	6	370
Spicy Penne Puttanesca	300	10	2	0	45	2	5	380
Broccoli & Pasta Parmesan	280	13	6	30	52	4	4	380
Moroccan Stew	150	3	0	0	29	5	11	400
Morningstar Farm Sesame Chik'n, 9.5 oz....	310	9	1	0	46	4	16	530
Organic Classics Chicken Cacciatore w/Pasta ..	340	11	2	50	43	3	6	410
Cajun Style Chicken Tetrazzini	370	12	5	55	43	3	4	470
Chicken Marsala w/Potatoes, 9.5 oz............	350	15	8	70	30	3	3	510
Thai Chicken Curry, 10.1 oz	420	17	6	40	50	3	4	510
Pritikin Coriander Scallops, 17.3 oz.............	150	1	0	15	24	7	11	170
Hungarian So-Soya, 8.8 oz........................	170	0	0	0	23	4	4	170
Lentil & Spinach Stew, 11.9 oz...................	210	2	0	0	39	9	8	200
Veggie Bolognaise w/Spaghetti, 7.8 oz........	300	5	0	0	38	13	4	240
Pasta w/Meatballs, 7.8 oz..........................	300	5	0	0	38	13	4	240
Lemon Mahi Mahi, 12.8 oz..........................	240	2	0	150	15	3	1	340
Putney Pasta Chicken Piccata Skillet, 9 oz ...	300	10	4	30	35	2	3	200
Rising Moon Organics Lasagna	380	10	2	0	56	6	4	460
Manicotti or Stuffed Shells.......................	370	10	2	0	54	6	4	470
Wegmans Italian Classics Pasta Marinara, 8.1 oz .	240	6	3	10	32	2	5	290
Italian Classics Eggplant Lasagna, 8.1 oz	280	17	6	25	23	2	6	310
Weight Watchers Smart Ones								
Mini Rigatoni w/Vodka Cream Sauce, 9.1 oz..	290	6	3	10	48	5	5	440
Fruit Inspirations Cranberry Turkey, 9.1 oz	250	2	0	30	43	4	19	460
Sweet & Sour Chicken, 9.1 oz....................	210	2	1	20	31	2	10	510
Roast Beef in Gravy, 9.1 oz	230	11	4	40	18	2	2	530
Lasagna Bake w/Meat Sauce, 9.1 oz...........	270	4	2	15	43	3	3	540
Lemon Herb Chicken Piccata, 9.1 oz	230	2	1	25	41	2	8	540

SKILLET MEALS, MEAL KITS AND HELPERS
REDUCED SODIUM (LESS THAN GENERIC):

	Cal	Fat	Sat	Chol	Carb	Fib	Sug	Sod
Blue Horizon Natural Pasta Twists, 8.1 oz	270	6	3	75	38	3	2	280
Natural Penne Marinara, 8.1 oz.................	270	6	3	20	38	3	2	280
Organic Penne Alla Vodka w/Shrimp	270	6	3	75	38	9	0	280
Skillet Meals:								
Natural Four Cheese Fettucine, 8.1 oz	430	22	8	90	39	2	0	380
Natural Pasta Shells & Pesto Sauce, 8.1 oz	280	6	2	40	38	3	1	420
Organic Penne Alfredo w/Shrimp.............	430	22	8	115	39	2	0	380
Organic Pesto Farfalle w/Shrimp	280	6	2	70	38	3	0	430
Contessa MicroSteam Chicken Alfredo, 6. oz ..	260	13	8	55	24	3	2	450
Sweet & Sour Chicken, prep, 9.5 oz............	400	12	3	35	61	2	22	480
Sweet & Sour Shrimp	250	1	0	65	48	4	16	490
Gourmet Dining Seafood Medley, 8 oz	220	4	1	60	28	3	4	440
Lean Cuisine Market Creations Chicken Primavera	260	6	3	40	32	3	3	550
Putney Pasta Chicken Alfredo Skillet, 9 oz ...	410	19	11	80	35	2	2	360
Shrimp Pesto Skillet, 9 oz	540	38	11	100	32	3	3	410
TGIF Friday's Complete Skillet Meals								
Chicken & Broccoli Alfredo, 8 oz	270	9	4	45	28	3	2	520
Tyson Skillet Creations Chicken Fajitas, 1/2 pkg	250	7	2	20	32	3	5	430
Asian Orange Chicken, 1/2 pkg	340	5	2	35	50	6	18	470

	Cal	Fat	Sat	Chol	Carb	Fib	Sug	Sod

DINNERS AND MEALS – SHELF-STABLE

(also see Pasta Fixings, pg 205)

	Cal	Fat	Sat	Chol	Carb	Fib	Sug	Sod
Macaroni and cheese, boxed, 1 cup	420	19	5	15	50	2	7	750
Meal kits and helpers:								
Hamburger mix/helper, cheese, 1 cup	310	15	2	60	30	1	2	920

Brands . . . *(10 oz serving unless noted)*
REDUCED SODIUM (LESS THAN GENERIC):
Meal Mart *Amazing Meals*

	Cal	Fat	Sat	Chol	Carb	Fib	Sug	Sod
Baked Ziti in Tomato Sauce, 12 oz	420	14	1	0	63	3	17	160
Fillet of Salmon, 12 oz	430	16	5	70	35	6	6	290
Eggplant Parmesan, 12 oz	320	14	2	0	44	2	17	290
Cheese Ravioli in Tomato Sauce, 12 oz	510	24	2	0	64	2	18	290
Beef Stuffed Cabbage, 12 oz	200	3	1	30	29	4	10	360
Beef Cholent, 12 oz	600	19	6	80	61	16	1	390
Beef Rib Steak, 12 oz	560	22	6	135	50	5	7	460
Bone-In Chicken, 12 oz	510	20	4	105	55	5	8	490
Beef & Lamb Kabob, 12 oz	620	18	6	50	83	10	2	510

SKILLET MEALS, MEAL KITS AND HELPERS

NOTE: Some of the following may require additional ingredients, which may raise the sodium content.

Delicaé Pantry *Slow Cooker Dinner*

	Cal	Fat	Sat	Chol	Carb	Fib	Sug	Sod
Country French Pork & White Bean	110	0	0	0	22	6	2	25
Homemade Turkey Barley	110	1	0	0	25	5	2	25
Italian Farm-Style Chicken	110	1	0	0	25	5	2	25
Big Easy Jambalaya	100	0	0	0	22	2	2	30
Italian Kitchen Osso Bucco	100	0	0	0	22	5	3	30
Grandma's Country Chicken & Rice	90	0	0	0	20	2	3	35
Mediterranean Lamb Shanks	120	1	0	0	24	6	4	35
Old Fashioned Pot Roast	80	0	0	0	17	3	4	45
French Bistro Short Ribs	60	0	0	0	13	2	3	45
Santa Fe Chicken w/Black Beans	100	0	0	0	19	3	4	60

REDUCED SODIUM (LESS THAN GENERIC):

	Cal	Fat	Sat	Chol	Carb	Fib	Sug	Sod
CookSimple New Orleans Jambalaya	130	1	0	0	28	2	3	190
Asian Burgers	150	5	1	0	25	3	2	280
Cranberry Wild Rice	140	0	0	0	32	3	11	280

Betty Crocker *Asian Hamburger Helper*

	Cal	Fat	Sat	Chol	Carb	Fib	Sug	Sod
Beef Fried Rice	90	0	0	0	19	0	1	300
Chicken Fried Rice	90	0	0	0	20	1	1	310

ENTREE/LIGHT MEALS

(also see specific prepared items in Ethnic Foods, pg 156-158, 163-170; Prepared Fish/Seafood, pg 176; Prepared Meats, pg 193, 195)

	Cal	Fat	Sat	Chol	Carb	Fib	Sug	Sod
Beef tamales in chili sauce, canned, 2	140	7	3	15	15	2	0	710
Beef stew, canned, 1 cup	220	12	5	37	16	4	2	947
Corned beef hash, canned, 1 cup	380	24	10	76	22	3	1	986

Brands . . . *(1 cup or 8 oz unless noted)*
The maximum serving size for the following entrees and light meals is 8 ounces. Items with more than 8 ounces are listed in Dinners/Meals, pg 138.

CANNED – *Most brands within generic average.*
FROZEN/REFRIGERATED

	Cal	Fat	Sat	Chol	Carb	Fib	Sug	Sod
Pritikin Veg Stuffed Shells, 3.9 oz	210	4	3	15	32	2	1	60
Roasted Turkey, 7.1 oz	260	1	0	95	24	3	16	70
Jamaican Curry Chicken, 6.6 oz	150	2	0	65	6	2	2	80

143

DINNERS, LIGHT MEALS AND ENTREES
Entree/Light Meals

	Cal	Fat	Sat	Chol	Carb	Fib	Sug	Sod
Seared Salmon w/Potato Hash, 5.7 oz	140	3	0	35	4	1	1	90
Poached Salmon w/Roasted Potato, 5.7 oz	140	3	0	35	4	1	1	90
Jerked Mahi Mahi, 4.3 oz	100	1	0	85	0	0	0	100
Mango & So Soya Stew	140	0	0	0	21	5	9	110
Spinach Ravioli, 7.8 oz	250	6	3	20	37	7	3	115
Braised White Fish w/Artichokes, 6.9 oz	150	3	0	35	7	1	4	130
REDUCED SODIUM (LESS THAN GENERIC):								
Amy's Kids Meals Baked Ziti	360	12	2	0	58	5	14	460
Light & Lean Pasta & Vegetables	210	5	2	5	33	3	3	470
Light & Lean Black Bean/Cheese Enchilada	240	5	2	5	44	4	5	480
Bird's Eye Voila! Garlic Shrimp, 1 cup	230	9	2	50	27	2	6	410
Blake's Mac & Cheese w/Chicken, 8 oz	360	17	5	80	34	3	5	320
Mac & Cheese w/Veggies, 8 oz	346	9	5	32	43	4	0	359
Macaroni & Beef, 8 oz	321	11	4	33	45	3	0	404
Farmhouse Mac & Cheese, 8 oz	370	18	5	50	45	4	0	480
Cincinnati Recipe Chili Spaghetti, 8 oz	260	10	4	30	29	0	1	500
Contessa MicroSteam Chicken Marsala, 6.8 oz	280	9	5	40	33	2	5	350
MicroSteam Garlic Chicken Penne, 6.8 oz	270	9	3	25	34	2	2	430
MicroSteam Shrimp Scampi Linguini, 6.8 oz	310	12	6	60	37	3	3	450
MicroSteam Chicken Florentine, 6.8 oz	340	14	8	60	38	2	2	450
MicroSteam Chicken Alfredo, 6.8 oz	260	13	8	55	24	3	2	450
Delitefuls (Walmart) Swai Caribbean BBQ	160	2	0	10	28	3	9	270
Bowtie Shrimp Scampi, 8 oz	210	6	1	45	26	4	2	300
Salmon Florentine Alfredo, 8 oz	201	5	3	30	28	3	6	320
Fillo Factory Eggplant/Red Pepper Fillo Pie	210	9	2	0	29	2	5	280
Broccoli & Cheese, 4.9 oz	290	16	8	40	25	2	2	330
Garden Lites Zucchini Souffle, 7 oz	140	1	0	0	26	3	5	320
Broccoli Souffle, 7 oz	140	1	0	0	26	4	5	340
Cauliflower Souffle, 7 oz	140	1	0	0	26	4	6	340
Roasted Veg Souffle, 7 oz	140	1	0	0	27	3	7	350
Spinach Souffle, 7 oz	140	1	0	0	25	4	5	390
Zucchini Portabella or Zucchini Marinara, 7 oz	110	4	1	0	19	4	3	390
Great Value Lasagna, 7.7 oz	280	9	5	20	36	2	8	420
Sesame Chicken, 8 oz	300	5	1	30	48	4	18	420
Ian's Chicken Nuggets, Kids Meal, 8 oz	440	14	2	50	60	2	21	320
Twisty Mac & Cheese, 8 oz	375	7	2	5	67	3	0	400
Kid Cuisine Deep Sea Fish Sticks, 7.7 oz	370	10	3	20	57	4	16	450
Chicken & Cheese Quesadillas, 7.6 oz	370	9	3	15	58	8	22	450
Last Minute Gourmet Chicken Alfredo Pasta	180	6	3	35	21	1	2	430
Meatloaf w/Mashed Potatoes, 6.1 oz	220	11	5	50	21	2	2	440
Chicken Artichoke Asiago w/Pasta, 5 oz	180	6	3	35	20	1	2	460
Lasagna w/Meat Sauce, 6.1 oz	230	10	5	50	19	1	4	500
Night Hawk Steak 'n Corn, 7 oz	340	21	8	55	21	3	3	330
Pritikin Jerked Chicken Breast, 5.9 oz	160	2	0	65	8	2	2	150
Vegetable Pizza, 7.3 oz	120	1	0	0	22	4	4	160
Shepherd's Pie, 5.8 oz	120	0	0	0	19	3	5	170
Turkey Lasagna, 5.9 oz	220	6	2	35	27	5	3	190
Vegetarian Crab Cakes, 4.9 oz	250	15	0	0	14	3	2	280
Tuv Tam Macaroni & Cheese, 6.1 oz	280	11	6	30	35	1	3	210
Fettuccini Alfredo, 6.1 oz	310	11	5	30	42	2	5	230
Lasagna w/Tomato Sauce, 6.1 oz	220	9	4	15	25	2	5	260
Vegetable Lo Mein, 6.1 oz	190	4	1	0	32	2	5	360
Baked Ziti, 6.1 oz	210	4	1	0	39	2	11	430

	Cal	Fat	Sat	Chol	Carb	Fib	Sug	Sod

SHELF-STABLE

REDUCED SODIUM (LESS THAN GENERIC):

	Cal	Fat	Sat	Chol	Carb	Fib	Sug	Sod
Celentano Vegetarian Penne w/Roasted Veg.	300	1	0	0	54	8	13	290
Good Earth Spicy Citrus Glazed Shrimp	180	1	0	0	38	4	14	250
Healthy Choice Mixers Sweet/Sour Chicken	390	3	1	25	78	3	20	400
Creamy Tomato Basil Penne, 1 pkg	290	5	1	5	50	6	5	490
Penne/Roasted Red Pepper Alfredo, 1 pkg	290	5	2	10	51	6	6	500
Spice Hunter Meal in a Cup								
Spinach & Garlic Risotto, 1 cup	240	2	1	5	47	1	2	460
Wild Mushroom Risotto, 1 cup	230	1	0	0	47	1	1	490
Garlic & Mushroom Potato, 1 cup	170	3	2	10	31	2	2	500

SKILLET MEALS, MEAL KITS AND HELPERS

SHELF-STABLE

REDUCED SODIUM (LESS THAN GENERIC):

	Cal	Fat	Sat	Chol	Carb	Fib	Sug	Sod
Annie's Homegrown								
Cheddar & Herb Chicken Skillet Meal	150	2	1	5	27	1	3	350
Romanos Marconi Grill Garlic Chicken	120	1	0	0	22	2	4	350
Chicken Marsala w/Linguini	150	1	0	0	30	1	2	390
Tony Chachere's Creole Gumbo Mix, 1/11.	70	0	0	0	15	0	1	380

ENTREES – ETHNIC

(see Asian–Entrees/Light Meals, pg 156; Hispanic/Latino–Entrees/Light Meals, pg 163; Mediterranean/Middle Eastern–Meals/Entrees, pg 169)

ENTREES – MEAT AND SEAFOOD

(see Fish/Seafood–Prepared Entrees, pg 176; Beef–Prepared Meals/Entrees, pg 193; Poultry–Prepared Meals/Entrees, pg 195)

ENTREES – PASTA/ITALIAN DISHES

(also see Entree/Light Meals, pg 143; Pasta Fixings, pg 205)

	Cal	Fat	Sat	Chol	Carb	Fib	Sug	Sod
Cheese tortellini, 1 cup	332	8	4	45	51	2	1	372
Spaghetti w/meat sauce, frozen, 1 cup	204	2	1	14	35	4	6	379
Macaroni and cheese, boxed, 1 cup prep	258	2	1	5	48	2	7	533
Macaroni and cheese, canned, 1 cup	200	6	2	15	28	1	1	1027
Spaghetti w/meatballs, canned, 1 cup	273	13	5	23	28	7	7	1035

Brands . . . *(1 cup or 8 oz serving unless noted)*

FROZEN/REFRIGERATED

	Cal	Fat	Sat	Chol	Carb	Fib	Sug	Sod
Armanino 4 Cheese Ravioli, 5.4 oz	330	9	5	45	45	2	2	130
Market Day Cheese Lasagna Rollups, 2.8 oz	140	3	2	10	22	1	1	110
Servioli Ricotta Cavatelli	170	2	0	5	35	2	1	5
SoyBoy Rosa Tofu Raviolis	180	3	1	0	29	4	2	125
Verde Tofu Raviolis	180	3	1	0	30	3	2	130
Original Tofu Raviolis	180	3	1	0	31	0	2	135

REDUCED SODIUM (LESS THAN GENERIC):

	Cal	Fat	Sat	Chol	Carb	Fib	Sug	Sod
Andrea Large Round Cheese Ravioli	270	3	1	15	49	2	4	210
Bite Size Cheese Ravioli	310	5	3	40	54	3	4	240
Armanino Cheese or Tri Color Tortellini, 4.2 oz	250	5	2	35	42	2	1	230
Barilla Tortellini, Ricotta & Spinach, 3/4 c	230	8	3	55	32	5	1	310
Tortellini, Cheese & Spinach, 3/4 c	240	8	3	35	32	3	1	310
Celentano Mini Cheese Ravioli, 4 oz	210	4	2	25	35	2	1	200
Large Cheese Ravioli, 4.4 oz	240	6	3	35	37	1	2	260
Large Beef Ravioli, 3 oz	180	6	3	35	24	2	1	260
Light Cheese Ravioli, 4.4 oz	200	3	1	20	34	2	3	270
Floresta Large Round Cheese Ravioli, 4.3 oz	190	3	2	20	33	2	2	230

DINNERS, LIGHT MEALS AND ENTREES
Entrees – Pasta/Italian Dishes

	Cal	Fat	Sat	Chol	Carb	Fib	Sug	Sod
Eating Right Italian-Style Meatballs, 5.........	90	3	1	25	5	0	1	180
Ian's Rotini & Mini Meatballs, 7 oz	290	8	4	13	41	4	4	280
Italian Village Square Cheese Ravioli, 4 oz ..	210	3	1	20	37	2	2	190
Mini Round Cheese Ravioli, 4.3 oz	200	3	1	20	35	2	2	210
Square Beef Ravioli, 3 oz	200	5	2	30	31	2	0	220
Large Round Cheese Ravioli, 4.3 oz.............	190	3	2	20	3	2	2	230
Meat Tortellini, 3.4 oz	300	8	3	25	45	2	2	230
Cheese Stuffed Rigatoni, 5 oz....................	270	8	5	30	38	2	3	260
Market Day Cheese Ravioli, 3.6 oz..............	210	7	4	35	28	5	4	170
Stuffed Eggplant, 3.5 oz	180	13	4	35	11	2	3	290
Michael Angelo's Stuffed Shells, 4 oz	210	9	6	40	18	1	1	260
Cheese Ravioli, 4 oz	218	8	4	35	27	2	7	273
Eggplant Parmesan, 6 oz...........................	280	19	3	40	23	4	5	330
Monterey Pasta Co Whole Wheat								
Chicken/Sun-Dried Tomato Ravioli	230	5	2	40	34	4	2	180
Tomato/Basil/Mozzarella Ravioli	250	7	4	35	34	4	1	250
Classic Italian Cheese Tortellini	290	6	3	35	48	5	1	290
Putney Pasta Sun-Dried Tomato Tortellini	330	7	3	45	50	1	3	240
Portobello & Grilled Onion Ravioli, 7 pcs	240	5	2	40	39	3	2	260
Butternut Squash/Maple Syrup Ravioli	200	4	2	30	35	1	6	270
Rosetto Italian Style Ravioli w/Sausage	240	5	2	10	39	2	1	210
Chicken & Herb Ravioli..............................	210	2	0	15	36	2	1	210
Cheese Tortellini	240	5	3	30	41	2	3	230
All Natural Beef Ravioli	220	4	1	10	39	2	1	250
Gourmet Butternut Squash Ravioli..............	240	3	1	5	45	3	4	260
Beef Ravioli...	240	4	2	10	40	2	1	280
Steam 'n Eat Cheese Ravioli, med square	230	4	2	15	37	2	2	290
All Natural Whole Wheat Cheese Ravioli	200	5	3	20	33	6	1	290
All Natural Cheese Ravioli	210	5	3	20	34	2	2	290
Cheese Ravioli...	230	4	2	15	37	2	2	290
Seviroli Stuffed Shells, 4.3 oz....................	220	5	3	25	30	2	1	210
Stuffed Rigatoni, 4 oz................................	370	8	4	65	60	4	2	220
Bite Size Cheese Ravioli, 3.6 oz	190	5	3	25	27	1	1	240
Shrimp & Roasted Garlic Ravioli, 3.6 oz.......	190	5	3	75	23	1	1	250
Spinach & Cheese Ravioli, 3.6 oz...............	200	5	3	20	27	2	1	250
Tortellini w/Meat	210	6	3	15	30	2	1	280
Large Cheese Ravioli, 3.6 oz......................	180	6	4	30	23	1	1	290
Tuv Tam Macaroni & Cheese, 6.1 oz	280	11	6	30	35	1	3	210
Fettuccini Alfredo, 6.1 oz...........................	310	11	5	30	42	2	5	230
Lasagna w/Tomato Sauce, 6.1 oz	220	9	4	15	25	2	5	260
Wegmans Cheese Stuffed Shells, 2.5 oz	140	7	4	45	12	1	2	160
Cheese Filled Manicotti, 2.5 oz...................	130	5	3	40	14	1	2	190
Small Round Cheese Ravioli.......................	240	8	5	50	36	1	3	250
Cheese Tortellini	240	4	3	30	37	2	2	250
SHELF-STABLE								
DeBoles Rice Pasta & Cheese, 1/2 cup	100	2	1	5	19	0	0	100
REDUCED SODIUM (LESS THAN GENERIC):								
Annie's Homegrown								
Cheddar & Herb Chicken Skillet Meal	150	2	1	5	27	1	3	350
Gluten-Free Rice Pasta & Cheese................	270	4	2	10	52	1	3	390
Lower Sodium Macaroni & Cheese	270	4	2	10	47	2	5	430
Eating Right *Kids* Pasta Rings......................	120	1	0	0	26	3	8	380
Namaste Foods Say Cheeze Pasta, 1/4 pkg ..	270	11	2	0	37	2	1	210
Pasta Pisavera Pasta Meal, 1/4 pkg.............	280	12	2	0	39	2	1	280
Taco Pasta Meal, 1/4 pkg	270	12	2	0	38	2	1	280

146

	Cal	Fat	Sat	Chol	Carb	Fib	Sug	Sod
Near East Basil & Herb Pasta	190	2	1	0	39	2	1	390
Road's End Organics Mac & Chreese, Alfredo	300	3	1	0	63	8	1	310
Penne & Chreese, Cheddar	310	3	1	0	62	6	1	340
Shells & Chreese or 123'z & Chreese (avg)	310	1	0	0	59	7	5	390
Mac & Chreese, Cheddar	320	2	0	0	56	9	2	400

PIZZA

	Cal	Fat	Sat	Chol	Carb	Fib	Sug	Sod
Pizza, cheese, 12", 1/4	391	18	6	20	42	3	5	653
Meat and veg, 12", 1/4	395	21	7	23	36	3	5	794
Pepperoni, 12", 1/4	432	22	7	22	42	3	5	902
Cheese, meat and veg, 12" rising crust, 1/4	404	18	6	28	43	3	5	954
Bread pizza, cheese, 6 oz	350	14	5	15	42	3	4	660

Brands . . . *(1/4 slice pizza unless noted)*

	Cal	Fat	Sat	Chol	Carb	Fib	Sug	Sod
Full of Life Flatbread Pizza Flax/Pistachio, 1/4.	119	6	1	1	13	1	0	125

REDUCED SODIUM (LESS THAN GENERIC):

A.C. LaRocco

	Cal	Fat	Sat	Chol	Carb	Fib	Sug	Sod
Ultra Thin Old World Veggie, 1/2	170	7	3	15	19	2	0	260
Ultra Thin Bruschetta Style, 1/2	170	8	4	16	17	1	0	290
Thin Crust Cheese & Garlic, 1/3	250	6	3	15	42	9	3	310
Thin Crust Garden Vegetarian, 1/3	250	7	3	13	41	10	3	310
Thin Crust Quattro Formaggio, 1/3	190	7	3	16	27	12	1	330
Ultra Thin Garlic Chicken Parmesan, 1/2	230	8	3	30	24	4	1	335
Thin Crust Tomato & Feta, 1/3	250	8	3	15	40	9	3	340
Thin Crust Greek Sesame, 1/3	250	8	3	17	40	9	3	350
Thin Crust Spinach & Artichoke, 1/3	210	8	4	20	27	12	1	390
America's Choice Cheese Pizza Slices	175	5	4	10	24	1	6	380
Amy's *Light in Sodium*, Spinach Pizza, 7.2 oz	440	18	6	20	54	3	5	390
Pesto, 1/3	310	12	4	10	39	2	3	480
Roasted Vegetable, No Cheese, 1/3	280	9	2	0	42	3	5	540
Margherita, 1/3	250	12	4	10	32	2	3	550
Better Bread Co Fresh Vegetable, 1/3	170	6	2	10	34	3	4	200
Roasted Garlic & Artichoke, 1/3	170	6	2	10	34	3	4	200
Margherita, 1/3	200	9	5	5	30	1	3	360
Betzio's Cheese Pan Pizza	160	5	3	10	22	1	4	320
Cheese Pizza Slices	175	5	4	10	24	1	6	380
Calif Pizza Kitchen *Crispy Thin Crust*								
Pesto Chicken, 1 pizza, 5.4 oz	420	18	6	30	44	4	3	490
Margherita, 1/3	290	13	5	20	31	2	3	520
Cheeseburger, 1/3	330	16	6	25	33	3	2	520
DiGiorno								
200 Calories Cheese & Tomato, 1/2	200	9	4	15	22	1	3	440
Deep Dish Four Cheese (small), 1/2	290	16	8	20	26	2	3	440
200 Calories Chicken w/Peppers/Onions, 1/2	200	9	4	20	22	1	2	470
200 Calories Pepperoni, 1/2	200	9	4	15	21	1	3	520
Ellio's Cheese Pizza, 2 slices	290	6	3	15	42	3	6	530
Epicurean Florentine Mushroom, 1/2	350	16	8	40	34	2	1	430
Frontera Roasted Vegetable, 1/3	220	6	3	10	31	2	2	360
Full of Life *Flatbread Pizza*								
Tomato Sauce w/3 Cheese, 9", 1/4	131	6	2	12	14	1	0	203
Mushroom, 9", 1/4	136	6	2	12	15	1	0	203
Olive & Feta Cheese, 9", 1/4	228	7	3	13	33	2	0	203
Cheese & Fresh Herb, 9", 1/4	140	6	2	12	16	1	0	206
Margherita, 9", 1/4	165	7	3	0	20	1	0	290
Thin Crust, Veggie, 1/5	250	5	0	20	30	3	5	480
Lean Cuisine Margherita Pizza-Wood Fire, 6 oz	310	7	3	15	46	3	7	460

DINNERS, LIGHT MEALS AND ENTREES
Pizza

	Cal	Fat	Sat	Chol	Carb	Fib	Sug	Sod
BBQ Chicken Pizza-Wood Fire, 6 oz	340	7	2	35	48	2	11	430
Spinach & Mushroom Deep Dish, 6.1 oz	340	7	3	10	52	2	5	430
Mushroom Pizza, 6 oz	300	5	2	5	50	4	5	470
Roasted Veg Deep Dish,6 oz	320	5	2	5	52	3	6	480
Deluxe Pizza, 6 oz	340	8	3	20	49	4	6	510
Life Choices/Living Right Cheese Mini, 1	240	7	3	10	33	3	4	320
Veggie Deluxe Mini, 1 pizza	220	5	2	5	33	4	5	345
Life Choices *OrganiCuisine* Veg No Cheese	150	5	2	5	21	4	2	440
OrganiCuisine, Mushroom/Onion, 1/4	150	5	2	5	21	4	2	440
OrganiCuisine, Chicken & Spinach, 1/4	140	4	2	10	21	4	1	460
OrganiCuisine 3 Cheese, 1/4	180	7	4	15	21	3	2	520
Macabee Kosher Foods Passover Pizza, 1/3	357	9	5	19	53	5	17	520
Market Day Cheese Pizza, 1/4	270	13	6	25	25	2	2	390
Margherita Flatbread, 1/3	240	8	4	15	31	1	2	490
Mystic Fire Roasted Veggie, 1/4	240	9	4	20	31	2	2	390
Cheese, 1/3	360	15	8	30	33	2	5	490
Supreme, 1/4	290	13	6	25	30	2	2	520
Newman's Own *Thin & Crispy*								
Roasted Garlic & Chicken, 1/3	270	10	4	30	31	2	3	540
O Organics Roasted Veg & Cheese, 1/2	250	7	4	15	39	2	5	460
Spinach & Cheese, 1/2	240	7	2	10	38	2	4	530
Pacifc Natural Foods BBQ Chicken, 1/3	270	9	5	25	30	1	3	520
Herb Garlic Chicken, 1/3	270	9	5	25	30	1	3	520
Reggio's Dinner Size, Cheese	330	12	5	20	41	2	2	420
Dinner Size, Grilled Vegetable	320	11	4	15	42	3	3	420
Dinner Size, Sausage	380	16	4	15	41	2	2	520
Rising Moon Organics Grilled Veggie, 1/2	360	15	9	20	41	7	3	480
Pesto & Buffalo Mozzarella, 1/2	380	16	9	30	43	6	3	500
Rustic Crust Old World Flatbread Pizza								
Basil Pesto & Roasted Red Pepper, 1/5	130	1	0	0	27	0	1	200
Ultimate Cheese & Herb, 1/8	140	3	2	5	23	0	1	210
Roasted Veg, 1/3	232	8	3	3	30	2	5	432
Safeway Select Ultra Thin Crust								
BBQ-Style Chicken, 1/4	250	10	5	35	23	1	5	430
Garlic Chicken, 1/3	320	12	5	35	31	1	1	460
ShopRite Cheese Pizza Slices, 1 slice	175	5	4	10	24	1	6	380
SuperFoodsRx Kitchen Turkey/Spinach, 1/3	260	7	3	20	41	10	3	320
Veggie, 1/3	260	8	3	15	41	10	3	360
Four Cheese, 1/3	270	9	3	20	40	9	3	380
Tofutti Pizza Pizzaz, 1 slice	175	5	2	0	24	0	11	320
Tombstone Light Veggie, 1/5	230	6	2	10	31	4	5	510
Uno Margherita Flatbread, 1/3	250	8	4	15	32	1	3	490
Wegmans *Italian Classics* Margherita, 1/3	270	9	4	20	33	1	3	380
Italian Classics Capicola & Salami, 1/3	290	11	5	30	32	1	3	510
Weight Watchers Smart Ones								
Veg Pizza Minis, 4	270	7	4	10	41	6	4	470
Cheese Pizza Minis, 4	270	7	4	10	38	5	4	480
Wild Harvest Organic Margherita, 1/3	230	9	5	25	27	2	3	260
Spinach & Feta, 1/3	260	11	6	30	28	2	3	350

BREAD PIZZA
(also see Pockets/Sandwiches/Wraps, pg 150)

REDUCED SODIUM (LESS THAN GENERIC):

	Cal	Fat	Sat	Chol	Carb	Fib	Sug	Sod
Ian's French Bread Pizza, Wheat Free	220	8	0	0	34	3	2	350
Macabee Kosher Foods Cheese Bagel Pizza, 1	150	5	3	12	18	0	1	340

	Cal	Fat	Sat	Chol	Carb	Fib	Sug	Sod
MacaBabies Mozzarella, 4	200	8	4	20	25	2	2	420
Mendelsohn's Pizza Bagel, 1	232	6	3	20	19	1	7	300

PIZZA FIXINGS

	Cal	Fat	Sat	Chol	Carb	Fib	Sug	Sod
Pizza crust, mix, 1/4	160	2	0	0	33	1	2	340
Refrig, thin crust, 1/5	180	5	1	0	29	1	3	360
Refrig, regular, 1/6	160	2	1	0	31	1	4	470
Pizza sauce, ready-to-use, 1/4 cup	40	2	0	0	9	1	3	410

Brands . . .

PIZZA KITS

	Cal	Fat	Sat	Chol	Carb	Fib	Sug	Sod
Gallo Lea Whole Wheat Pizza Kit, 1/4 pizza	160	1	0	0	32	4	3	6

PIZZA CRUST AND DOUGH

FROZEN/REFRIGERATED

	Cal	Fat	Sat	Chol	Carb	Fib	Sug	Sod
Better Bread Co Dough Ball, 1/6	110	3	0	0	30	1	3	95
Kinnikinnick 10" Pizza, 1 slice	110	3	1	20	20	1	4	110
Longo's Tavern Style Crusts, 1/8	70	1	0	0	11	1	0	45
Sicilian Crusts, 1/8	160	1	0	0	32	2	1	85

REDUCED SODIUM (LESS THAN GENERIC):

	Cal	Fat	Sat	Chol	Carb	Fib	Sug	Sod
Kinnikinnick Personal Size Pizza Crust, 1/2	248	7	1	26	41	5	4	180

CRUST MIXES

	Cal	Fat	Sat	Chol	Carb	Fib	Sug	Sod
Authenic Foods Pizza Crust, 1/8 of 11"	130	2	1	0	27	2	1	90
Chébé Pizza Crust Mix, 1/10	70	0	0	0	17	0	0	103
Gallo Lea LS Pizza Kit (includes sauce), 1/4	160	1	0	0	32	4	3	63
Lucini Cinque e Cinque, all varieties, 1/6	160	3	0	0	24	5	5	25

REDUCED SODIUM (LESS THAN GENERIC):

	Cal	Fat	Sat	Chol	Carb	Fib	Sug	Sod
'Cause Your Special, 1/6 of 10"	130	0	0	0	31	1	2	231
Low Carbolicious Sauce & Crust Mix, 1/8	120	8	1	0	4	1	1	190
Namaste Foods Pizza Crust Mix, 1 slice	90	0	0	0	22	1	0	190

READY-TO-USE CRUSTS

Some of the following crusts may be in the refrigerated section.

	Cal	Fat	Sat	Chol	Carb	Fib	Sug	Sod
Better Bread Co Pizza Crust, 1/3	10	0	0	0	2	0	0	25
Ener-G Rice Shell, 1/8 of 10" or 1/4 of 6"	60	3	0	0	7	2	1	65
Yeast-Free Rice Shell, 6", 1/4	70	3	0	0	11	1	0	85
Yeast-Free Rice Shell, 10", 1/8	90	3	0	0	14	1	0	105
Kinnikinnick Gluten Free 10" Pizza Crust, sl	110	3	1	20	20	1	4	110
Mama Mary's 12" 100% Whole Wheat, 1/6	90	3	1	0	16	3	0	125
12" Thin & Crispy, 1/6	120	4	1	0	18	1	0	135
Meijer 7" Thin Pizza Crust, 1/2	90	1	0	0	17	1	1	115
12" Thin Pizza Crust, 1/6	100	1	0	0	18	1	1	120
Rustic Crust Napoli Herb, 1/8	80	3	0	0	12	1	2	115

REDUCED SODIUM (LESS THAN GENERIC):

	Cal	Fat	Sat	Chol	Carb	Fib	Sug	Sod
Birrittella's Pizza Dough, 1/8	150	2	1	0	30	2	1	190
Boboli 12" Whole Wheat Thin Crust, 1/6	120	3	1	0	22	4	2	230
Deli-catessan								
Pizza/Focaccia Thin Crusts, 1/3	80	3	0	0	9	3	1	40
Mama Mary's 7" Thin & Crispy, 1/2	130	4	1	0	21	0	0	150
12" Brick Oven Style, 1/6	154	5	0	0	23	1	0	153
7" Original, 1/2	187	6	1	0	28	1	0	185
Meijer Classic 7" Pizza Crust, 1/2	150	2	0	0	27	1	1	180
Classic 12" or Square Pizza Crust, 1/6	150	2	0	0	27	1	1	180
Whole Wheat, 1/6	140	2	0	0	27	2	1	190
Rustic Crust								
Napoli Herb (Gluten Free), 1/8	80	3	0	0	12	1	2	115
Pizza Originale, 1/8	120	2	0	0	25	1	1	160

DINNERS, LIGHT MEALS AND ENTREES
Pockets, Sandwiches and Wraps

	Cal	Fat	Sat	Chol	Carb	Fib	Sug	Sod
Ultimate Whole Grain, 1/8	110	1	0	0	25	4	0	160
Classic Sourdough, 1/8	140	1	0	0	28	0	1	170
Great Grains, 1/8	140	2	0	0	28	5	0	190
Italian Herb, 1/8	140	2	1	0	25	0	1	200
Cheesy Herb or Tuscan 6 Grain, 1/8 (avg)	135	2	1	5	25	1	1	210

PIZZA SAUCE *(1/4 cup unless noted)*

	Cal	Fat	Sat	Chol	Carb	Fib	Sug	Sod
Casa Visco Pizza Sauce	40	3	1	0	6	1	3	110
Cento Fully Prepared Pizza Sauce	30	0	0	0	5	1	3	140
DeLallo Italian Style	30	0	0	0	7	2	4	105
Gefen Classic Italian	40	2	0	0	6	2	4	120
FF Pizza Sauce	34	0	0	0	7	2	4	120
Palmieri Pizza Sauce	50	3	0	0	5	1	4	60

REDUCED SODIUM (LESS THAN GENERIC):

	Cal	Fat	Sat	Chol	Carb	Fib	Sug	Sod
Dei Fratelli								
Pizza Sauce or Presto! Pizza Sauce	30	0	0	0	5	1	4	230
Don Pepino Pizza Sauce	45	3	0	0	4	1	2	230
Eden Organic Pizza - Pasta Sauce	33	2	0	0	5	3	2	150
Enrico's All Natural	35	2	0	0	6	0	5	150
Food Club Pizza Sauce	40	1	0	0	7	2	3	220
Furmano's Chunky Deep Dish Style	15	0	0	0	3	1	1	190
Giant Pizza Sauce	40	1	0	0	7	2	3	220
LE Roselli's Pizza Sauce	20	1	0	0	3	1	1	150
Meijer Pizza Sauce (canned)	40	1	0	0	7	2	3	220
Muir Glen Pizza Sauce	40	1	0	0	6	2	3	230
Pastene California Pizza Sauce	30	1	0	0	5	1	3	230
Rosa Fully Prepared Pizza Sauce	45	2	0	0	6	2	4	190
Sclafani Special Pizza Sauce	45	3	0	0	4	1	2	230

POCKETS, SANDWICHES AND WRAPS

	Cal	Fat	Sat	Chol	Carb	Fib	Sug	Sod
Pocket sandwich, cheese, 4.5 oz	290	9	4	20	38	3	5	450
Beef and cheese, 4.5 oz	360	18	9	50	36	1	5	830
Croissant sandwich w/chicken/broccoli/cheese	300	11	4	35	37	5	5	640
Wrap, chicken caesar	230	11	4	55	22	14	1	820
Panini, roast beef and cheddar, 6 oz	430	21	9	55	39	4	3	1070

Brands . . . *(4.5 oz serving unless noted)*
FROZEN/REFRIGERATED
REDUCED SODIUM (LESS THAN GENERIC):

	Cal	Fat	Sat	Chol	Carb	Fib	Sug	Sod
Amy's Broccoli/Cheese Pocket Sandwich, 4.5 oz	300	12	3	10	40	5	3	350
Cheese Pizza Pocket Sandwich, 4.5 oz	300	10	4	15	42	4	5	450
Spinach Pizza Pocket Sandwich, 4.5 oz	280	4	0	15	47	3	3	460
Aunt Trudy's Fillo Pocket Sandwich								
Roasted Sweet Potato, 5 oz	310	12	2	0	45	4	0	270
Roasted Veg, 5 oz	240	11	1	0	33	3	1	280
3 Bean Veggie, 5 oz	260	7	1	0	42	5	0	300
Eggplant & Roasted Peppers, 5 oz	210	7	1	0	34	3	0	310
Samosa, 5 oz	260	10	2	0	39	3	2	320
Mexicali Veg, 5 oz	230	7	1	0	38	3	0	350
Mushroom & Leek, 5 oz	190	6	1	0	32	3	0	380
Spinach & Potato, 5 oz	250	9	1	0	40	4	0	380
Asian Vegetable, 5 oz	240	10	2	0	34	3	2	390
Bob Evans Pretzel Pigs in a Blanket, 1	130	8	-	15	11	0	-	260
Pigs in a Blanket, Sausage & Cheese	160	6	-	10	23	1	-	380
Dr Praeger's Veggie Pocket, 2.8 oz	150	5	0	0	22	5	2	240
Tex Mex Veggie Pocket, 2.8 oz	150	5	0	0	24	5	5	320

	Cal	Fat	Sat	Chol	Carb	Fib	Sug	Sod
Foster Farms *Great Bites*								
Santa Fe Mini Cheeseburger, 1	100	4	0	15	9	0	1	180
All Am Mini Chicken Cheeseburger, 1	90	4	0	15	9	0	1	200
Guiltless Gourmet								
Mediterranean Spinach Wrap, 5.8 oz	220	6	2	5	39	6	2	410
Black Bean Chipotle Wrap, 5.8 oz	230	6	1	0	47	7	5	450
Ian's Mini Chicken Sandwich, 2.5 oz	184	5	1	20	27	1	3	305
Lean Cuisine Philly Style Steak/Cheese Panini	320	9	4	30	39	4	4	540
Lean Pockets Four Cheese Pizza	270	5	3	20	42	2	10	490
Smucker's *Uncrustables*								
PB & Honey, Grape Jelly, or Strawberry	210	9	2	0	26	3	9	230
Peanut Butter & Grape Jelly or Strawberry	210	9	2	0	25	2	9	240
Vennitti's *Stuffed Sandwich* Classic Meatball	290	9	4	20	39	1	2	350
Stuffed Sandwich Cheese Pizza	280	6	4	15	41	2	3	420
Stuffed Sandwich Beef Tacp	331	11	6	40	39	4	-	423
Stuffed Sandwich Pepperoni Pizza	340	12	5	25	42	2	2	460
Weight Watchers Smart Ones								
Mini Cheeseburger, 1	200	9	4	25	20	3	4	360
Chicken/Mushroom Smart Mini Wrap, 1	220	5	2	15	30	7	4	510
White Castle Hamburgers, 2	260	13	5	25	25	1	3	350

QUICHES, PIES AND SOUFFLES

	Cal	Fat	Sat	Chol	Carb	Fib	Sug	Sod
Pot pie, turkey, 7 oz	350	18	6	32	35	2	-	695
Beef, 7 oz	449	24	9	38	44	2	1	737
Chicken, 7 oz	434	26	9	37	39	2	7	745
Souffle, spinach, 8 oz	234	18	8	160	8	1	3	770
Quiche loraine, 6.5 oz	380	25	7	175	22	1	4	770

Brands . . . *(7 oz serving unless noted)*

FROZEN/REFRIGERATED

	Cal	Fat	Sat	Chol	Carb	Fib	Sug	Sod
Garden Lites Butternut Squash Souffle, 7 oz	180	2	1	60	34	5	18	100
REDUCED SODIUM (LESS THAN GENERIC):								
Blake's All Natural Chicken Pot Pie, 8 oz	370	17	7	25	40	3	2	380
All Natural Turkey Pot Pie	370	16	6	20	40	3	2	380
All Natural Chicken or Turkey Pie (all meat)	360	18	7	25	34	1	2	380
Chicken Pot Pie, 8 oz	340	17	8	30	34	5	1	470
Fillo Factory Eggplant/Red Pepper Fillo Pie, 5 oz	230	9	2	0	35	3	5	310
Broccoli & Cheese Fillo Pie, 4.9 oz	290	16	8	40	25	2	2	330
Garden Lites Zucchini Souffle, 7 oz	140	2	0	20	24	3	5	320
Broccoli Souffle, 7 oz	140	2	0	20	23	5	5	340
Roasted Vegetable Souffle, 7 oz	140	2	0	20	24	3	8	350
Lean on Me Baking Co Gluten Free Quiche								
Mushroom & Swiss 5 oz	120	4	2	15	3	0	2	300
Spinach & Swiss, 5 oz	120	4	2	15	3	0	2	310
Tomato, Basil, Onion & Mozzarella, 5 oz	130	5	3	15	4	0	2	340
Broccoli & Cheddar, 5 oz	130	5	4	15	3	0	2	350

SIDE DISHES

(also see Pasta/Noodles–Side Dishes, pg 205)

Potatoes and onion rings:

	Cal	Fat	Sat	Chol	Carb	Fib	Sug	Sod
Mashed potatoes, instant, 1/3 cup mix	80	0	0	0	18	1	0	21
w/butter, instant, 1/4 cup mix	90	1	0	0	20	1	1	420
Hash browns, plain, frozen, 1/2 cup	86	1	0	0	19	2	1	23
Potato pancake, mix, 1 med	99	5	1	35	10	1	1	283
French fries, seasoned, frozen, 3 oz	120	4	1	20	20	2	1	360

151

DINNERS, LIGHT MEALS AND ENTREES
Side Dishes

	Cal	Fat	Sat	Chol	Carb	Fib	Sug	Sod
Onion Rings, breaded, frozen, 3 oz	220	11	2	0	27	1	5	390
Stuffed potato, cheese, 5 oz	200	9	3	0	24	1	9	550
Scalloped potatoes, mix, 1 oz	100	1	0	0	21	1	1	570
Salads:								
Cole slaw, prepared, 1/2 cup	146	9	2	4	14	2	12	194
Tuna salad, 1/3 cup	192	9	3	13	10	0	5	412
3 bean salad, 1/2 cup	113	0	0	0	26	3	18	495
Potato salad, 1/2 cup	179	10	1	86	14	2	8	661
Macaroni salad, prepared, 3/4 cup	330	22	5	15	28	2	8	800
Mix, 2/3 cup	180	1	0	0	37	2	5	920
Vegetables:								
Green beans and almonds, frozen, 1/2 cup	60	3	0	0	5	2	2	95
Corn in butter sauce, frozen, 1/2 cup	150	3	1	0	28	2	5	260
Succotash, canned, 1/2 cup	80	1	0	0	18	3	0	282
Broccoli w/butter sauce, frozen, 1/2 cup	50	2	1	5	7	2	2	330
Spinach, creamed, frozen, 1/2 cup	169	13	4	16	9	2	3	335
Peas and onions in sauce, frozen, 1/2 cup	60	0	0	0	11	3	0	340
Broccoli w/cheese sauce, frozen, 1/2 cup	90	5	3	5	8	1	4	490

Brands . . . *(1/2 cup serving unless noted)*

PASTA SIDES *(see Pasta/Noodles–Sides Dishes, pg 205)*

POTATOES AND ONION RINGS
FROZEN/REFRIGERATED

	Cal	Fat	Sat	Chol	Carb	Fib	Sug	Sod
Hash browns – Most brands within generic average (23mg).								
Alexia Sweet Potato Julienne Fries, 3 oz	150	6	1	0	24	3	4	140
Betty Crocker Quicksides								
Sour Cream & Chives, 2/3 cup	210	12	6	20	23	2	1	135
Cascadian Farm Organic								
Crinkle or Straight Cut French Fries, 3 oz	100	4	1	0	17	2	1	10
Shoe String Fries, 3 oz	110	5	1	0	17	2	1	10
Wedge Cut Oven Fries, 3 oz	100	3	0	0	17	2	1	10
Country Style, 3 oz	50	0	0	0	12	1	0	10
Dr Praeger's Sweet Potato Pancakes, 1	80	2	0	0	12	3	6	140
Golden Sweet Potato Pancakes, 1	80	4	1	0	10	0	4	20
Hanover Candied Sweet Potatoes, 5 oz	300	1	1	0	73	3	47	130
Ian's Alphatoes Potato Fries, 3 oz	130	6	1	0	20	1	1	135
Kineret Potato Latke, 1.5 oz	80	4	1	0	10	1	1	115
Ore-Ida Steam n' Mash Sweet Potatoes, 4.3 oz	90	0	0	0	20	3	7	30
Potatoes O'Brien, 3 oz	60	0	0	0	14	2	1	40
Simply Potatoes Homestyle Slices, 2/3 cup	90	0	0	0	21	2	0	75
Wegmans Sweet Potato Fries, 3 oz	140	3	1	0	23	4	7	115
Woodstock Crinkle Cut Oven Fries, 3 oz	140	4	0	0	25	2	1	25
REDUCED SODIUM (LESS THAN GENERIC):								
Alexia Sweet Potato Julienne Fries, 3 oz	150	6	1	0	24	3	4	140
Oven Crinkles, Classic, 3 oz	120	4	0	0	19	3	0	170
Yukon Gold Julienne Fries, 3 oz	130	4	0	0	22	2	0	180
Oven Crinkles, Onion & Garlic, 3 oz	110	4	0	0	18	3	0	190
Betty Crocker Quicksides Red Potato, 2/3 c	170	7	5	20	23	2	2	200
Dr Praeger's Potato Pancakes, 1	100	4	0	15	13	3	1	190
Golden Potato Pancakes, 1	70	3	0	5	10	1	2	190
McCain Sweet Potato	160	7	1	0	25	3	6	190
Meijer Potato Sticks, 2/3 cup	170	11	2	0	15	2	0	150
Ore-Ida Onion Ringers, 3 oz	180	10	2	0	2	2	3	160
Golden Patties, 2.4 oz	170	8	2	0	15	2	1	170
Simply Potatoes Mashed Sweet, 1/2 cup	110	1	0	5	22	2	14	160

	Cal	Fat	Sat	Chol	Carb	Fib	Sug	Sod
Diced Potatoes w/Onion, 2/3 cup	80	0	0	0	19	2	0	170
Country Style Mashed, 1/2 cup	110	4	2	10	17	2	2	180

MIXES

Mashed potatoes – *Most brands within generic average (21mg), flavored varieties may contain added sodium.*

	Cal	Fat	Sat	Chol	Carb	Fib	Sug	Sod
Gefen Potato Pancake Latke Mix, SF	90	1	0	0	19	0	1	20
Potato Pancake Mix, 1/7	30	1	1	21	5	1	0	81
Kineret Potato Latke Mix, NSA	130	1	0	0	30	1	2	115
Streits LS Potato Pancake Mix, 1.5 oz	100	1	0	0	20	1	1	140

PREPARED SALADS

	Cal	Fat	Sat	Chol	Carb	Fib	Sug	Sod
Hanover 3 Bean Salad, 3.1 oz	100	1	0	0	22	3	14	120
Vegetable Salad, 3.1 oz	80	0	0	0	17	3	15	120

VEGETABLE SIDES

(also see Vegetables–Frozen, pg 189)

FROZEN/REFRIGERATED

	Cal	Fat	Sat	Chol	Carb	Fib	Sug	Sod
Birds Eye *Steamfresh* Long Grain White Rice w/Mixed Vegetables	190	1	0	0	42	2	3	15
Green Giant Green Beans & Almonds, 3/4 c	40	2	0	0	4	1	1	80

REDUCED SODIUM (LESS THAN GENERIC):

	Cal	Fat	Sat	Chol	Carb	Fib	Sug	Sod
Alexia Onion Rings, 3 oz (6)	240	13	2	0	27	2	2	150
Roasted Potatoes w/Mushrooms, 4.8 oz	140	8	1	0	15	3	0	190
Roasted Sweet Potatoes & Veg, 4.4 oz	160	6	1	0	21	5	6	190
Birds Eye Tuscan Vegs in Tomato Sauce	50	2	0	0	7	2	3	180
Steamfresh Lightly Sauced Corn w/Butter	110	2	0	0	21	1	5	210
Dr. Praeger's Broccoli Pancakes, 2 oz	80	4	0	0	9	2	1	170
Spinach Pancakes, 1.3 oz	80	4	0	0	9	2	0	190
Golden Black Bean Pancakes, 1.4 oz	70	3	1	0	10	0	1	180
Baja or Texas Corn Fritters, 1.4 oz	100	4	1	10	14	1	2	200
Broccoli or Spinach Pancakes, 1.4 oz	70	3	1	0	10	1	1	210
Veg or Aucchini Pancakes, 1.4 oz	70	3	1	0	10	1	1	210
Wegmans *Food You Feel Good About, Special Blends* Artichokes/Asparagus w/Lemon Butter	50	2	1	0	7	3	2	150
Brussels Sprouts in Butter Sauce, 2/3 cup	70	2	1	5	9	3	4	200

ETHNIC FOODS

See RESOURCES, page 305, for a partial list of manufacturers and retailers offering low-salt products online or visit **LowSaltFoods.com** *for additional sources.*

ETHNIC FOODS

ASIAN – ADDITIVES AND SEASONINGS

	Cal	Fat	Sat	Chol	Carb	Fib	Sug	Sod
Rice vinegar, 1 tbsp	0	0	0	0	0	0	0	0
Seasoned, 1 tbsp	20	0	0	0	5	0	5	240
Mirin sweet cooking wine, 1 tbsp	20	0	0	0	5	0	3	55
Curry paste, 1 tsp	8	0	0	0	1	0	0	210
Fried rice seasoning mix, 1 1/3 tbsp	30	0	0	0	6	0	0	490
Miso/soybean paste, 1 tbsp	28	1	0	0	4	1	1	522

Brands . . . *(1 tsp unless noted)*

	Cal	Fat	Sat	Chol	Carb	Fib	Sug	Sod
Ginger People Pickled Sushi Ginger, 1 oz	20	0	0	0	5	0	5	0
Mitsukan Mirin Sweet Cooking Seasoning, 1 tbsp	35	0	0	0	8	0	4	15
Sambal Oelek Ground Fresh Chili Paste	0	0	0	0	0	0	0	110
Tiger Tiger Minced Red or Green Chili Paste	13	0	0	0	3	1	1	100
Minced Coriander or Ginger Paste (avg)	11	0	0	0	3	1	1	100
Minced Garlic Paste	16	0	0	0	2	1	1	100

REDUCED SODIUM (LESS THAN GENERIC):

	Cal	Fat	Sat	Chol	Carb	Fib	Sug	Sod
A Taste of Thai Panang Curry Paste, 1 tsp	10	0	0	0	2	0	1	150

SEASONING MIXES

	Cal	Fat	Sat	Chol	Carb	Fib	Sug	Sod
A Taste of Thai Spicy Peanut Bake, 1/4 envl	50	2	1	0	8	1	7	140
NOH Korean Kim Chee Mix	10	0	0	0	2	0	1	80
Sun-Bird Mongolian Beef Seasoning Mix, 2 tsp	25	0	0	0	6	0	4	0
Phad Thai Mix, 1 tbsp	25	0	0	0	6	0	4	45

ASIAN – CONDIMENTS

	Cal	Fat	Sat	Chol	Carb	Fib	Sug	Sod
Wasabi, powder, 1 tsp	0	0	0	0	0	0	0	0
Paste or prepared, 1 tsp	15	1	0	0	3	0	0	100
Chinese mustard, 1 tsp	10	0	0	0	1	0	0	75

Brands . . . *(1 tsp unless noted)*

	Cal	Fat	Sat	Chol	Carb	Fib	Sug	Sod
Dynasty Sweet & Hot Mustard	15	0	0	0	2	0	2	35
Chinese-Style Mustard	5	0	0	0	1	0	0	45
Mee Tu Chinese Style Mustard	2	0	0	0	1	0	0	40
Polynesian Chinese Style Mustard	2	0	0	0	1	0	0	40
Roland Chinese Hot Mustard	2	0	0	0	1	0	0	40
Sun Luck Hot Mustard Paste	10	0	0	0	1	0	0	50

ASIAN – DINNERS AND MEALS

(also see Dinners/Meals–Frozen, pg 138)

	Cal	Fat	Sat	Chol	Carb	Fib	Sug	Sod
Sweet and sour chicken, 10 oz	408	6	2	21	69	3	32	708
Chow mein, chicken, w/egg roll, 9 oz	210	7	4	30	28	3	3	850
Rice bowl w/chicken, 10 oz	357	4	1	45	63	2	12	943
Oriental beef, 9 oz	250	7	4	30	31	3	3	960
Fried rice, shrimp, 10 oz	224	2	0	56	40	6	6	976
Stir fry, shrimp, 9.8 oz	200	2	0	105	28	5	17	1330
Lo mein, shrimp, 10 oz	458	15	3	54	67	4	20	1617

Brands . . . *(10 oz serving unless noted)*
The minimum serving size for the following items is 8.1 ounces. Serving sizes 8 ounces or less are listed in Asian–Entrees and Light Meals, pg 156.

FROZEN/REFRIGERATED

REDUCED SODIUM (LESS THAN GENERIC):

	Cal	Fat	Sat	Chol	Carb	Fib	Sug	Sod
Amy's Brown Rice & Vegetable Bowl, 10 oz	260	9	1	0	36	5	7	270
Thai Stir-Fry, 9.5 oz	310	11	7	0	45	5	2	420

155

ETHNIC FOODS
Asian – Dinners and Meals

	Cal	Fat	Sat	Chol	Carb	Fib	Sug	Sod
An-Joy Gen'l Tsao's Chicken, 10.1 oz	540	17	5	95	70	2	28	360
Sesame Chicken, 10.1 oz.............................	500	19	5	95	56	1	19	510
Healthy Choice								
Cafe Steamers Sesame Chicken, 10.4 oz.....	340	5	1	30	55	4	19	330
Cafe Steamers Sweet/Spicy Orange Chicken	310	3	1	30	52	4	16	380
Cafe Steamers Pineapple Chicken, 10.6 oz ..	330	5	1	30	53	4	21	400
Cafe Steamers Gen'l Tso's Chicken, 10.9 oz.	300	3	1	30	53	4	12	500
Cafe Steamers Thai-Style Chicken & Veg.....	260	5	1	35	36	4	10	500
Cafe Steamers Lemongrass Chicken/Shrimp	280	4	1	45	42	6	11	530
Lean Cuisine Thai Chicken Spring Rolls, 8 oz	200	7	2	25	23	1	4	390
Garlic Chicken Spring Rolls, 8 oz	200	8	2	20	24	2	4	420
Hunan Stir Fry w/Beef, 8.5 oz....................	280	8	2	20	36	5	12	460
Sweet & Sour Chicken, 10 oz.....................	300	3	0	30	51	2	16	490
Beef & Broccoli, 9 oz	270	5	2	20	43	2	9	520
Beef Chow Fun, 9 oz	320	5	2	20	54	3	18	520
Asian-Style Pot Stickers, 9 oz	260	4	1	10	49	2	9	530
Chicken Fried Rice, 9 oz...........................	260	5	1	25	41	4	5	530
Lemongrass Chicken, 9 oz.........................	260	6	1	25	33	5	7	550
Szechuan Style Stir Fry w/Shrimp, 9 oz	210	2	0	50	37	5	11	550
Chicken Chow Mein w/Rice, 9 oz	240	4	1	25	39	3	3	550
Chicken in Peanut Sauce, 9 oz	280	6	1	25	35	5	5	550

SKILLET MEALS, MEAL KITS AND HELPERS
Some brands require added ingredients, which may raise sodium content.

FROZEN/REFRIGERATED
REDUCED SODIUM (LESS THAN GENERIC):

	Cal	Fat	Sat	Chol	Carb	Fib	Sug	Sod
Contessa Sweet & Sour Chicken, prep, 9.5 oz	400	12	3	35	61	2	22	480
Sweet & Sour Shrimp, 10 oz	250	1	0	65	48	4	16	490
Kahiki Sweet & Sour Chicken....................	310	8	-	-	54	1	-	430
Orange Chicken....................................	330	5	-	-	62	2	-	530
Tai Pei *Stir Fry Creations* Sweet/Sour Pork .	470	7	2	30	85	7	27	340
Skillet Meals Sweet/Sour Chicken, 12 oz ...	460	8	1	25	82	2	31	430

SHELF-STABLE
REDUCED SODIUM (LESS THAN GENERIC):

	Cal	Fat	Sat	Chol	Carb	Fib	Sug	Sod
Wanchai Ferry Sweet & Sour Chicken	170	0	0	0	41	1	13	270
Spicy Garlic Chicken..............................	150	1	0	0	34	1	10	340
Cashew Chicken	200	4	1	0	38	1	8	450
Orange Chicken....................................	210	1	0	0	48	1	15	460

(ASIAN – ENTREES AND LIGHT MEALS)

	Cal	Fat	Sat	Chol	Carb	Fib	Sug	Sod
*Sushi, cucumber roll, 4 pc	98	0	0	0	22	1	4	203
Vegetable roll, 4 pc	212	1	0	0	44	2	4	255
Shrimp and avocado, 4 pc.........................	300	5	1	44	38	1	4	283
Spicy shrimp, 4 pc	240	4	0	30	38	1	2	440
Eel roll, 4 pc..	300	3	1	22	58	1	4	460
California Roll, 4 pc	195	1	0	0	45	1	6	480
Crab Roll, 4 pc.......................................	220	2	1	4	42	2	6	520
Egg roll, pork, 3 oz.................................	189	6	1	12	25	2	5	446
Chicken, 3 oz...	168	3	0	12	24	3	6	459
Vegetable, 3 oz......................................	167	4	1	0	27	2	6	477
Fried rice, 1 cup.....................................	228	3	1	32	43	2	1	554
Mix, 1 cup prep......................................	25	1	0	0	47	1	3	1095

While sushi numbers are an average, the sodium content varies widely and is based on ingredients used.

	Cal	Fat	Sat	Chol	Carb	Fib	Sug	Sod

Brands ▮▮▮ (1 cup or 8 oz unless noted)

The serving size for the following items is 8 ounces or less. Items with more than 8 ounces are listed in Asian–Dinners and Meals, pg 155.

FROZEN/REFRIGERATED

	Cal	Fat	Sat	Chol	Carb	Fib	Sug	Sod
Contessa Shanghai Stir-Fry Veg, 4 oz	60	0	0	0	13	2	8	250
InnovAsian Sweet & Sour Chicken, 6.1 oz	310	7	1	15	55	1	27	250
Last Minute Gourmet Sesame Chicken w/Rice	220	6	1	25	35	0	9	450
Tai Pei Sweet & Sour Shrimp, 6.1 oz	230	3	1	15	46	1	20	95
Sweet & Sour Chicken, 6.1 oz	220	4	1	10	41	1	17	180
Garlic Shrimp or Gen'l Tso's Chicken, 5.1 oz	70	2	0	15	10	2	5	290
Bourbon Street Chicken, 6 oz	180	3	0	10	34	2	13	330
Kung Pao Chicken, 7.1 oz	220	5	1	20	34	2	10	330

EGG ROLLS AND SPRING ROLLS

FROZEN/REFRIGERATED

REDUCED SODIUM (LESS THAN GENERIC):

	Cal	Fat	Sat	Chol	Carb	Fib	Sug	Sod
Blue Horizon Thai-Style Shrimp Spring Rolls	130	4	2	0	16	1	1	210
Chinese-Style Shrimp Spring Rolls, 2.1 oz.	110	4	2	0	16	1	1	210
Thai-Style Vegetable Spring Rolls, 2.1 oz.	130	4	2	0	15	1	1	250
Indian-Style Vegetable Spring Rolls, 2.1 oz	110	4	2	0	15	1	1	250
Lucky Pot Stickers, all varieties	70	1	0	0	14	1	1	170
Original Rangoon Chicken/Cheese Roll	80	4	2	20	5	0	0	160
Pagoda Asian Style Sensations								
White Meat Chicken Mini Egg Rolls	100	5	1	3	12	1	2	200
Shanghai Kitchen Shrimp Spring Rolls, 3	100	4	1	1	20	3	5	148
Vegetable Spring Rolls, size (3)	88	3	1	0	20	3	5	149
Tai Pei Pork Egg Roll w/o sauce, 3 oz	130	6	2	15	13	2	2	330
Chicken Egg Roll w/o sauce, 3 oz	120	6	1	15	12	2	2	350
Wegmans Classics Pork/Veg Potsticker	40	2	0	5	4	0	0	70
Asian Classics Vegetable Potstickers, 0.7 oz	30	1	0	0	6	0	1	75
Asian Classics Chicken & Veg Potstickers	30	1	0	5	4	0	0	75
Asian Classics Pork & Shrimp Wontons, 2	68	2	1	14	7	0	0	96

RICE AND NOODLE DISHES

FROZEN/REFRIGERATED

	Cal	Fat	Sat	Chol	Carb	Fib	Sug	Sod
Spaa Natural Foods Fried Rice Sizzling Thai	329	5	3	0	65	1	1	101

SHELF-STABLE

REDUCED SODIUM (LESS THAN GENERIC):

	Cal	Fat	Sat	Chol	Carb	Fib	Sug	Sod
A Taste of China Szechuan Noodles, 1/2	216	6	1	0	40	1	3	338
Sweet & Sour Rice, 1/2 pkg	260	3	1	0	53	2	6	340
A Taste of Thai Pad Thai Noodles, 1/2 pkg	260	4	1	0	51	1	13	261
Coconut Ginger Noodles, 1/2 pkg	226	5	2	0	38	1	1	271
Peanut Noodles, 1/2 pkg	331	7	5	0	54	1	13	342
Pad Thai for Two, 1/2 pkg	380	2	0	0	85	3	15	340
Yellow Curry Noodles, 1 cup prep	250	6	4	0	48	1	5	350
Red Curry Noodles, 1/2 pkg	290	8	4	0	52	1	10	360
Annie Chun's Noodle Express Thai Peanut	200	7	1	0	29	1	5	300
Peanut Sauce Noodle Bowl, 1/2 bowl	280	11	1	0	40	1	5	340
Peanut Sesame Chow Mein, 1/3 pkg	280	8	1	0	42	1	6	390
Teriyaki Noodle Bowl, 1/2 bowl	200	3	0	0	38	1	5	440
Sushi Wraps Brown Rice, 1/2 pkg	150	1	0	0	30	2	0	460
Sushi Wraps White Rice, 1/2 pkg	170	1	0	0	35	1	1	460
Noodle Express, Spicy Szechuan, 1/2 pkg	170	3	0	0	29	1	4	470
Fortune Brand Yakisoba Sweet 'N' Sour								
Stir-Fry Noodles, 1/2 pkg	225	2	0	0	46	1	1	225

	Cal	Fat	Sat	Chol	Carb	Fib	Sug	Sod
POT STICKERS AND WONTONS								
FROZEN/REFRIGERATED								
Lotus Restaurant Cr Cheese Wonton	120	8	2	10	9	0	0	110
REDUCED SODIUM (LESS THAN GENERIC):								
Lucky Pot Stickers, all varieties (3)............	70	1	0	0	14	1	1	170
SUSHI								
FROZEN/REFRIGERATED								
Wegmans Tuna Pacific Sushi, 5.6 oz............	210	4	1	15	32	2	1	115
Vegetable Roll, 5 oz................................	190	4	1	0	34	3	3	115
Salmon California Roll, 5.6 oz	240	8	2	15	32	2	1	120
REDUCED SODIUM (LESS THAN GENERIC):								
Wegmans Wasabi Roll, 6 oz	300	12	2	30	31	1	2	200
Avocado Roll, 4 oz	460	10	2	0	71	16	2	200

ASIAN – FORTUNE COOKIES

	Cal	Fat	Sat	Chol	Carb	Fib	Sug	Sod
Fortune cookie, 1...	30	0	0	0	7	0	4	22

Brands . . . *Most brands within generic average.*

ASIAN – FRIED RICE

(see Asian–Entrees/Light Meals, pg 156)

ASIAN – NOODLES

	Cal	Fat	Sat	Chol	Carb	Fib	Sug	Sod
Bean thread/Cellophane noodles, 2 oz	200	0	0	0	46	2	0	3
Rice noodles (rice sticks)................................	193	0	0	0	48	0	0	110
Chow mein/Soba noodles, 2 oz	200	1	0	0	39	2	1	390
Udon noodles, 2 oz..	190	2	0	0	37	3	5	660
Somen noodles, 2 oz	203	1	0	0	42	3	1	1049

Brands . . . *(2 oz unless noted)*
FROZEN/REFRIGERATED

	Cal	Fat	Sat	Chol	Carb	Fib	Sug	Sod
House Foods Black or White Shirataki Noodles .	5	0	0	0	2	1	0	0
Tofu Shirataki, 4 oz	20	1	0	0	3	2	0	15
Orchids Shirataki, White, 1.8 oz....................	6	0	0	0	2	0	0	5

SHELF-STABLE
Bean thread/cellophane noodles – *Most brands within generic average (3mg).*
Annie Chun's

	Cal	Fat	Sat	Chol	Carb	Fib	Sug	Sod
Maifun or Pad Thai Rice Noodles....................	210	0	0	0	50	0	0	75
Eden Kuzu Pasta, Japanese	200	0	0	0	48	2	0	0
100% Buckwheat Soba or Bifun Wheat-free Pasta.	200	1	0	0	43	3	2	5
Hausame (mung bean) Pasta	190	0	0	0	47	0	0	5
Kamut or Spelt Soba (avg)	200	1	0	0	38	3	1	120
Kamut or Spelt Udon (avg)..........................	200	2	0	0	38	3	0	120
Whole Grain or Wheat & Rice Udon (avg)	200	2	0	0	38	3	0	120
Hakubaku Cha Soba (Green Tea) Noodles	200	1	0	0	40	3	0	4
Itsuki Inaka Soba Noodles, 2.9 oz	280	2	0	0	54	0	0	59
JFC White Shirataki (Yam) Noodles................	0	0	0	0	1	0	0	0
Brown Shirataki (Yam) Noodles....................	5	0	0	0	2	0	0	5
Minokuni Buckwheat Noodles, 2.8 oz.............	220	2	0	0	44	2	0	60
Orchids Buckwheat Noodles, 3 oz..................	430	2	0	0	59	0	0	0
Chuka Soba, 3 oz..	227	1	0	0	47	0	0	47
Shirayuki Udon, 3.5 oz................................	100	1	0	2	20	1	0	45
Sun Luck Tomoshiraga Somen, 3 oz..............	330	15	2	0	65	2	0	70
Chuka Soba, 3 oz..	310	2	0	0	61	0	0	140
REDUCED SODIUM (LESS THAN GENERIC)								
China Boy Chow Mein Noodles....................	130	5	2	0	16	1	0	160

	Cal	Fat	Sat	Chol	Carb	Fib	Sug	Sod
Roland Low Mein or Udon Noodles	190	1	0	0	40	1	0	170
Buckwheat Soba Noodles	190	1	0	0	40	1	0	170

ASIAN – PICKLED FOODS

	Cal	Fat	Sat	Chol	Carb	Fib	Sug	Sod
Pickled ginger, 1 tbsp	30	0	0	0	7	0	5	65
Kimchee (kimchi), 2 tbsp	10	0	0	0	2	0	1	550
Brands . . .								
The Ginger People Natural Pickled Sushi Ginger	20	0	0	0	5	0	5	0
Roland Sushi Ginger, 1 tbsp	0	0	0	0	0	0	0	70
Well-Pac Kimchee, 1 oz	10	0	0	0	3	1	1	135

ASIAN – SAUCES

	Cal	Fat	Sat	Chol	Carb	Fib	Sug	Sod
Sweet and sour sauce, 1 tbsp	18	0	0	0	5	0	4	95
Duck sauce, 1 tbsp	40	0	0	0	10	1	6	130
Peanut sauce, 1 tbsp	40	2	1	0	4	1	4	135
Pad thai sauce, 1 tbsp	35	1	0	0	8	0	7	150
Chili sauce, 1 tsp	5	0	0	0	1	0	1	150
Hoisin sauce, 1 tbsp	25	1	0	0	5	0	5	245
Chinese barbecue sauce, 1 tbsp	30	1	0	0	5	0	5	250
Curry sauce, 1 tbsp	25	0	0	0	4	1	0	250
Mix, 1/5 pkg	110	7	4	0	8	1	2	860
Plum sauce, 1 tbsp	50	0	0	0	13	0	12	260
Kung pao sauce, 1 tbsp	30	1	0	0	4	0	3	350
Szechuan sauce, 1 tbsp	50	1	0	0	10	0	6	550
Stir-fry sauce, 1 tbsp	15	0	0	0	3	0	3	570
Teriyaki sauce, 1 tbsp	15	0	0	0	3	0	2	690
Lite, 1 tbsp	15	0	0	0	3	0	3	320
Oyster sauce, 1 tbsp	25	0	0	0	5	0	4	850
Bean sauce, 1 tbsp	30	0	0	0	5	1	4	875
Soy sauce, 1 tbsp	8	0	0	0	1	0	0	902
Reduced sodium, 1 tbsp	10	0	0	0	2	0	0	600
Fish sauce, 1 tbsp	15	0	0	0	1	0	0	1730
Brands . . . *(1 tbsp unless noted)*								
BEAN SAUCE								
House of Tsang Brown Bean Sauce	15	0	0	0	3	0	2	140
Sharwood's Black Bean & Red Pepper Sauce ..	9	0	0	0	1	0	1	95
Black Bean Stir-Fry Sauce	20	0	0	0	4	0	4	90
CHILI/GARLIC SAUCE								
A Taste of Thai								
Sweet Red Chili Sauce, 1 tsp	5	0	0	0	1	0	1	95
Garlic Chili Pepper Sauce, 1 tsp	5	0	0	0	1	0	1	95
Aroma Chef Thai Sweet Chili Sauce, 1 tsp	15	0	0	0	3	0	2	115
Asian Gourmet Spicy Chili & Garlic, 1 tsp	0	0	0	0	1	0	1	70
Dynasty								
Thai Style Sweet Chili Sauce, 1 tsp	15	0	0	0	3	0	2	115
Heaven & Earth								
Dragon Fire Chili Sauce	25	0	0	0	6	0	6	50
Huy Fong Foods Chili, Sriracha Hot, 1 tsp	5	0	0	0	1	0	1	100
Chili Garlic Sauce, 1 tsp	0	0	0	0	0	0	0	115
Robbie's Garlic Sauce, 1 tsp	5	0	0	0	1	0	1	70
Robert Rothschild Farm								
Thai Sweet Chili Dipping Sauce, 2 tbsp	50	0	0	0	12	0	12	55
Roland Sweet Chili Sauce, Thai Style, 1 tsp	10	0	0	0	3	0	2	60

	Cal	Fat	Sat	Chol	Carb	Fib	Sug	Sod
Sriracha Chili Sauce, 1 tsp	5	0	0	0	1	0	1	125
Sharwood's Sweet Chili & Red Pepper, 1 tsp	4	0	0	0	1	0	1	16
Sun Luck Hot Chili Sauce, 1 tsp	0	0	0	0	1	0	1	125

CURRY SAUCE/PASTE

	Cal	Fat	Sat	Chol	Carb	Fib	Sug	Sod
Ginger People Thai Green Curry Sauce	15	0	0	0	2	0	2	80
Sable & Rosenfeld Cashew Curry Sauce	35	3	0	5	3	0	1	85
Coconut Curry Sauce, 2 tbsp	60	5	2	0	3	0	1	85
Sharwood's Curry Stir-Fry Sauce	25	2	1	0	2	0	1	140
Steel's All Natural Mango Curry Sauce	19	0	0	0	5	0	5	0
World Foods								
Thai Masaman Curry, 2 tbsp	36	3	2	0	3	0	2	112
Malaysian Vegetable Curry, 2 tbsp	23	2	1	0	2	0	1	112
Malaysian Rendang Curry, 2 tbsp	64	5	4	0	4	1	3	112
Thai Red Curry, 2 tbsp	28	2	2	0	2	0	1	140

DUCK SAUCE (see Sweet/Sour Sauce, pg 161)

HOISIN/PLUM SAUCE

	Cal	Fat	Sat	Chol	Carb	Fib	Sug	Sod
Heaven & Earth Raspberry Hoisin	20	0	0	0	4	0	4	140
Jok 'n' Al Plum Sauce	8	0	0	0	2	0	1	42
Robert Rothschild Farm								
Thai Plum Garlic Dipping Sauce, 2 tbsp	60	0	0	0	15	0	14	75
Sharwood's Hoisin & Plum Sauce	13	0	0	0	3	0	2	118
REDUCED SODIUM (LESS THAN GENERIC):								
Polynesian Hoisin Sauce, 2 tbsp	40	0	0	0	10	0	8	160
Premier Japan Organic, Wheat-free	15	0	0	0	3	0	2	160

KUNG PAO/SZECHUAN SAUCE

	Cal	Fat	Sat	Chol	Carb	Fib	Sug	Sod
Sharwood's Kung Pao Sauce	25	0	0	0	6	0	4	101

LEMON SAUCE/ORANGE SAUCE

	Cal	Fat	Sat	Chol	Carb	Fib	Sug	Sod
Asian Gourmet Orange Sauce, 2 tbsp	50	0	0	0	11	0	11	75
Iron Chef Orange Sauce Glaze w/Ginger	60	0	0	0	15	0	13	100
Lee Kum Kee Orange Sauce & Glaze, 2 tbsp	80	0	0	0	19	2	15	50
Wegmans Spicy Orange Sauce,	30	0	0	0	7	0	7	105

OYSTER/FISH SAUCE

	Cal	Fat	Sat	Chol	Carb	Fib	Sug	Sod
REDUCED SODIUM (LESS THAN GENERIC):								
Orchids Oyster Sauce	10	0	0	0	3	0	2	250
Mushroom Vegetarian Oyster Sauce	18	0	0	0	5	0	2	300

PAD THAI SAUCE Most brands within generic average (150mg)

PEANUT SAUCE

	Cal	Fat	Sat	Chol	Carb	Fib	Sug	Sod
A Taste of Thai Peanut Satay Sauce	40	3	2	0	5	1	3	90
Big Acres Chipotle Peanut Sauce, 2 tbsp	60	3	0	0	6	1	3	115
Heaven & Earth Peanut Sauce	100	16	0	0	5	0	1	90
King of Siam Thai Peanut Sauce, 2 tbsp	90	5	1	0	11	1	7	100
Mr. Spice SF Thai Peanut Sauce/Marinade	25	1	0	0	3	0	2	0
Stonewall Kitchen Garlic Peanut, 2 tbsp	60	3	0	0	8	0	6	95
Thai Kitchen Satay or Spicy Satay, 2 tbsp	80	5	1	0	6	1	4	130

PLUM SAUCE (see Hoisin/Plum Sauce above)

SOY, TAMARI AND PONZU SAUCES

	Cal	Fat	Sat	Chol	Carb	Fib	Sug	Sod
REDUCED SODIUM (LESS THAN GENERIC):								
Chef Myron's Ponzu Sauce	30	2	0	0	3	0	3	220
Eden Foods Ponzu Sauce	5	0	0	0	1	0	0	340
House of Tsang LS Soy Sauce	0	0	0	0	0	0	0	320
LS Ginger Soy Sauce	10	0	0	0	2	0	0	330
Kikkoman Ponzu Lime	10	0	0	0	2	0	2	360
Ponzu	10	0	0	0	2	0	2	400

	Cal	Fat	Sat	Chol	Carb	Fib	Sug	Sod
Premier Japan Organic Ginger Tamari........	5	0	0	0	2	0	1	390
World Harbors Angostura Lite Soy..............	10	0	0	0	2	0	2	390

STIR-FRY SAUCE

	Cal	Fat	Sat	Chol	Carb	Fib	Sug	Sod
Mr. Spice SF Ginger Stir-Fry Sauce/Marinade ..	15	0	0	0	4	0	3	0
World Foods Pineapple Lemon, 1/4 jar	70	0	0	0	18	1	14	10
Burmese Pineapple Stir Fry, 2 tbsp	23	1	0	0	4	0	3	140
Tamarind Chilli Dipping/Stir-Fry, 2 tbsp	25	0	0	0	6	0	5	140

REDUCED SODIUM (LESS THAN GENERIC):

	Cal	Fat	Sat	Chol	Carb	Fib	Sug	Sod
Annie Chun's Shiitake Soy Ginger Sauce	15	0	0	0	4	0	3	180

SWEET AND SOUR SAUCE

	Cal	Fat	Sat	Chol	Carb	Fib	Sug	Sod
Ah-So Chinese-Style Duck, 2 tbsp..................	50	0	0	0	13	0	10	15
Asian Gourmet Duck Sauce, 2 tbsp.............	50	0	0	0	7	0	7	60
Dynasty Chinese Duck Sauce, 2 tbsp	80	0	0	0	19	0	10	95
Heaven and Earth Tangerine, 2 tbsp...........	25	0	0	0	6	0	6	5
House of Tsang Sweet & Sour Stir-Fry	35	0	0	0	9	0	8	75
Iron Chef Pineapple Duck Sauce, 2 tbsp........	30	0	0	0	11	0	7	65
Mr. Spice SF Sweet & Sour Sauce, 2 tbsp	45	0	0	0	10	1	9	0
Orient Chef Sweet & Sour Sauce, 2 tbsp	50	0	0	0	14	0	12	25
Rice Road Sweet & Sour w/Peanuts..............	30	0	0	0	7	0	7	35
Robbie's Sweet & Sour Sauce, 2 tbsp	50	0	0	0	12	0	12	5
Rocky Mt Mandarin Sweet n' Spicy, 2 tbsp	90	0	0	0	21	1	17	20
Sun Luck Restaurant Sweet & Sour, 1 tbsp	30	0	0	0	7	0	7	35

TERIYAKI SAUCE

	Cal	Fat	Sat	Chol	Carb	Fib	Sug	Sod
Garlic Survival Co Roasted Garlic Teriyaki......	10	0	0	0	2	0	2	125
Sable & Rosenfeld Tipsy Teriyaki, 2 tbsp	70	3	0	0	10	0	9	135

MISC SAUCES

	Cal	Fat	Sat	Chol	Carb	Fib	Sug	Sod
Ah-So Ham Glaze, 2 tbsp.............................	50	0	0	0	13	0	10	15
Bull-Dog 50% Less Salt Chuno Sauce	15	0	0	0	3	0	3	120
ChinaBlue Tangy Ginger Sauce	25	0	0	0	6	0	6	15
Ginger People Ginger Lemon Grass, 2 tbsp	100	10	0	0	4	0	3	105
Ginger Wasabi Sauce, 2 tbsp	80	7	0	0	4	0	2	115
Heaven & Earth Ginger Mint Sauce	35	0	0	0	9	1	9	10
Four Fruit..	20	1	0	0	9	0	9	10
Mee Tu All-Purpose Chinese Marinade	25	0	0	0	7	0	6	120
Neera's Spicy Tamarind Sauce, 1 tsp	15	0	0	0	5	0	5	98
Asian Tamarind Sauce, 2 tsp........................	61	0	0	0	16	0	10	110
Robt Rothschild Farm Ginger Wasabi Sauce..	10	1	0	0	1	0	1	10
Lemon Wasabi Sauce, 1 tsp.........................	20	2	1	0	1	0	0	30
Sharwood's Gen'l Tsao's Stir-Fry Sauce	20	0	0	0	4	0	3	140
Stonewall Kitchen Wasabi Ginger, 2 tbsp	50	0	0	0	13	0	12	140
World Foods Singapore Nyonya Laksa, 2 tbsp...	24	2	1	0	2	0	1	84
Malaysian Noodle Sauce, 2 tbsp	22	1	0	0	3	1	2	140

ASIAN – SEASONING MIXES

(see Asian–Additives/Seasonings, pg 155)

ASIAN – SEAWEED

	Cal	Fat	Sat	Chol	Carb	Fib	Sug	Sod
Agar, fresh, 1 oz..	0	0	0	0	2	-	0	3
Nori, fresh, 1 oz..	10	0	0	0	1	-	0	14
Spirulina, fresh, 1 oz	7	0	0	0	1	-	0	28
Spirulina, dried, 1 oz	83	2	1	0	7	-	0	309

Brands . . . *Most brands within generic average.*

	Cal	Fat	Sat	Chol	Carb	Fib	Sug	Sod

ASIAN – SOUPS

	Cal	Fat	Sat	Chol	Carb	Fib	Sug	Sod
Ramen, most flavors, 1/2 block (avg)	190	7	4	0	28	1	0	880
Miso soup, 1 cup	60	2	0	0	7	1	1	1170

Brands . . .
REDUCED SODIUM (LESS THAN GENERIC):

	Cal	Fat	Sat	Chol	Carb	Fib	Sug	Sod
Edward & Sons Miso-Cup, Reduced Sodium .	25	1	0	0	3	1	1	270

ASIAN – TEMPURA BATTER

(see Bread Crumbs/Coating Mixes, pg 25)

ASIAN – VEGETABLES

	Cal	Fat	Sat	Chol	Carb	Fib	Sug	Sod
Water chestnuts, 1/4 cup..............................	25	0	0	0	6	2	1	12
Bamboo shoots, 1/2 cup...............................	25	0	0	0	3	2	1	15
Bean sprouts, 1/2 cup..................................	25	0	0	0	3	2	1	270
Asian stir-fry vegetables, seasoned, frozen, 1/2 c	50	0	0	0	9	2	5	300
w/o seasoning, 1/2 cup..............................	30	0	0	0	5	2	2	15
Baby corn, 1/2 cup	10	0	0	0	6	4	6	340
Mushrooms, canned, 1/2 cup	20	0	0	0	3	2	0	380
Chow mein vegetables, canned, 1/2 cup..........	20	0	0	0	4	1	0	422
Chop suey vegetables, canned, 1/2 cup..........	15	0	0	0	3	1	2	630

Brands . . . *(1/2 cup unless noted)*
CANNED

Bamboo shoots – *Most brands within generic average (15mg).*
Water chestnuts – *Most brands within generic average (12mg).*

	Cal	Fat	Sat	Chol	Carb	Fib	Sug	Sod
Asian Gourmet Baby Corn Whole Spears	30	2	1	0	4	3	1	30
Ka-Me Stir Fry Veg	20	0	0	0	4	2	0	10
La Choy Bean Sprouts or Fancy Mixed Veg......	15	0	0	0	3	1	1	60
Polar Bean Sprouts....................................	30	0	0	0	4	0	4	15
Season Baby Corn Stir-Fry Cut......................	30	1	0	0	4	3	1	35
Sun Luck Mushrooms, Straw........................	10	0	0	0	8	0	0	0
Baby Sweet Corn or Stir-Fry Baby Corn.........	5	0	0	0	1	2	1	10
Tiger Tiger Stir-Fry Vegetables, 1 cup............	50	0	0	0	9	2	0	20

FROZEN/REFRIGERATED *(also see Vegetables – Frozen, pg 189)*

	Cal	Fat	Sat	Chol	Carb	Fib	Sug	Sod
Wegmans Food Feel Good About Baby Corn ...	70	1	0	0	16	2	3	15

ASIAN – WRAPPERS

	Cal	Fat	Sat	Chol	Carb	Fib	Sug	Sod
Wonton wrapper, 1	23	0	0	1	5	0	0	46
Egg roll wrapper, 1	93	0	0	3	19	1	0	183

Brands . . . *(1 wrapper unless noted)*

	Cal	Fat	Sat	Chol	Carb	Fib	Sug	Sod
Blue Dragon Spring Roll Wrapper..................	38	0	0	0	9	0	0	110
Dynasty Wonton Wrapper............................	17	0	0	0	4	0	0	18
Egg Roll Wrapper.....................................	57	0	0	2	12	0	0	60
Fortune Brand Gyoza (Potsticker) Wrapper	19	0	0	0	4	0	0	37
Egg Roll Wrapper.....................................	66	0	0	0	15	1	0	138
Frieda's Wonton Wrapper............................	20	0	0	0	4	0	0	37
Twin Dragon Gyoza (Potsticker) Wrapper	19	0	0	0	4	0	0	37
Shu Mai Wrappers....................................	20	0	0	0	4	0	0	40
Egg Roll Wrapper	66	0	0	0	15	1	0	138

HAWAIIAN/CARIBBEAN

	Cal	Fat	Sat	Chol	Carb	Fib	Sug	Sod
Sashimi, 1 slice...	10	0	0	4	0	0	0	3
Poi, 1 cup...	269	0	0	0	65	1	0	29
Lau lau, pork, 1	413	26	9	142	3	2	0	147

	Cal	Fat	Sat	Chol	Carb	Fib	Sug	Sod
Portuguese sausage, 2 oz	203	17	5	50	0	0	0	449
Kalua pork, 3 oz	211	15	5	67	0	0	0	1487
Lomi salmon, 1 cup	152	4	1	19	14	2	–	1643

Brands . . . *Most brands within generic range.*

HISPANIC/LATINO – DINNERS AND MEALS

(also see Dinners/Meals–Frozen, pg 138)

	Cal	Fat	Sat	Chol	Carb	Fib	Sug	Sod
Beef tamale/beef enchilada w/beans/rice, 13.4 oz	460	14	5	0	69	5	2	1210
Beef enchiladas w/beans and rice, 11 oz	360	11	5	20	55	9	7	1390

Brands . . . *(10 oz serving unless noted)*
The minimum serving size for the following items is 8.1 ounces. Serving sizes 8 ounces or less are listed in Hispanic/Latino–Entrees/Light Meals below.

FROZEN

REDUCED SODIUM (LESS THAN GENERIC):

	Cal	Fat	Sat	Chol	Carb	Fib	Sug	Sod
Amy's *Lite in Sodium Bowls*								
Mexican Casserole, 9.5 oz	370	16	5	20	48	7	4	390
Lean Cuisine Fajita-Style Chicken Spring Rolls	200	7	2	30	20	2	3	510

HISPANIC/LATINO – ENTREES AND LIGHT MEALS

	Cal	Fat	Sat	Chol	Carb	Fib	Sug	Sod
Beef and cheese chimichanga, 4 oz	320	11	3	20	41	2	3	470
Bean and cheese burrito, 5.1 oz	280	8	3	5	44	5	4	630
Tamales, beef in chili sauce, canned, 5 oz	140	7	3	15	15	2	0	710
Beef and bean burrito, 5.1 oz	294	10	3	7	43	5	8	723
Spanish rice, canned, 1/2 cup	90	2	0	0	15	1	1	770
Mix, 1/2 cup prep	240	1	0	0	54	1	3	870

Brands . . . *(1 cup or 8 oz unless noted)*
The serving size for the following items is 8 ounces or less. Items with more than 8 ounces are listed in Hispanic/Latino–Dinners/Meals above.

REDUCED SODIUM (LESS THAN GENERIC):

	Cal	Fat	Sat	Chol	Carb	Fib	Sug	Sod
Amy's *Lite in Sodium* Black Bean Enchilada	160	6	1	0	22	3	2	190
Lite in Sodium Bean & Cheese Burrito, 6 oz	330	9	3	10	51	7	2	290
Lite in Sodium Bean/Cheese Burrito	320	8	1	0	52	8	2	290
Vegetable Enchilada, 4.8 oz (1)	320	12	1	0	44	6	4	380
Black Bean Veg Enchilada, 4.8 oz	160	6	1	0	22	3	2	390
Cedarlane Garden Veg Enchilada, 4.5	140	3	2	10	20	3	4	310
Don Miguel Beef Tacos, 2 oz	160	8	3	5	19	3	0	220
Spicy Beef Tacos, 2 oz	160	8	3	5	18	3	0	230
Bean & Cheese Tacos, 2 oz	130	6	2	5	19	3	0	230
Beef, Beean & Cheese Tacos, 2 oz	170	8	3	5	18	3	0	230
Chicken Tacos, 2 oz	120	5	1	5	17	2	0	230
Eating Right Kids Chicken/Cheese Quesadilla	260	7	2	30	30	5	2	310
El Monterey Tornados SW Chicken, 2.8 oz	170	6	2	5	22	1	1	250
Bean & Cheese Burrito, 4 oz	240	7	2	5	35	2	1	270
Beef/Bean/Red Chili Burrito, 4 oz	300	14	5	15	34	2	1	270
Beef & Bean Burrito, 4 oz	300	14	5	15	33	2	1	300
Beef/Bean/Green Chili Burrito, 4 oz	290	14	5	15	32	2	1	300
Beef & Bean Chimichanga, 4 oz	310	15	5	15	33	2	1	300
SW Chicken Taquitos in Butter, 2.8 oz	170	8	3	10	20	1	0	330
Tornados Chicken Club, 2.8 oz	210	10	3	20	21	0	1	330
Spicy Taco Picante Burrito, 4 oz	290	14	5	15	31	1	1	340
Supreme Steak/Cheese Chimichanga, 5 oz	330	15	5	30	35	1	1	350
Glutenfreeda Gluten-Free Burrito								
Chicken & Cheese, 4 oz	227	6	2	17	36	3	0	173

	Cal	Fat	Sat	Chol	Carb	Fib	Sug	Sod
Vegetarian Bean & Cheese, 4 oz	196	7	2	12	29	3	0	188
Vegetarian & Dairy Free, 4.6 oz	177	3	0	0	33	4	0	261
Las Campanas								
Chicken/Rice/Bean Burrito	250	6	2	10	35	2	1	370
Tina's Spicy Beef & Bean Burrito, 4 oz	290	9	3	10	40	8	2	350

HISPANIC/LATINO – SAUCES

	Cal	Fat	Sat	Chol	Carb	Fib	Sug	Sod
Hot sauce, 1 tsp	0	0	0	0	0	0	0	30
Salsa, 2 tbsp	9	0	0	0	2	1	1	198
Fresh, refrg, 2 tbsp	10	0	0	0	2	0	1	250
Taco sauce, 2 tbsp	10	0	0	0	2	1	1	230
Enchilada sauce, red, 1/4 cup	25	1	0	0	5	1	4	310
Enchilada sauce, green, 1/4 cup	25	2	0	0	3	1	0	340
Chili sauce, 2 tbsp	29	0	0	0	6	2	3	375
Nacho/cheese sauce, 2 tbsp	70	5	1	0	6	0	2	450
Mole paste, 2 tbsp	230	15	2	0	12	2	7	460

Brands . . . *(2 tbsp unless noted)*

CHILI SAUCE

	Cal	Fat	Sat	Chol	Carb	Fib	Sug	Sod
505 Southwestern Chipotle Green Chile	10	0	0	0	2	0	1	80
Green Chili Sauce	5	0	0	0	2	0	1	95
Big Acres Mango Peach Chili Sauce	35	0	0	0	8	1	6	50

ENCHILADA SAUCE

REDUCED SODIUM (LESS THAN GENERIC):

	Cal	Fat	Sat	Chol	Carb	Fib	Sug	Sod
La Preferida Green Chili Enchilada, 1/4 c	25	2	0	0	2	1	0	250

HOT SAUCE *(see Hot Pepper Sauce, pg 93)*

MOLE

REDUCED SODIUM (LESS THAN GENERIC):

	Cal	Fat	Sat	Chol	Carb	Fib	Sug	Sod
Big Acres Milago Mole Sauce	45	2	0	0	6	1	3	70
Robert Rothschild Farm								
Spicy Mexican Mole Simmer Sauce, 2 tbsp	10	0	0	0	2	0	1	50
Mexican Mole Simmer Sauce, 2 tbsp	30	1	0	0	5	0	4	80

QUESO/NACHO CHEESE SAUCE

REDUCED SODIUM (LESS THAN GENERIC):

	Cal	Fat	Sat	Chol	Carb	Fib	Sug	Sod
Mrs Renfro's Nacho Cheese Sauce	30	2	0	0	4	0	2	150
Santa Fe Salsa Con Queso	45	4	1	5	3	0	1	200

SALSA/TACO SAUCE

FRESH (REFRIGERATED)

	Cal	Fat	Sat	Chol	Carb	Fib	Sug	Sod
Emerald Valley Mango Salsa	15	0	0	0	3	0	2	95
Green Salsa	10	0	0	0	2	1	1	110
Fiesta Salsa	20	0	0	0	4	1	1	125
Salsa, Hot, Med, or Mild	10	0	0	0	2	0	1	140
Frieda's Mild Salsa	10	0	0	0	1	0	1	75
La Mexicana Mild or Hot Salsa	10	0	0	0	0	0	0	75
Melissa's Fire Roasted Salsa	5	0	0	0	1	0	1	75
Muir Glen Garlic Cilantro Salsa	10	0	0	0	2	0	1	130
Medium or Mild Salsa	10	0	0	0	3	0	1	130
Black Bean & Corn Salsa	20	0	0	0	4	1	1	135
Chipotle Salsa, medium	10	0	0	0	2	0	1	140
Santa Barbara								
Mango & Peach Salsa	20	0	0	0	5	0	3	85
Grilled Pineapple–Chipotle Salsa	15	0	0	0	4	0	1	95
Roasted Chili Salsa	10	0	0	0	2	1	1	110
Roasted Garlic Salsa	10	0	0	0	2	0	1	115

	Cal	Fat	Sat	Chol	Carb	Fib	Sug	Sod
Black Bean & Corn, Medium	20	0	0	0	4	0	2	120
Artichoke Salsa...................................	15	1	1	0	2	0	1	140

SHELF-STABLE

501 Southwestern

	Cal	Fat	Sat	Chol	Carb	Fib	Sug	Sod
Chipotle Honey Roasted Green Chile...........	10	0	0	0	2	0	1	80
Green Chile Sauce.................................	5	0	0	0	2	0	1	95
Alberto's Jalapeño Relish	3	0	0	0	7	0	6	0
American Spoon Corn Salsa	20	0	0	0	4	1	1	35
Mango Habanero Salsa............................	35	0	0	0	9	1	8	70
Smoky Southwest Salsa..........................	10	0	0	0	2	0	1	75
Kiwi Lime Salsa Verde............................	30	0	0	0	7	0	5	65
Tomatillo Salsa...................................	15	0	0	0	3	0	1	110
Cherry Peach Salsa	25	0	0	0	7	0	5	115
Apple Chipotle Salsa..............................	30	0	0	0	7	0	4	120
Arriba! *Fire Roasted*								
Mexican Green Salsa, all heats..................	10	0	0	0	2	0	0	100
Black Bean & Corn Salsa.........................	15	0	0	0	2	2	0	125
Better Than Fred's Caribbean Salsa	15	0	0	0	4	1	3	25
Just Peachy Salsa	15	0	0	0	4	1	3	25
Salsa Hot...	15	0	0	0	3	1	1	70
Medium or Mild...................................	15	0	0	0	3	1	1	75
Cannon's Cannon Fire Salsa, Hot or Med	15	0	0	0	3	0	1	20
Clint's Texas Salsa, Mild or Med.................	5	0	0	0	1	0	1	70
Dei Fratelli Chipotle Salsa Medium..............	10	0	0	0	2	1	1	135
Desert Pepper Peach Mango	15	0	0	0	4	0	3	25
Roasted Tomato Chipotle Corn Salsa...........	100	0	0	0	2	0	0	85
Diana's Veggie Pineapple Salsa	15	0	0	0	3	0	1	0
Black Bean w/Corn...............................	15	0	0	0	3	0	0	20
Three Bean Salsa.................................	20	0	0	0	3	0	2	45
Eat Smart Garden Style Sweet Salsa	20	0	0	0	5	0	4	95
El Pato Jalapeño Salsa	0	0	0	0	0	0	0	30
Salsa de Chile Fresca.............................	5	0	0	0	1	0	1	135
El Pinto Mild Green Chile Taco Sauce...........	10	0	0	0	2	0	1	55
Enrico's Chunky Style Salsa NSA, Mild or Hot	10	0	0	0	3	0	2	60
Frontera Corn & Poblano Salsa	10	0	0	0	2	0	1	135
Chipotle Salsa	10	0	0	0	2	1	1	140
Mango Key Lime Salsa............................	15	0	0	0	3	0	2	140
Frog Ranch Salsa, all varieties....................	10	0	0	0	2	1	1	40
Garlic Survival Co. Tomatillo Garlic Salsa	20	0	0	0	4	1	0	15
Garlic or Triple Garlic Salsa.....................	10	0	0	0	2	1	1	70
Gloria's Roasted Garlic & Pineapple Salsa	40	0	0	0	10	0	9	5
Santiam Ridge Peach Mango Salsa	50	0	0	0	12	0	10	15
Happy Valley Apple Salsa	20	0	0	0	4	0	3	45
Goldwater's Cochise Corn & Black Bean	30	2	0	0	4	1	1	80
Papago Peach Salsa..............................	15	0	0	0	3	0	1	85
Ruby Raspberry Salsa............................	20	0	0	0	5	0	5	90
Sedona Red Salsa	10	0	0	0	2	0	1	100
Paradise Pineapple Salsa.........................	15	0	0	0	3	0	3	115
Grande Sweet Garden Salsa	20	0	0	0	5	0	4	120
Great Value Peach Pineapple Chipotle Salsa .	15	0	0	0	4	1	3	105
Green Mt Gringo Salsa, all heats................	10	0	0	0	2	0	1	90
Roasted Garlic Salsa..............................	10	0	0	0	2	0	1	90
Gunther's Tomatillo Salsa Verde	10	0	0	0	2	0	0	50
Spicy Ginger Pineapple Salsa....................	10	0	0	0	2	0	2	50

ETHNIC FOODS
Hispanic/Latino – Sauces

	Cal	Fat	Sat	Chol	Carb	Fib	Sug	Sod
Fiery Cranberry Habanero Salsa	10	0	0	0	2	0	0	70
Fiery Peri Peri Dark Cherry Salsa	10	0	0	0	2	0	0	70
Lime Mango Salsa	10	0	0	0	4	0	2	80
Peach Salsa	10	0	0	0	2	0	2	80
Spicy Chipotle & Smoked Corn Salsa	10	0	0	0	2	0	2	90
Jalapeno Salsa Fresca	10	0	0	0	2	0	2	130
Black & White Bean Salsa	10	0	0	0	4	0	0	130
Chesapeake Bay Crab Salsa	10	0	0	0	2	0	0	130
Salsa Fresca	10	0	0	0	2	0	2	130
Huskies Salsa Hot or Mild	10	0	0	0	3	0	2	110
Jardine's *7J Ranch* Chipotle Med Salsa	10	0	0	0	2	1	0	105
Campfire Roasted Med Salsa	10	0	0	0	2	0	0	130
LaVictoria Salsa Bravia Hot Sauce, 1 tbsp	0	0	0	0	0	0	0	25
Green Taco Sauce, Mild or Med, 1 tbsp	0	0	0	0	1	0	0	70
Salsa Supreme, Mild	10	0	0	0	2	0	1	105
Salsa Victoria, Hot	10	0	0	0	2	1	0	110
Salsa Supreme, Medium	5	0	0	0	1	0	0	135
Thick 'n Chunky Salsa Verde, Medium	10	0	0	0	2	0	1	140
Miguel's Stowe Away Salsa Mild or Med	10	0	0	0	2	0	1	85
Mrs Renfro Raspberry Chipotle Salsa	15	0	0	0	4	0	3	70
Pomegranate Salsa	20	0	0	0	5	0	3	90
Pineapple Salsa	15	0	0	0	4	0	2	105
Tequila Salsa	15	0	0	0	4	0	2	140
Neera's Caribbean Salsa, 1 tbsp	25	0	0	0	7	0	6	60
Newman's Own Organic Cilantro	10	0	0	0	3	0	2	85
Chunky Peach Salsa	25	0	0	0	6	1	5	90
Chunky Pineapple Salsa	15	0	0	0	3	1	3	90
All Natural Chunky Salsa, all heats	10	0	0	0	2	1	1	105
Black Bean & Corn or Mango Salsa	20	0	0	0	5	2	1	140
OrganicVille Pineapple Salsa	15	0	0	0	4	0	3	135
Medium or Mild Salsa	15	0	0	0	3	0	1	135
Pace Pineapple Mango Chipotle Salsa	20	0	0	0	4	0	4	130
Palmieri Salsa, all varieties	10	0	0	0	2	0	2	65
Red Cactus Country Sweet Med Salsa	20	0	0	0	4	0	3	70
Robert Rothschild Farm Mango Salsa	30	0	0	0	8	1	7	15
Tequila Lime Salsa	10	0	0	0	2	1	1	90
Roasted Corn & Black Bean	20	0	0	0	4	1	1	95
Raspberry Salsa	45	0	0	0	9	1	9	105
Raspberry Chipotle Salsa	45	0	0	0	9	1	9	105
Salsa Patria Chunky, all heats	5	0	0	0	1	0	0	70
Salpica Habanero Lime Salsa	15	0	0	0	4	0	3	50
Roasted Corn & Bean Salsa	20	0	0	0	4	1	0	90
Chipotle Black Bean Salsa	15	0	0	0	3	1	0	90
Spring Break Salsa (seasonal)	15	0	0	0	3	0	2	110
Fall Harvest Salsa (seasonal)	15	0	0	0	4	0	3	140
Cabin Fever Salsa (seasonal)	20	0	0	0	4	0	0	140
Singing Pig Sweet Onion Salsa	25	0	0	0	6	0	5	20
Roasted Garlic Salsa	10	0	0	0	2	0	0	85
Southern Delight								
Savory Apple & Honey Salsa, all	15	0	0	0	4	0	4	5
Spike Santa Fe All Natural Black Bean/Corn	15	0	0	0	4	0	2	105
Stonewall Kitchen Peach Salsa	10	0	0	0	2	0	1	30
Mango Lime Salsa	15	0	0	0	3	0	2	35
Papaya Salsa	20	0	0	0	4	0	4	75
Pineapple Chipotle Salsa	20	0	0	0	5	0	4	85

	Cal	Fat	Sat	Chol	Carb	Fib	Sug	Sod
Spicy Tomato Salsa	5	0	0	0	2	0	1	115
Salsa Verde	10	0	0	0	2	1	1	135
Texas Pepper Works Alamo Select Salsa	10	0	0	0	2	0	1	70
Raspberry Chipotle Salsa	20	0	0	0	5	0	4	115
Trigger's Peach Salsa	15	0	0	0	4	0	3	55
Garden Salsa	10	0	0	0	2	0	1	65
Pineapple Salsa	20	0	0	0	5	0	5	80
Voodoo Bayou Salsa, Mild or Med	10	0	0	0	2	0	0	125
Walnut Acres Sweet SW Peach Salsa	20	0	0	0	5	0	4	85
Midnight Sun Salsa	15	0	0	0	3	1	2	125
Fiesta Cilantro Salsa	10	0	0	0	2	0	2	135

MISC SAUCES

	Cal	Fat	Sat	Chol	Carb	Fib	Sug	Sod
Rosa Mexicano Veracruzana Sauce, 1 tbsp	5	0	0	0	1	0	1	45
Ranchera Sauce, 1 tbsp	10	1	0	0	1	0	1	60
Mestiza Sauce, 1 tbsp	5	0	0	0	1	0	0	75
Granadilla Sauce, 1 tbsp	10	0	0	0	2	0	1	85

HISPANIC/LATINO – SEASONING MIXES AND CONDIMENTS

	Cal	Fat	Sat	Chol	Carb	Fib	Sug	Sod
Sofrito, 1 tsp	0	0	0	0	1	0	0	45
Recaito, 1.5 tsp	0	0	0	0	0	0	0	85
Guacamole seasoning mix, 1/8 pkt	15	0	0	0	2	0	0	160
Enchilada sauce mix, 1/6 pkt	20	0	0	0	4	0	1	250
Chili seasoning mix, 1/4 pkt	30	1	0	0	5	2	1	310
Mole, ready-to-use, 2 tbsp	100	13	2	0	10	2	6	400
Burrito seasoning mix, 1/6 pkt	15	0	0	0	4	0	0	410
Fajita seasoning mix, 1/6 pkt	15	0	0	0	3	0	0	450
Taco seasoning mix, 1/6 pkt	20	0	0	0	5	0	0	550
30% less sodium	20	0	0	0	3	1	2	330

Brands . . . *(1 tsp unless noted)*

CANNED

	Cal	Fat	Sat	Chol	Carb	Fib	Sug	Sod
Frontera Guacamole Mix, 1 tbsp	5	0	0	0	1	0	0	35

MIXES

	Cal	Fat	Sat	Chol	Carb	Fib	Sug	Sod
Ancho Mama's Chile Seasoning	0	0	0	0	0	0	0	0
Cedar Hill Seasonings Taco Chili Mix	115	3	0	0	24	9	3	30
Chipotle Del Sol SW Seasoning	0	0	0	0	0	0	0	0
Concord Foods Salsa Seasoning Mix, Hot or Mild	10	0	0	0	1	0	0	100
Guacamole Mix, 1.5 tsp	10	0	0	0	3	0	0	130
Frontier SF Taco Seasoning, 1/4 tsp	10	0	0	0	2	0	0	0
New Traditions Fajita Seasoning, 1/4 tsp	0	0	0	0	2	0	0	0
Simply Organic Guacamole Dip Mix, 1/2 tsp	5	0	0	0	1	0	0	95

HISPANIC/LATINO – TORTILLAS AND TACO SHELLS

	Cal	Fat	Sat	Chol	Carb	Fib	Sug	Sod
Corn tortilla, 6" diam, 1	58	1	0	0	12	1	0	3
Corn taco shell, shelf-stable, 1	55	3	1	0	8	3	0	80
Flour tortilla, 6", 1	94	2	1	0	15	1	1	191
10", 1	218	5	1	0	36	2	1	445
Whole wheat tortilla, 1	120	2	1	0	20	1	0	280

Brands . . .

TORTILLAS

	Cal	Fat	Sat	Chol	Carb	Fib	Sug	Sod
Boghosian *Valley Bread* Plain Lavash	130	3	0	0	23	1	2	125
Food for Life Sprouted Grain	150	4	1	0	24	5	0	140
French Meadow Fat Flush Tortilla, 6"	100	1	0	0	18	3	1	105
Wheat & Sprouted Grain Tortilla	110	1	0	0	21	3	1	110
Hemp Tortilla	90	3	0	0	12	3	1	130

	Cal	Fat	Sat	Chol	Carb	Fib	Sug	Sod
Garden of Eatin' Whole Wheat Tortillas	110	1	0	0	22	3	0	130
La Tapatia Organic Flax & Whole Wheat	90	3	0	0	14	3	0	140
Pepito Flour Tortillas (8 oz pkg)	80	2	1	0	14	1	1	65
Flour Tortillas (16 oz pkg)	170	4	1	0	29	1	2	130
Sol de Oro Low Carb High Fiber	45	2	0	0	10	8	1	80
Multi-Graine Whole Wheat Gorditas	120	3	1	0	20	5	2	70
Tumaro's Premium White Flour	120	2	0	0	23	1	1	130
Pesto & Garlic or Honey Wheat (avg)	110	1	0	0	23	1	1	135
Garden Spinach/Veg or Sun-Dried Tomato/Basil	110	2	0	0	23	1	1	140
REDUCED SODIUM (LESS THAN GENERIC):								
Azteca Salad Shells	210	11	2	0	23	1	0	150
Boghosian Garlic & Herb Lavash	110	3	0	0	18	1	1	190
Great Value Fajita Size Flour Tortillas	80	1	0	0	15	2	0	150
Joseph's *Mexicali*, all varieties	175	3	1	0	31	1	2	170
La Jalisciense Tortilla Factory Flour	90	2	0	0	17	1	1	150
La Tortilla Whole Wheat, Garlic & Herb	50	2	0	0	11	8	0	180
Whole Wheat, Low Carb, Original	50	2	0	0	10	7	0	210
Rudi's Organic Bakery Spelt Tortillas	140	3	0	0	27	1	1	200
Whole Spelt Tortillas	150	3	0	0	28	3	1	210
TACO SHELLS (SHELF-STABLE)								
Bearitos Tostada Shells, 2 shells	140	7	1	0	17	1	0	5
Taco Shells, blue or yellow, 2 shells	140	7	1	0	17	1	0	5
Casa Fiesta Jumbo Taco Shell	160	7	5	5	23	3	0	5
All Natural Taco Shells, 3	150	6	5	0	21	2	0	10
Garden of Eatin' Blue or Yellow Corn, 2	140	7	1	0	17	1	0	5
Mission Taco Shells, 2	100	4	1	0	14	1	0	0
Jumbo Taco Shells, 1	90	4	1	0	13	1	0	0
Rio Rancho Tostada Bowls	180	9	2	0	22	3	0	5
Taco Bell Taco Shells, 3	150	6	3	0	21	2	0	5

HISPANIC/LATINO – VEGETABLES

	Cal	Fat	Sat	Chol	Carb	Fib	Sug	Sod
Vegetables:								
Tomatillos, raw, diced, 1/2 cup	21	1	0	0	4	1	0	1
Tomatillos, canned, 2.1 oz	15	0	0	0	3	2	1	15
Nopalitos (cactus), canned, 2 tbsp	5	0	0	0	1	0	0	560
Peppers:								
Whole green chiles, 1 pepper (1.3 oz)	15	0	0	0	3	1	1	100
Diced green chiles, 2 tbsp	5	0	0	0	1	1	0	110
Chipotle peppers in adobo, 2 tbsp	30	1	0	0	5	3	1	260
Jalapeños, diced, 2 tbsp	8	0	0	0	1	1	0	468
Refried beans:								
Refried beans, canned, 1/2 cup	100	1	0	0	17	6	1	540
Mix, prep, 1/2 cup	160	1	0	0	29	11	1	610
Brands . . . *(2 tbsp unless noted)*								
PEPPERS								
Alberto's Sweet Jalapeno Relish, all, 2 tbsp	30	0	0	0	7	0	0	0
Cannon Sweet Hots, all, 2 tbsp	25	0	0	0	6	0	6	10
Just Plain Green Chile, Hot or Mild, 2 tbsp	10	0	0	0	2	0	0	0
El Pato Hot Chile Peppers, 1	6	0	0	0	1	1	0	27
Casa Fiesta Diced or Whole Green Chiles, 2 tbsp	5	0	0	0	1	0	0	85
El Rio Chopped Green Chiles, 2 tbsp	5	0	0	0	1	0	0	75
Embassa Chipotle Peppers in Adobo, 2 tbsp	15	1	0	0	2	1	1	140
Great Value Chopped Green Chiles, 2 tbsp	5	0	0	0	2	1	0	75
LaPreferida Diced Green Chiles, 2 tbsp	10	0	0	0	2	1	0	75

	Cal	Fat	S.F.	Chol	Carb	Fib	Sug	Sod
LaVictoria Diced Fire Roasted Green Chiles, 2 tbsp	5	0	0	0	1	0	1	75
Meijer Whole Green Chiles, 1 pepper	10	0	0	0	1	1	0	75
Chopped & Peeled Green Chiles, 2 tbsp	5	0	0	0	1	1	0	75
Natural Value Whole or Diced, 2 tbsp............	10	0	0	0	2	1	1	40
Ortega Diced Jalapeños, 2 tbsp	10	0	0	0	2	0	1	25
Diced Green Fire Roasted Chiles, 1 oz	10	0	0	0	2	0	1	70

GUACAMOLE (see Dips/Spreads, pg 220)

REFRIED BEANS (1/2 cup unless noted)

CANNED

	Cal	Fat	S.F.	Chol	Carb	Fib	Sug	Sod
Amy's Light in Sodium Refried Beans	140	3	0	0	22	6	1	190
Light in Sodium Refried Black Beans..........	140	3	0	0	21	6	1	220
Bearitos LF, NSA....................................	140	3	0	0	23	9	2	5
Eden Black Soy & Black Beans Refried..........	90	3	1	0	13	6	1	170
Kidney Beans Refried.................................	80	1	0	0	15	6	0	180
Pinto Beans or Spicy Pinto Beans Refried.....	90	1	0	0	19	7	1	180
Black Beans or Spicy Black Beans Refried....	110	2	0	0	18	7	0	180
Full Circle Refried Black Beans...................	120	2	0	0	22	8	2	330
La Sierra Refried Pinto	150	5	1	0	19	7	2	310
Natural Value Refried Black	123	0	0	0	22	2	0	259
Refried Pinto	134	0	0	0	26	10	0	261
Seneca FF Spicy....................................	120	0	0	0	22	8	1	290
Shari's Organic, Refried Black	110	0	0	0	20	4	0	330
Refried Pintos.......................................	110	0	0	0	20	4	0	330
Refried w/Roasted Garlic...........................	110	0	0	0	20	4	0	330

MIXES

REDUCED SODIUM (LESS THAN GENERIC):

	Cal	Fat	S.F.	Chol	Carb	Fib	Sug	Sod
Fantastic World Foods Refried Beans.......	130	2	0	0	21	7	0	270
Mexicali Rose FF Refried Beans, Instant....	100	0	0	0	19	5	1	280

MEDITERRANEAN/MIDDLE EASTERN – MEALS AND ENTREES

Entrees:

	Cal	Fat	S.F.	Chol	Carb	Fib	Sug	Sod
Lentils w/fresh veg (madras sambar), 4 oz	80	3	1	0	11	1	1	390
Peas and cheese (matar-paneer), 4 oz	140	11	4	15	9	2	3	510
Potato dumplings (jaipur karhi), 4 oz	70	4	1	0	8	1	3	520
Knish, potato, 1 pc....................................	200	4	0	0	38	2	0	530
Pierogies, potato/broccoli/cheddar, 4 oz (3) ...	190	5	1	5	32	2	2	530
Masala noodles, mix, 1/2 pkg	220	8	4	0	32	2	1	765
Rice pilaf w/veg and nuts, mix, 1 cup............	290	12	5	15	39	1	2	880
Mashed veg curry (pav bhaji), mix, 1/2 cup...	210	15	3	30	16	2	3	920

Meals:

	Cal	Fat	S.F.	Chol	Carb	Fib	Sug	Sod
Chicken tikka masala, 10 oz	260	6	2	45	37	3	4	680
Chicken korma, 10 oz	340	9	1	40	44	3	4	720
Palak paneer, 10 oz	240	11	6	35	23	4	5	810
Chicken biryani, 10 oz	390	12	2	20	54	4	7	1080

Brands . . .

ENTREES

FROZEN

REDUCED SODIUM (LESS THAN GENERIC):

	Cal	Fat	S.F.	Chol	Carb	Fib	Sug	Sod
Golden Gourmet Potato/Onion Pierogies, 3	182	3	1	36	35	1	9	195
Potato & Cheese Pierogies, 4 oz (3)..........	240	5	2	5	39	1	2	250
Life Choices/Living Right								
Cheese & Potato Pierogies, 4 oz	240	7	1	0	39	2	1	330
Cheese, Potato & Broccoli Pierogies, 4 oz ..	240	5	1	0	39	2	1	330
Cheese/Potato/Soy Bacon Pierogies, 4.3 oz .	250	7	1	0	40	2	1	340

169

	Cal	Fat	Sat	Chol	Carb	Fib	Sug	Sod
Old Fashioned Kitchen								
Potato & Onion Pierogies, 4 oz (3)	180	3	1	0	35	1	9	200
MIXES								
Neera's Urad & Channa Dal, 1 cup prep	104	1	0	0	18	9	0	4
Dal & Seasoning Mix, 1 cup prep	140	1	0	0	23	12	0	4
Biryani Rice Mix, 1 cup prep	132	1	0	0	29	1	0	4
Shahi Pilau Rice Mix, 1 cup prep	286	8	1	0	48	2	0	6
REDUCED SODIUM (LESS THAN GENERIC):								
Kohinoor *Rice Treat*								
Madurai Lemon Rice, 1/2 pkg	237	5	1	2	44	13	1	400
Veg Pilaf, 1/2 pkg	248	8	1	0	38	14	4	475
Sadaf Falafel Mix, 1/8 pkg	140	2	0	0	25	2	5	190
Basmati Rice, Sweet Harmony, 1/3 pkg	210	2	0	0	43	3	4	250
Shamiana Punjabi Mix, 1 oz mix	141	8	4	0	12	1	1	190
SHELF-STABLE								
Tasty Bite								
Meal Inspirations Zany Multigrain, 4.4 oz	180	5	1	0	28	4	2	270
Paneer Makhani, 5 oz	190	15	6	30	8	1	3	310
Meal Inspirations Chunky Chickpeas, 4 oz	210	7	1	0	30	10	5	350
Meal Inspirations Barley Medley, 4 oz	210	2	0	0	41	9	6	350
Peas Paneer, 5 oz	150	10	5	13	7	6	5	350
MEALS								
FROZEN								
REDUCED SODIUM (LESS THAN GENERIC):								
A Taste of India								
Masala Rice/Lentils, 1/2 pkg	260	5	3	0	47	2	4	310
Spice Rice w/Raisins, 1/2 pkg	330	12	5	0	51	2	8	320
Amy's *Indian* Mattar Paneer, 10 oz	370	11	4	20	54	6	8	390
Paneer Tikka, 9.5 oz	320	7	0	20	36	5	6	550
Sukhi's *Lean Fare* Chicken Jalfrezi, 11 oz	290	2	0	50	44	3	2	320
Lean Fare Chicken Saag, 11 oz	280	3	0	35	43	3	2	340
Lean Fare Channa Masala, 11 oz	340	4	0	0	69	9	12	380
Lean Fare Chicken Tikka Masala, 11 oc	330	3	1	60	47	2	2	390
Lean Fare Dal Saag, 11 oz	300	3	0	0	60	8	4	390
Tandoor Chef Vegetable Korma	330	11	3	0	46	8	4	500
MEAL KITS AND HELPERS								
SHELF-STABLE								
CookSimple Punjabi Curry	190	3	2	0	39	5	12	15
REDUCED SODIUM (LESS THAN GENERIC):								
CookSimple Tibetan Dal	140	1	0	0	25	7	2	270

MEDITERRANEAN/MIDDLE EASTERN – SAUCES

	Cal	Fat	Sat	Chol	Carb	Fib	Sug	Sod
Curry paste, ready-to-use, 1 tbsp	10	0	0	0	2	0	1	270
Jalfrezi, 1/2 cup	100	7	1	0	11	2	5	380
Korma sauce, 4 oz	372	35	15	19	13	1	9	480
Curry sauce, ready-to-use, 1/4 cup	90	6	4	0	6	0	4	510
Tandoori paste, 2 tbsp	40	1	0	0	7	1	5	1200
Brands . . . *(1/4 cup sauce unless noted)*								
FROZEN/REFRIGERATED								
Opaa! Harissa, 2 tbsp	35	4	0	0	2	0	1	125
READY-TO-USE								
Chef Shaikh's								
Curry Sauce, Hot or Med	50	2	0	0	7	5	2	110
Curry Sauce, Mild	45	1	0	0	7	3	3	120

	Cal	Fat	Sat	Chol	Carb	Fib	Sug	Sod
Mr. Spice Organic								
SF Indian Curry Sauce	30	0	0	0	6	0	4	0
Neera's								
Kashmiri Marinade, 1 tbsp	18	1	0	0	5	0	3	69
Tamarind Sauce, 1 tbsp	15	0	0	0	3	0	0	98
Asian Tamarind Sauce, 2 tbsp	61	0	0	0	16	0	10	110
Steel's Mango Curry Sauce, 1 tbsp	19	0	0	0	5	0	5	0
Stonehouse 27 Cooking Sauce								
Tomato & Chilies	90	6	0	0	8	1	4	0
Dates & Tamarind	130	7	1	0	15	2	10	10
Spicy Cashews & Cream	110	9	4	15	6	1	2	15
Cilantro & Coconut	100	6	3	0	10	2	5	25
Tamarind & Garlic	80	5	2	0	8	2	4	25
Cashews & Cream, Hot or Mild	200	16	6	25	9	1	3	30
Tamarind & Garlic, 1/2 cup	140	9	3	0	12	3	6	40

MEDITERRANEAN/MIDDLE EASTERN – SEASONING MIXES

	Cal	Fat	Sat	Chol	Carb	Fib	Sug	Sod
Garam marsala, 1 tsp	5	0	0	0	2	0	0	5
Grape leaves, 1	0	0	0	0	0	0	0	60
Raita, 2.3 oz	41	1	1	0	6	0	4	100
Vindaloo paste, 2 tbsp	96	9	1	0	5	4	1	449
Tandoori paste, 2 tbsp	40	1	0	0	7	1	5	1200
Brands . . .								
Neera's Garam Masala, 1/4 tsp	2	0	0	0	0	0	0	0
Yogurt Seasoning Raita Mix, 1 tbsp	6	0	0	0	2	0	0	2
Tandoori Paste, 2 tsp	19	2	0	0	3	1	0	156

FISH AND SEAFOOD

See RESOURCES, page 305, for a partial list of manufacturers and retailers offering low-salt products online or visit **LowSaltFoods.com** *for additional sources.*

FISH AND SEAFOOD

ANCHOVY PASTE

	Cal	Fat	Sat	Chol	Carb	Fib	Sug	Sod
Anchovy paste, 1 tbsp	30	3	1	55	0	0	0	940

Brands . . . *Most brands within generic average.*

CLAM JUICE

	Cal	Fat	Sat	Chol	Carb	Fib	Sug	Sod
Clam juice, 1/4 cup	1	0	0	0	0	0	0	280

Brands . . . *(1/4 cup unless noted)*

	Cal	Fat	Sat	Chol	Carb	Fib	Sug	Sod
Bar Harbor Clam Juice	0	0	0	0	0	0	0	120
Look's Atlantic Clam Juice	0	0	0	0	0	0	0	120

FISH AND SEAFOOD – CANNED

	Cal	Fat	Sat	Chol	Carb	Fib	Sug	Sod
Oysters, 2 oz	70	3	1	45	3	0	0	140
Smoked, 2 oz	120	7	2	35	6	0	0	240
Sardines, boneless/skinless in water, 1.8 oz	75	5	1	30	0	0	0	195
In tomato sauce, 1.8 oz	85	5	1	50	1	1	0	220
Brisling in oil, 1.5 oz	105	8	2	33	1	1	0	250
Salmon, sockeye, 2 oz	94	4	1	25	0	0	0	204
Pink, 2 oz	79	3	1	31	0	0	0	314
Mackerel, jack, 2 oz	88	4	1	45	0	0	0	215
Tuna, packed in oil, 2 oz	105	5	2	18	0	0	0	224
Light, packed in water, 2 oz	66	0	0	17	0	0	0	192
Mussels, smoked, 2 oz	90	5	2	50	3	0	0	250
Crab, 2 oz	30	0	0	45	1	0	0	300
Imitation crab (surimi), 2 oz	45	0	0	3	8	0	2	252
Gefilte fish, 2 oz	64	3	0	9	5	0	4	345
Clams, chopped/minced, 2 oz	30	0	0	12	2	0	1	370
Herring, pickled, 1.6 oz	119	8	1	6	4	0	4	395
Smoked, kipper, 1.6 oz	95	7	1	30	0	0	0	395
Caviar, black or red, 1 oz	71	5	1	167	1	0	0	425
Shrimp, 2 oz	57	1	0	143	0	0	0	441
Anchovies in oil, 1 oz	47	2	0	19	0	0	0	825

Brands . . . *(2 oz unless noted)*

ANCHOVIES – *Most brands within generic average (825mg).*

CAVIAR – *Most brands within generic average (425mg).*

CLAMS

	Cal	Fat	Sat	Chol	Carb	Fib	Sug	Sod
Crown Prince Natural Boiled Baby Clams, 2 oz	50	1	0	50	1	0	0	105

REDUCED SODIUM (LESS THAN GENERIC)

	Cal	Fat	Sat	Chol	Carb	Fib	Sug	Sod
Bumble Bee Fancy Whole Baby Clams, 3 oz	50	1	1	40	2	0	0	270
Cento Whole Shelled Baby Clams, 3 oz	50	2	1	25	1	0	0	290

CRAB

	Cal	Fat	Sat	Chol	Carb	Fib	Sug	Sod
Natural Value Leg & Body Crab Meat, 2 oz	70	1	0	30	1	0	0	140

REDUCED SODIUM (LESS THAN GENERIC)

	Cal	Fat	Sat	Chol	Carb	Fib	Sug	Sod
Miller's Select Jumbo Lump, 3.3 oz	60	1	0	75	0	0	0	160
Phillips Crabmeat, 2 oz	40	0	0	45	0	0	0	180

GEFILTE FISH

	Cal	Fat	Sat	Chol	Carb	Fib	Sug	Sod
Mrs. Adler's No Salt, 1 pc	50	2	1	20	3	1	1	40

REDUCED SODIUM (LESS THAN GENERIC)

	Cal	Fat	Sat	Chol	Carb	Fib	Sug	Sod
Mother's Gefilte Fish, 4 oz pc	70	3	1	20	3	1	0	220
Mrs Adler's Gefilte, 2 oz	50	2	1	20	3	1	1	200
Old Jerusalem Gefilte, 2 oz	50	3	1	25	5	1	2	210

FISH AND SEAFOOD
Fish and Seafood – Canned

	Cal	Fat	Sat	Chol	Carb	Fib	Sug	Sod
Rokeach Old Vienna Gefilte fish, 4 oz pc.....	60	3	1	30	3	1	2	240
Ungar's								
Gefilte, No Sugar Added, 1.9 oz.................	70	4	1	15	3	0	1	180
Gefilte Fish, Lite, 2.5 oz (2 slices)	80	3	0	20	5	2	3	190
HERRING AND KIPPER SNACKS								
Alstertor Herring Fillets in Tomato Sauce, 1 pc	190	14	1	25	4	0	3	110
Brunswick								
Fish Steaks in Spring Water, 1.7 oz..............	75	4	1	58	0	0	0	120
Fish Steaks w/Tabasco Peppers, 1.7 oz..........	100	7	2	40	1	0	0	120
Crown Prince Kipper Snacks, NSA, 1.6 oz......	55	7	1	30	0	0	0	35
Season Kipper Snacks, NSA, 1.6 oz	95	7	1	30	0	0	0	40
MACKEREL								
Season Fillet of Mackerel, NSA, 2 oz	90	5	2	25	0	0	0	55
REDUCED SODIUM (LESS THAN GENERIC)								
Geisha Jack Mackerel...................................	78	2	1	45	0	0	0	152
MISC FISH								
REDUCED SODIUM (LESS THAN GENERIC)								
Mother's								
All Whitefish in Jelled Broth, 1 pc	50	3	1	20	2	1	0	220
Vitarroz Octopus in Soya Oil, 2oz................	80	3	1	45	3	0	0	150
MUSSELS								
Pacific Pearl Smoked, 2 oz.......................	120	7	1	13	2	0	1	95
Polar Mussels, 2 oz	60	3	0	15	1	0	0	90
OYSTERS								
REDUCED SODIUM (LESS THAN GENERIC)								
Polar Oysters or Pieces Oysters....................	70	3	2	3	4	0	0	150
SALMON								
Crown Prince Natural Alaskan Pink, 2 oz........	80	5	1	15	0	0	0	50
Miramonte	70	3	0	30	0	0	0	45
Natural Sea Wild Alaskan Pink	90	5	0	40	0	0	0	60
Raincoast Trading								
Pink Salmon, NSA, 2 oz	90	4	1	40	0	0	0	25
Wild Sockeye, NSA, 2 oz	110	7	2	45	0	0	0	35
Season Pink, NSA.......................................	90	5	1	40	0	0	0	40
Trident Seafoods								
Sea Alaska Chum Salmon, 4 oz	130	4	1	70	0	0	0	65
SARDINES								
Beach Cliff Sardines in Soybean Oil	95	7	2	55	0	0	0	125
Small Sardines in Soybean Oil......................	100	7	2	58	0	0	0	130
Sardines in Water....................................	95	6	1	50	1	0	0	135
Bela Olhao Portugal Sardines	130	9	2	20	0	0	0	115
Sardines in Olive Oil	120	7	2	20	0	0	0	130
Brunswick Sardines in Water, NSA	70	4	1	50	0	0	0	100
Sardines in Olive Oil	95	7	1	55	0	0	0	125
Sardines w/Hot Tabasco Peppers	95	6	1	55	0	0	0	140
Crown Prince Brisling in Oil, NSA.................	115	9	3	23	0	0	0	62
Sardines in Water.....................................	95	6	2	28	1	0	0	75
Fish Steaks or Sardines w/Green Chilies........	100	6	2	28	0	0	0	85
Fish Steaks or Sardines in Louisiana Hot Sauce..	115	8	4	33	0	0	0	95
Skinless & Boneless Sardines in Olive Oil.......	110	6	1	8	0	0	0	140
Crown Prince Natural Brisling in Water..........	105	9	4	30	0	0	0	45
Skinless & Boneless Sardines in Water	70	3	1	15	1	0	0	100
Skinless & Boneless Sardines in Olive Oil	110	6	1	8	0	0	0	140
El Mexicana Sardines in Tomato Sauce, 2 oz...	70	2	0	30	3	0	3	95

	Cal	Fat	Sat	Chol	Carb	Fib	Sug	Sod
Gefen Sardines in Water, NS	75	5	1	30	0	0	0	28
King Oscar Sardines in Water, NSA	70	5	2	55	0	0	0	50
Sardines in Soybean Oil, NSA	70	5	2	55	0	0	0	50
Martel Fancy Plain Sardines	70	4	1	28	0	0	0	130
Ocean Prince								
Fish Steak or Sardines w/Chili	100	6	2	28	0	0	0	85
Fish Steaks or Sardine in Louisiana Hot Sauce	115	8	4	33	0	0	0	95
Fish Steaks or Sardines in Olive Oil	105	6	2	33	0	0	0	105
Polar Sardines in Water, 3 oz	100	3	0	50	1	0	1	140
Reese Skinless/Boneless in Water, LS	105	9	2	25	0	0	0	100
Brisling in Tomato Sauce & Sherry	110	9	3	40	1	1	1	135
Season Skinless/Boneless in Water, NSA	65	3	1	17	0	0	0	25
Sardines in Olive Oil, NSA	73	5	2	55	0	0	0	35
Sardines in Spanish Sauce	185	16	4	23	4	1	0	40
Sardines in Hot Sauce, NSA, 2 oz	75	3	1	70	1	1	0	60
Sardines in Tomato Sauce, NSA, 2.2 oz	110	6	4	45	1	0	0	95
Skinless/Boneless in Tomato Sauce, 2 oz	80	3	1	25	1	0	1	100
SHRIMP								
Geisha Tiny Shrimp, 2.1 oz	42	0	0	182	1	0	1	215
TUNA (ALBACORE)								
American Tuna Wild Albacore, NSA	100	5	2	10	0	0	0	20
Bumble Bee Chunk Albacore in Water, Very LS	70	1	0	30	0	0	0	35
Chicken of the Sea Chunk Albacore, Very LS..	60	1	0	25	0	0	0	35
Chunk Light in Water, LS	60	1	0	30	0	0	0	90
Chunk Light in Spring Water, 50% Less Salt...	60	1	0	30	0	0	0	125
Crown Prince Natural NSA Albacore in Water	60	0	0	20	0	0	0	30
NSA Tongol Tuna in Spring Water	70	0	0	35	0	0	0	35
Albacore in Spring Water	60	0	0	25	0	0	0	105
Deep Sea Chunk Light Tongol	60	0	0	35	0	0	0	50
Gefen Fancy Albacore Chunk White LS	60	1	0	25	0	0	0	35
Henry & Lisa's Solid White Albacore, 3 oz	150	8	3	30	0	0	0	113
Miramonte Light Chunk Tuna in Water, NSA....	60	0	0	30	0	0	0	5
Natural Sea Chunk, NSA	60	0	0	20	0	0	0	120
Natural Value Albacore in Water, NSA	70	1	0	30	1	0	0	140
Chunk Tongol or Yellowfin Tuna in Water, NSA	60	0	0	30	0	0	0	140
Rainforest Trading Solid White Albacore, NSA	90	3	1	30	0	0	0	15
StarKist Chunk White Albacore, Very LS	60	1	0	25	0	0	0	35
LS Albacore White Tuna (pouch)	90	1	1	30	0	0	0	70
Chunk Light, LS	60	1	0	25	0	0	0	100
LS Chunk Light (pouch)	80	1	0	30	1	1	0	130
Wegmans *Food You Feel Good About*								
Light Yellowfin Tuna in Water	60	1	0	15	0	0	0	140
Whole Foods Market 365 Tongol, NSA	60	0	0	35	0	0	0	50
Albacore, NSA	65	1	0	30	0	0	0	80

FISH AND SEAFOOD – FRESH

	Cal	Fat	Sat	Chol	Carb	Fib	Sug	Sod
Monkfish, 3 oz	65	1	0	21	0	0	0	15
Trout, rainbow, farmed, 3 oz	117	5	1	50	0	0	0	30
Tuna (albacore), yellowfin, 3 oz	92	1	0	38	0	0	0	31
Pike, northern, 3 oz	75	1	0	33	0	0	0	33
Salmon, chinook or sockeye, 3 oz	152	9	3	43	0	0	0	40
Atlantic, farmed, 3 oz	177	11	3	47	0	0	0	50
Pink, 3 oz	99	3	0	44	0	0	0	57
Smoked, 3 oz	99	4	1	20	0	0	0	666

FISH AND SEAFOOD
Fish and Seafood – Frozen

	Cal	Fat	Sat	Chol	Carb	Fib	Sug	Sod
Catfish, wild, 3 oz	81	2	1	49	0	0	0	37
Eel, 3 oz	156	10	2	107	0	0	0	43
Cod, atlantic, 3 oz	70	1	0	37	0	0	0	46
Pacific, 3 oz	70	1	0	31	0	0	0	60
Halibut, 3 oz	94	2	0	27	0	0	0	46
Sturgeon, 3 oz	89	3	1	51	0	0	0	46
Clams, 3 oz	63	1	0	29	2	0	0	48
Crayfish, farmed, 3 oz	61	1	0	91	0	0	0	53
Perch, 3 oz	77	1	0	77	0	0	0	53
Snapper, 3 oz	85	1	0	31	0	0	0	54
Haddock, 3 oz	74	1	0	48	0	0	0	58
Bass, sea 3 oz	82	2	0	35	0	0	0	58
Freshwater, 3 oz	97	3	1	58	0	0	0	60
Orange roughy, 3 oz	65	1	0	51	0	0	0	61
Sole (flounder), 3 oz	77	1	0	41	0	0	0	69
Pollock, atlantic, 3 oz	78	1	0	60	0	0	0	73
Walleye, 3 oz	69	1	0	60	0	0	0	84
Mackerel, pacific or jack, 3 oz	134	7	2	40	0	0	0	73
Atlantic, 3 oz	174	12	3	60	0	0	0	77
King, 3 oz	89	2	0	45	0	0	0	134
Swordfish, 3 oz	103	3	1	33	0	0	0	77
Anchovies, 3 oz	111	4	1	51	0	0	0	88
Oysters, pacific, 3 oz	69	2	0	43	4	0	0	90
Eastern, farmed, 3 oz	50	1	0	21	5	0	0	151
Shrimp, 3 oz	90	1	0	129	1	0	0	126
Scallops, 3 oz	75	1	0	28	2	0	0	137
Lobster, spiny, 3 oz	95	1	0	60	2	0	0	150
Northern, 3 oz	77	1	0	81	0	0	0	252
Mussels, 3 oz	73	2	0	24	3	0	0	243
Crab, blue or dungeness, 3 oz	74	1	0	68	0	0	0	250
Alaskan king, 3 oz	71	1	0	36	0	0	0	711
Cuttlefish, 3 oz	67	1	0	95	1	0	0	316
Seafood substitutes:								
Shrimp, imitation, 3 oz	86	1	0	31	8	0	-	599
Scallop, imitation, 3 oz	84	0	0	18	9	0	-	676
Crab, imitation, 3 oz	81	0	0	13	0	0	5	715

Brands . . . *(3 oz unless noted)*
Most fresh fish and seafood within generic average.

FISH AND SEAFOOD – FROZEN

Most frozen fish and seafood is comparable to fresh, however, prepared fish (i.e. battered or breaded) may contain added sodium.

FISH AND SEAFOOD – MEAL KITS AND HELPERS

	Cal	Fat	Sat	Chol	Carb	Fib	Sug	Sod
Tuna mix/helper, cheese, 1 cup	290	11	2	20	32	1	2	890

Brands . . . *Most brands within generic average.*

FISH AND SEAFOOD – PREPARED ENTREES

(also see Dinners/Meals–Frozen, pg 138)

	Cal	Fat	Sat	Chol	Carb	Fib	Sug	Sod
Fish sticks, breaded, 3 oz	209	11	2	27	18	1	2	354
Fish fillet, battered or breaded, 3 oz	211	13	3	31	15	1	4	484
Popcorn shrimp, 3.2 oz	240	12	4	55	24	0	2	630
Crab cakes, 3 oz	242	16	3	125	8	0	0	745

	Cal	Fat	Sat	Chol	Carb	Fib	Sug	Sod

Brands . . . *(3 oz serving unless noted)*

	Cal	Fat	Sat	Chol	Carb	Fib	Sug	Sod
Goose Point Steamers in 5 Clams, 14 clams...	70	4	2	25	3	0	0	70
SeaPak Coconut Shrimp, 3.7 oz	310	14	4	65	36	1	19	140
Wildcatch Sockeye Salmon Burgers, 4 oz	200	10	2	70	1	0	0	130

REDUCED SODIUM (LESS THAN GENERIC)

	Cal	Fat	Sat	Chol	Carb	Fib	Sug	Sod
Blue Horizon Bites, all varieties, 2 oz (2).....	80	2	1	15	7	1	4	210
Tempura Shrimp, 3.5 oz............................	160	2	0	85	22	1	0	290
Disney Cheddar Treasures	120	6	3	25	3	0	0	230
Dr. Praeger's Potato-Crusted Fishies, 3	90	4	1	10	9	0	1	210
Potato-Crusted Fishies or Fish Sticks, 3.......	80	4	1	25	7	1	0	220
Lightly Breaded Fish Fillets, 1	100	4	1	15	12	0	1	250
Lightly Breaded Fish Sticks, 3	150	6	2	15	16	1	1	290
Salmon Cakes, 1.....................................	190	10	1	15	15	3	0	350
Fisher Boy Fish Filets, 2 oz	170	9	2	20	16	0	1	260
Fish Portions, Crunchy, 2.7 oz...................	170	10	2	20	15	0	1	320
Crab Cakes, 1..	140	5	1	10	16	1	3	350
Gorton's Grilled Tilapia, Garlic & Butter, 3.2 oz	80	3	1	50	1	0	0	150
Grilled Tilapia, Signature Grilled, 3.2 oz	80	3	1	50	1	0	0	250
Grilled Fillets, Classic Grilled, 3.9 oz	100	3	1	65	1	0	0	260
Grilled Salmon, Classic Grilled, 3.2 oz	100	3	1	35	1	0	0	270
Grilled Fillets, Lemon Pepper or Garlic Butter..	100	3	1	70	1	0	0	290
Grilled Fillets, Italian Herb, 3.9 oz	100	3	1	60	1	0	0	300
Grilled Salmon, Lemon Butter, 3.2 oz..........	100	3	1	40	1	0	0	300
Great Value Breaded Fish Sticks, 3.4 oz	230	12	3	25	19	3	2	290
Henry & Lisa's Salmon Burger, 3.2 oz	120	4	1	30	9	2	3	210
Bay Scallops w/Japanese Marinade, 4.5 oz ..	140	3	0	57	14	0	12	273
Kineret Crunchy Fish Portions, 2	260	10	2	35	29	1	1	270
Life Choices Whole Fillet Fish Sticks, 3	190	4	0	20	27	5	1	290
Mrs. Pauls Lightly Breaded Flounder Fillets	160	7	2	25	11	0	1	150
Lightly Breaded Haddock Fillets, 4 oz...........	230	10	3	40	17	1	1	210
Lightly Breaded Tilapia Fillets, 4 oz	230	11	3	35	17	1	1	220
Deviled Crab Cakes, 2.9 oz........................	220	12	2	60	12	3	1	320
Xtra Large Crunchy Fish Sticks, 3 oz (4)......	190	9	2	30	18	1	1	370
Phillips Coastal Crab Cakes	220	17	3	90	7	0	1	380
Steamer Creations Garlic/Herb Shrimp, 4 oz	180	9	5	160	3	0	1	390
Sea Cuisine Coconut Crusted Tilapia, 5 oz....	320	15	6	20	26	3	7	290
SeaPak Herb Butter Salmon, 5 oz...............	350	26	11	105	3	0	1	280
Trident Salmon Burgers, 2.8 oz	130	7	1	30	1	0	0	230
Natural Ultimate Fish Sticks, 3.3 oz	170	7	1	40	15	1	0	240
Panko Breaded Cod, 3 oz	160	6	0	20	16	0	1	300
Panko Breaded Tilaplia, 4 oz......................	240	10	2	30	21	0	1	350
Naturals SW Style Tilapia, 6 oz	170	6	1	65	3	0	1	360
Baja Style Breaded Cod Fillets, 4.2 oz.........	220	8	1	25	22	1	0	390
Naturals Mediterranean Style Cod Fillets, 6 oz	200	9	1	45	5	1	0	390
Naturals Lemon Herb Tilapia, 6 oz..............	190	5	1	65	4	1	0	400
Van de Kamp's Lightly Breaded Tilapia, 4 oz	240	11	3	35	17	1	1	280
Wegmans Salmon Burgers, 4.4 oz	310	15	3	90	7	1	0	200

177

FRUITS AND VEGETABLES

*See RESOURCES, page 305, for a partial list of manufacturers and retailers offering low-salt products online or visit **LowSaltFoods.com** for additional sources.*

FRUITS AND VEGETABLES

FRUIT JUICE

(see Fruit/Fruit-Blended Juices/Drinks, pg 42)

FRUITS – CANNED

	Cal	Fat	Sat	Chol	Carb	Fib	Sug	Sod
Pineapple, light syrup, 1/2 cup	66	0	0	0	17	1	16	1
Grapefruit sections, light syrup, 1/2 cup	76	0	0	0	20	1	19	3
Apricots, halves, light syrup, 1/2 cup	80	0	0	0	21	2	19	5
Pears, halves, light syrup, 1/2 cup	72	0	0	0	19	2	15	6
Fruit cocktail, light syrup, 1/2 cup	69	0	0	0	18	1	17	7
Peaches, halves, heavy syrup, 1/2 cup	97	0	0	0	26	2	26	8
Light syrup, 1/2 cup	68	0	0	0	18	2	17	6
Mandarin oranges, light syrup, 1/2 cup	77	0	0	0	20	1	20	8
Fruit salad, light syrup, 1/2 cup	73	0	0	0	19	1	17	8
Cherries, sweet, heavy syrup, 1/2 cup	100	0	0	0	26	1	19	10
Plums, light syrup, 1/2 cup	79	0	0	0	21	1	19	25
Applesauce, 1/2 cup	97	0	0	0	25	2	21	36
Unsweetened, 1/2 cup	51	0	0	0	14	1	11	2

Brands . . . *Most brands within generic average.*

FRUITS – DRIED

	Cal	Fat	Sat	Chol	Carb	Fib	Sug	Sod
Apple, 1 ring	16	0	0	0	4	1	4	6
Apricot, 1 half	8	0	0	0	2	0	2	0
Currants (raisins), 1/2 cup	204	0	0	0	53	5	48	6
Dates, 1	23	0	0	0	6	1	5	0
Fig, 1	21	0	0	0	5	1	4	1
Prunes, 1	20	0	0	0	5	1	3	0

Brands . . . *Most brands within generic average.*

FRUITS – FRESH

	Cal	Fat	Sat	Chol	Carb	Fib	Sug	Sod
Apple, 1 med	72	0	0	0	19	3	14	1
Apricot, 1	17	0	0	0	4	1	3	0
Banana, 1 med	105	0	0	0	27	3	14	1
Blackberries, 1 cup	62	0	0	0	14	8	7	1
Blueberries, 1 cup	83	0	0	0	21	4	14	1
Cantaloupe, med, 1/4	47	0	0	0	11	1	11	22
Cherries, sweet with pits, 1 cup	74	0	0	0	19	3	15	0
Cranberries, 1 cup	44	0	0	0	12	4	4	2
Grapefruit, 1/2	52	0	0	0	13	2	9	0
Grapes, 1 cup	110	1	0	0	29	1	25	3
Guava	37	1	0	0	8	3	5	1
Honeydew, med, 1/4	90	0	0	0	23	2	20	45
Kiwi, 1 med	46	0	0	0	11	2	7	2
Kumquat	13	0	0	0	3	1	2	2
Lemon	17	0	0	0	5	2	1	1
Lime	20	0	0	0	7	2	1	1
Lychee (litchi), 1	6	0	0	0	2	0	1	0
Mango, 1 cup	107	0	0	0	28	3	24	3
Nectarine, med	60	0	0	0	14	2	11	0
Orange, med	62	0	0	0	15	3	12	0
Papaya, 1 cup	55	0	0	0	14	2	8	4

179

FRUITS AND VEGETABLES
Fruits – Frozen

	Cal	Fat	Sat	Chol	Carb	Fib	Sug	Sod
Peach, med	38	0	0	0	9	2	8	0
Pear, med	96	0	0	0	26	5	16	2
Persimmon, japanese, 1	118	0	0	0	31	6	21	2
Pineapple, 1 cup	74	0	0	0	20	2	14	2
Plum	30	0	0	0	8	1	7	0
Pomegranate	105	0	0	0	26	1	25	5
Raspberries, 1 cup	64	1	0	0	15	8	5	1
Rhubarb, 1 cup	26	0	0	0	6	2	1	5
Strawberries, halves, 1 cup	49	0	0	0	12	3	7	2
Tangerine, med	45	0	0	0	11	2	9	2
Watermelon, 1/16 wedge	86	0	0	0	22	1	18	3

FRUITS – FROZEN

	Cal	Fat	Sat	Chol	Carb	Fib	Sug	Sod
Apples, unsweetened slices, 1 cup	83	1	0	0	21	3	-	5
Apricots, sweetened, 1 cup	237	0	0	0	61	5	-	10
Blackberries, unsweetened, 1 cup	97	1	0	0	24	8	16	2
Blueberries, unsweetened, 1 cup	79	1	0	0	19	4	13	2
Boysenberries, unsweetened, 1 cup	66	0	0	0	16	7	9	1
Cherries, sour, unsweetened, 1 cup	71	1	0	0	17	3	14	2
Cherries, sweet, usweetened, 1 cup	90	0	0	0	22	3	18	0
Mixed fruit, unsweetened, 1 cup	80	0	0	0	21	3	16	0
Melon balls, 1 cup	57	0	0	0	14	1	-	54
Peaches, unsweetened slices, 1 cup	67	0	0	0	17	3	12	0
Raspberries, sweetened, 1 cup	258	0	0	0	65	11	54	3
Rhubarb, 1 cup	29	0	0	0	7	3	2	3
Strawberries, sliced, sweetened, 1 cup	200	0	0	0	51	3	44	0

Brands . . . *Most brands within generic average.*

FRUITS – JAMS, JELLIES & FRUIT SPREADS

(see Jams/Jellies/Fruit Spreads, pg 78)

LEGUMES / BEANS – CANNED

(also see Refried Beans, pg 169)

	Cal	Fat	Sat	Chol	Carb	Fib	Sug	Sod
Soybeans, 1/2 cup	149	8	1	0	9	5	3	204
Fava beans (broad beans), 1/2 cup	100	0	0	0	17	5	0	250
Cannellini beans, 1/2 cup	153	0	0	0	29	6	0	270
Black-eyed peas, 1/2 cup	70	1	0	0	12	3	6	320
Aduki beans (adzuki beans), 1/2 cup	109	0	0	0	20	5	0	323
Great northern beans, 1/2 cup	100	1	0	0	28	5	0	330
Pinto beans, 1/2 cup	103	1	0	0	18	6	0	353
Lower sodium, 1/2 cup	80	0	0	0	18	7	0	220
Garbanzo beans (chickpeas), 1/2 cup	143	1	0	0	27	5	0	359
50% less salt/lower sodium, 1/2 cup	110	3	0	0	15	3	2	220
Kidney beans (red beans), 1/2 cup	108	0	0	0	19	7	0	379
50% less salt/lower sodium, 1/2 cup	120	1	0	0	20	6	4	220
Lima beans, 1/2 cup	95	0	0	0	18	6	0	405
Black beans, 1/2 cup	109	0	0	0	20	8	0	461
50% less salt/lower sodium,1/2 cup	110	1	0	0	17	6	1	240
Pork and beans, 1/2 cup	134	1	0	9	25	7	16	524
Baked beans, 1/2 cup	150	1	0	0	29	7	5	550
Navy beans, 1/2 cup	148	1	0	0	27	7	0	587

Brands . . . *(1/2 cup unless noted)*

	Cal	Fat	Sat	Chol	Carb	Fib	Sug	Sod
ADUKI (ADZUKI) BEANS								
Eden Organic Aduki	110	0	0	0	19	5	0	10
BAKED BEANS/PORK AND BEANS								
Eden Organic Baked w/Sorghum /Mustard	150	0	0	0	27	7	6	130
BLACK BEANS (TURTLE BEANS)								
365 Black, NSA	110	1	0	0	19	7	1	10
Eden Organic Black	110	1	0	0	18	6	0	15
Caribbean Black	90	1	0	0	20	7	1	135
Full Circle Organic Black	130	0	0	0	24	6	5	130
Goya Black LS	100	0	0	0	18	8	0	125
Kuner's Black, NSA	110	1	0	0	19	7	1	10
LaPreferida Organic Black	110	1	0	0	18	6	0	140
Meijer Organics Black	120	0	0	0	22	5	1	85
Mrs Grimes Black, NSA	110	1	0	0	19	7	1	10
Natural Value Organic Black	100	0	0	0	19	5	4	140
Nature's Promise Organic Black	120	0	0	0	21	6	0	130
O Organics Organic Black	130	0	0	0	24	6	5	130
Private Select Organic Black	130	0	0	0	24	6	5	130
Westbrae Natural Organic Black	100	0	0	0	19	5	4	140
Wild Harvest Organic Black	130	0	0	0	24	6	5	130
BLACK-EYED PEAS								
Eden Organic	90	1	0	0	16	4	1	25
BROAD BEANS (see Fava Beans below)								
BUTTER BEANS (see Lima Beans, pg 182)								
CANNELLINI (WHITE KIDNEY) BEANS								
Carmelina Brand Cannellini	125	1	0	0	23	6	0	80
Eden Organic, NSA	100	1	0	0	17	5	1	40
CHICKPEAS (see Garbanzo Beans below)								
CHILI BEANS								
Kuner's NSA Chili Beans in Chili Sauce	120	2	0	0	21	5	0	15
Mrs Grimes Chili Beans in Chili Sauce, NSA	120	2	0	0	21	5	0	15
REDUCED SODIUM (LESS THAN GENERIC):								
Westbrae Natural	100	0	0	0	19	5	2	150
CRANBERRY BEANS (BORLOTTI)								
Carmelina Brand Borlotti	121	1	0	0	22	9	0	80
FAVA BEANS (BROAD BEANS) – Most brands within generic average (250mg).								
GARBANZO BEANS (CHICKPEAS)								
365 NSA	90	2	0	0	15	4	1	10
Carmelina Brand Garbanzo	135	2	0	0	23	6	4	80
Eden Organic Garbanzo	130	1	0	0	23	5	1	30
Full Circle Organic Garbanzo	120	2	0	0	21	3	4	120
Goya LS Garbanzo	100	0	0	0	23	5	1	120
Kuner's NSA Garbanzo	90	2	0	0	15	4	1	10
LaPreferida Organic Garbanzo	130	1	0	0	20	7	0	120
Natural Value Organic Garbanzo	110	2	0	0	18	5	3	140
Private Select Organic Garbanzo	120	2	0	0	21	3	4	120
Westbrae Natural Organic Garbanzo	110	2	0	0	18	5	3	140
Wild Harvest Organic Garbanzo	120	2	0	0	21	3	4	120
REDUCED SODIUM (LESS THAN GENERIC):								
Nature's Promise Garbanzo	120	1	0	0	20	7	0	150
GREAT NORTHERN BEANS								
Eden Organic	110	1	0	0	20	8	1	45
Westbrae Natural Organic	100	0	0	0	19	6	2	140

	Cal	Fat	Sat	Chol	Carb	Fib	Sug	Sod
GREEN BEANS *(see Green Beans, pg 186)*								
KIDNEY BEANS (RED BEANS)								
365 Everyday Value NSA	110	1	0	0	20	7	1	10
Bush's Best Reduced Sodium Dark Red	105	0	0	0	22	8	3	130
Eden Organic Kidney	100	0	0	0	18	10	1	15
Small Red	100	1	0	0	17	5	1	25
Full Circle Organic, Dark Red	120	0	0	0	22	6	2	120
Goya Red Kidney, LS	110	0	0	0	19	8	0	110
Kuner's Dark Red Kidney, NSA	110	1	0	0	27	7	1	10
Meijer Organics Dark Red Kidney	110	0	0	0	19	4	1	100
Mrs Grimes Dark Red Kidney, NSA	110	1	0	0	20	7	1	10
Natural Value Organic Kidney or Red (avg)	100	0	0	0	18	5	2	140
Private Select Organic, Dark Red	120	0	0	0	22	6	2	120
Westbrae Natural Organic Red or Kidney (avg)	100	0	0	0	19	7	2	140
LENTILS								
REDUCED SODIUM (LESS THAN GENERIC):								
Westbrae Natural Organic	100	0	0	0	17	9	2	150
LIMA BEANS (BUTTER BEANS)								
Carmelina Brand Butter Beans	105	1	0	0	19	6	0	80
Eden Organic Butter Beans	100	1	0	0	17	4	0	35
MISC/MIXED BEANS								
Private Select Tri-Bean Blend	130	0	0	0	24	7	3	120
Westbrae Natural Organic Soup Beans	100	0	0	0	10	6	2	140
REDUCED SODIUM (LESS THAN GENERIC):								
Westbrae Natural Organic Salad Beans	100	1	0	0	19	5	2	150
NAVY BEANS								
Eden Organic	110	0	0	0	20	7	0	15
PINK BEANS								
Goya Pink, LS	100	0	0	0	19	7	0	110
PINTO BEANS								
365 NSA	110	0	0	0	20	7	1	10
Eden Organic Pinto	110	1	0	0	18	6	1	15
Full Circle Organic Pinto	120	0	0	0	23	9	2	120
Kuner's NSA Pinto	110	1	0	0	20	7	1	10
Goya Pinto, LS	100	0	0	0	18	7	0	115
Natural Value Organic Pinto	100	0	0	0	19	7	2	140
Private Select Organic Pinto	120	0	0	0	23	9	2	120
Westbrae Natural Organic Pinto	100	0	0	0	19	7	2	140
Wild Harvest Organic Pinto	120	0	0	0	23	9	2	120
REFRIED BEANS *(see Hispanic/Latino–Refried Beans, pg 169)*								
RICE & BEANS								
Eden Organic Rice & Caribbean Black Beans	120	1	0	0	23	4	1	100
Cajun Rice & Beans	110	1	0	0	23	3	1	115
Brown Rice & Green Lentils	120	1	0	0	23	2	0	120
Brown Rice w/Chick Peas or w/Kidney Beans	110	1	0	0	23	2	0	135
Brown Rice & Pinto Beans	120	1	0	0	24	3	1	140
REDUCED SODIUM (LESS THAN GENERIC):								
Eden Organic Curried Rice & Lentils	130	1	0	0	21	1	1	200
SOY BEANS								
Eden Organic Black	120	6	1	0	8	7	1	30
Westbrae Natural Organic	150	7	1	0	11	3	3	140
WAX BEANS *(see Wax Beans, pg 188)*								
WHITE BEANS *(see Cannellini Beans, pg 181)*								

	Cal	Fat	Sat	Chol	Carb	Fib	Sug	Sod

LEGUMES/BEANS – DRIED/RAW

Soybeans, 1/2 cup	415	19	3	0	28	9	7	2
Black beans, 1/2 cup	331	1	0	0	60	15	2	5
Navy beans, 1/2 cup	350	2	0	0	63	25	4	5
Lentils, 1/2 cup	339	1	0	0	58	29	2	6
Fava beans (broad beans), 1/2 cup	256	1	0	0	44	19	4	10
Kidney beans (red beans), 1/2 cup	310	1	0	0	56	14	2	11
Pinto beans, 1/2 cup	335	1	0	0	60	15	2	12
Great northern beans, 1/2 cup	310	1	0	0	57	19	2	13
Lima beans (butter beans), 1/2 cup	301	1	0	0	56	17	8	16
Garbanzo beans (chickpeas), 1/2 cup	364	6	1	0	61	17	11	24

Brands . . . *Most brands within generic average.*

LEGUMES/BEANS – FROZEN

Edamame, 1/2 cup	90	2	0	0	9	8	0	30
Lima beans, fordhook, 1/2 cup	85	0	0	0	16	4	1	46
Lima beans, baby, 1/2 cup	110	0	0	0	20	5	2	240
With butter sauce, 1/2 cup	133	3	2	5	18	6	1	330

Brands . . . *(1/2 cup unless noted)*

EDAMAME

Birds Eye Edamame in the Pod	110	4	0	0	12	9	2	0
Edamame	120	5	0	0	8	6	2	5

LIMA BEANS

Birds Eye Fordhook	100	0	0	0	18	3	4	5
Giant Fordhook	100	0	0	0	18	4	3	5
Hanover Silver Line Baby Lima Beans	100	0	0	0	20	8	2	80
McKenzie's Speckled Butter Beans	100	0	0	0	19	6	1	130
Pictsweet Fordhook	100	0	0	0	18	4	3	5
ShopRite Fordhook Lima Beans	100	0	0	0	18	4	3	5

LEGUMES/BEANS – PACKAGED MIX

Bountiful Pantry Boston Baked Beans	200	1	0	0	39	1	9	0

TOMATOES – CANNED

Whole tomatoes, 1/4 cup	10	0	0	0	3	1	2	90
Stewed tomatoes, 1/4 cup	17	0	0	0	4	1	2	141
Diced or chopped tomatoes, 1/4 cup	13	0	0	0	3	1	2	145
Seasoned, 1/4 cup	25	0	0	0	6	1	4	325
Crushed tomatoes, 1/4 cup	20	0	0	0	3	1	3	170
Tomato paste, 1/4 cup	54	0	0	0	12	4	8	180
Tomato puree, 1/4 cup	24	0	0	0	6	1	3	249
Tomato sauce, 1/4 cup	20	0	0	0	5	1	3	390

Brands . . .

CRUSHED AND STRAINED *(1/4 cup unless noted)*

Bionaturae Crushed or Strained	15	0	0	0	3	1	2	10
Cento Crushed	35	0	0	0	7	2	4	20
Dei Fratelli No Salt Crushed	20	0	0	0	4	1	3	15
No Salt Crushed w/Basil & Herbs	20	0	0	0	4	1	3	15
Eden Organic Crushed or Crushed w/Basil	20	0	0	0	3	1	2	0
Crushed w/Onion & Garlic	20	0	0	0	3	1	2	0
Full Circle Crushed, NSA	20	0	0	0	5	1	2	20
Furmano's Crushed w/Garlic/Olive Oil, 1/2 cup	40	0	0	0	8	2	4	85
Chunky Crushed Tomatoes, 1/2 cup	35	0	0	0	8	2	4	100
Chunky Crushed w/Basil/Garlic/Oregano, 1/2 cup	40	0	0	0	8	2	4	120

FRUITS AND VEGETABLES
Tomatoes – Canned

	Cal	Fat	Sat	Chol	Carb	Fib	Sug	Sod
LaSquisita Crushed	25	0	0	0	5	2	3	68
Pomi Strained	25	0	0	0	5	1	4	85
Progresso Crushed	20	0	0	0	4	1	2	95
Red Pack Crushed in Thick Puree	20	0	0	0	4	1	2	120
S&W Crushed, Italian Style	20	0	0	0	4	1	2	95
Crushed in Rich Puree	20	0	0	0	4	1	2	125
Tuttorossa Crushed w/Basil	10	0	0	0	4	1	4	120
Woodstock Farms Organic Crushed w/Basil	25	0	0	0	5	1	4	85
DICED AND CHOPPED *(1/2 cup unless noted)*								
Bionaturae Diced	30	0	0	0	6	1	4	20
Carmelina 'e... San Marzano Italian Chopped	25	0	0	0	6	2	4	20
Organic Italian Chopped	25	0	0	0	6	2	4	20
Dei Fratelli Low Sodium	25	0	0	0	7	1	5	100
Eden Organic Diced or Diced w/Basil	30	0	0	0	6	2	4	5
Diced w/Roasted Onion	30	0	0	0	6	2	4	5
Diced w/Green Chilies	30	0	0	0	5	2	3	35
Furmano's Diced or Petite Diced	25	0	0	0	5	1	3	125
Petite Diced w/Green Chilies	25	0	0	0	5	1	3	125
Lucini Tuscan Harvest Plum Diced Tomatoes	19	0	0	0	4	1	4	80
Muir Glen Diced, NSA	30	0	0	0	6	1	4	15
Pomi Chopped	20	0	0	0	4	3	4	10
S&W Ready-Cut Diced, NSA	25	0	0	0	6	2	4	50
Safeway Diced, NSA	25	0	0	0	5	1	3	20
Woodstock Farms Organic Diced, NSA	25	0	0	0	5	1	4	45
REDUCED SODIUM (LESS THAN GENERIC):								
Furmano's								
Italian Diced w/Basil/Garlic/Oregano	35	0	0	0	7	1	5	150
TOMATO PASTE *(2 tbsp unless noted)*								
Bionaturae Tomato Paste	30	0	0	0	6	1	4	20
Cento Tomato Paste	30	0	0	0	7	2	5	25
Contadina Tomato Paste	30	0	0	0	6	1	3	20
Full Circle Organic Tomato Paste	30	0	0	0	6	1	3	35
Hunt's Tomato Paste, NSA	30	0	0	0	6	2	4	15
La Squisita Tomato Paste	30	0	0	0	6	1	3	0
Muir Glen Organic Tomato Paste	30	0	0	0	6	1	3	20
Our Family Tomato Paste	30	0	0	0	6	1	3	20
S&W Tomato Paste	30	0	0	0	6	1	3	20
Whole Foods Market 365 Tomato Paste	33	0	0	0	6	1	3	20
Woodstock Farms Organic Tomato Paste	30	0	0	0	6	1	3	20
TOMATO PUREE AND SAUCE *(1/4 cup unless noted)*								
Carmelina 'e... San Marzana Italian Tomato Puree	13	0	0	0	3	1	2	10
Cento Tomato Puree	25	0	0	0	5	1	3	15
Contadina Puree	20	0	0	0	4	1	1	15
Dei Fratelli No Salt Puree	20	0	0	0	4	1	3	15
Furmano's Puree	20	0	0	0	4	1	3	40
Great Value Puree, NSA	25	0	0	0	5	1	3	15
Hunt's, Sauce, NSA	15	0	0	0	4	1	3	15
Muir Glen Organic Puree	20	0	0	0	5	1	3	20
Sauce, NSA	20	0	0	0	5	1	3	30
Progresso Puree	25	0	0	0	5	1	3	15
Rokeach Sauce w/Mushrooms, NSA	40	1	0	0	7	1	0	25
S&W Puree	30	0	0	0	6	2	3	15
Safeway Sauce, NSA	20	0	0	0	4	1	2	25
Woodstock Farms Organic Tomato Sauce	20	0	0	0	5	1	1	30

	Cal	Fat	Sat	Chol	Carb	Fib	Sug	Sod
WHOLE, PEELED AND STEWED TOMATOES *(1/2 cup unless noted)*								
Academia Barilla Peeled Cherry	30	0	0	0	6	12	4	0
Bel Aria Plum (Pomodori Pelati Italian)	25	0	0	0	6	2	4	20
Bella Terra Organic Italian Whole Peeled	30	0	0	0	5	2	5	35
Bionaturae Whole	30	0	0	0	6	1	4	20
Carmelina 'e... San Marzano Italian Cherry	30	0	0	0	6	2	4	20
Italian Peeled or Organic Italian Peeled	25	0	0	0	6	2	4	20
Cento Whole Cherry Tomatoes	20	0	0	0	4	1	3	15
Peeled Tomatoes, Italian or San Marzano	25	0	0	0	5	2	4	20
Dei Fratelli No Salt Whole Tomatoes	20	0	0	0	5	1	4	10
No Salt Whole Tomatoes in Puree	30	0	0	0	7	2	4	20
Eden Organic Whole Roma or Whole Roma w/Basil	30	0	0	0	4	1	2	10
Furmano's Whole Peeled, NSA	25	0	0	0	5	1	3	10
Italian Style Plum Tomatoes	25	0	0	0	5	1	3	100
Whole Peeled	25	0	0	0	5	1	3	125
Stewed Tomatoes	40	0	0	0	9	1	6	130
Hunt's NSA Whole or NSA Stewed	20	0	0	0	5	1	3	25
LaSquisita Peeled w/Basil	25	0	0	0	6	2	4	20
Lucini Tuscan Harvest Plum Whole Tomatoes	19	0	0	0	4	1	4	80
S&W Stewed, NSA	35	0	0	0	9	2	7	50
Sclafani Whole	20	0	0	0	8	2	4	20
TOMATO AND VEGETABLE MIX								
REDUCED SODIUM (LESS THAN GENERIC):								
Glory *Sensibily Seasoned*								
Lower Sodium Tomatoes & Okra, 1/2 cup	35	0	0	0	8	2	4	150

TOMATOES – DRIED

	Cal	Fat	Sat	Chol	Carb	Fib	Sug	Sod
Tomato halves, dried, 2-3	15	0	0	0	3	1	0	5
Seasoned, dried, 2-3	15	0	0	0	3	1	0	25

Brands . . . *Most brands within generic average.*

VEGETABLES – CANNED

(also see Pickled/Specialty Vegetables, pg 96)

	Cal	Fat	Sat	Chol	Carb	Fib	Sug	Sod
Garlic, crushed or chopped, 1 tsp	10	0	0	0	1	0	0	0
Onions, cocktail, 1 onion	0	0	0	0	0	0	0	30
French fried, 2 tbsp	45	4	2	0	3	0	0	60
Yam, 1/2 cup	130	1	0	0	29	2	23	30
Sweet potato, 1/2 cup	101	0	0	0	24	3	18	50
Beets, 1/2 cup (4 oz)	37	0	0	0	9	1	8	176
Pickled beets, 1 oz	15	0	0	0	4	1	4	60
Harvard beets, 1/2 cup	90	0	0	0	22	3	0	199
Spinach, 1/2 cup	30	0	0	0	3	2	0	200
Mixed vegetables, peas and onions, 1/2 cup	31	0	0	0	5	1	0	265
Corn, whole kernel, 1/2 cup	82	1	0	0	20	2	4	286
50% less sodium, 1/2 cup	80	1	0	0	16	1	4	180
Creamed, 1/2 cup	92	1	0	0	23	2	4	365
Carrots, 1/2 cup	28	0	0	0	7	2	3	295
Greens, collard, 1/2 cup	50	0	0	0	7	3	3	300
Green beans, 1/2 cup	18	0	0	0	4	2	2	311
50% less sodium, 1/2 cup	20	0	0	0	4	1	2	200
Greens, turnip, 1/2 cup	16	0	0	0	3	2	0	324
Potatoes, 1 cup	88	0	0	0	15	2	0	326
Peas and carrots, 1/2 cup	48	0	0	0	11	3	3	332
Mushrooms, 1/2 cup	20	0	0	0	4	2	2	332

	Cal	Fat	Sat	Chol	Carb	Fib	Sug	Sod
Asparagus, 1/2 cup	18	0	0	0	3	1	0	360
50% less salt, 1/2 cup	15	0	0	0	2	1	1	210
Wax beans, 1/2 cup	23	0	0	0	5	2	2	360
Peas, 1/2 cup	66	0	0	0	12	4	4	390
50% less sodium, 1/2 cup	60	0	0	0	11	3	4	200
Artichoke hearts, 1/2 cup (4 oz)	35	0	0	0	6	4	1	420
Artichoke hearts, marinated, 1 oz	25	2	0	0	2	1	0	105
Zucchini, italian style, 1/2 cup	33	0	0	0	8	0	1	424
Cabbage, red, 1/2 cup	80	0	0	0	20	0	16	440
Sauerkraut, 1/2 cup	15	0	0	0	4	3	1	720
Reduced sodium, 1/2 cup	20	0	0	0	4	4	0	480
Brands . . . *(1/2 cup unless noted)*								
ARTICHOKE								
Cento Quartered/Marinated Artichoke Hearts	20	2	0	0	2	0	0	80
Napoleon Quartered Marinated Artichoke Hearts	25	2	0	0	2	1	0	90
Vigo Quartered Marinated Artichoke Hearts, 1 oz	30	2	0	0	3	1	1	90
ASPARAGUS								
Star Fine Foods Marinated Green, 1 oz	13	0	0	0	2	0	1	100
Tillen Farms Pickled Crispy, all, 3 spears	10	0	0	0	1	0	0	75
BEETS								
Freshlike Selects Sliced Pickled Beets, 1 oz	20	0	0	0	4	0	4	20
Wegmans Foods Feel Good NSA Sliced Beets	40	0	0	0	8	1	6	25
CABBAGE – *Most brands within generic average (440mg).*								
CARROTS								
The Allens Tiny Tender Sliced Carrots	35	0	0	0	8	3	3	40
Tillen Farms Pickled Crispy, 1 oz	30	0	0	0	7	1	6	5
Wegmans Foods You Feel Good About Sliced Carrots, NSA	30	0	0	0	6	2	4	55
REDUCED SODIUM (LESS THAN GENERIC):								
Freshlike Crinkle Sliced Carrots	45	0	0	0	11	3	3	180
COLLARD GREENS *(see Greens–Collard/Turnip/Other Greens, pg 187)*								
CORN *(also see Asian Vegetables, pg 162)*								
Butter Kernel Whole Kernel Corn, NSA	70	1	0	0	10	2	3	10
Del Monte Whole or Cream Style Sweet, NSA	60	1	0	0	11	3	7	10
Freshlike Whole Kernel, NSA	130	2	0	0	27	2	8	10
Great Value Whole Kernel, NSA	60	1	0	0	13	3	1	10
Green Giant Niblets, NSA	60	1	0	0	13	1	3	0
Our Family Whole, NSA	60	2	0	0	9	2	7	10
Pride Whole Kernel Golden Corn, NSA	70	1	0	0	10	2	3	10
Safeway Whole, NSA	80	1	0	0	17	2	6	20
Wegmans Foods You Feel Good About Whole Kernel, NSA	80	1	0	0	17	2	4	15
Wylwood Whole Kernel, NSA	70	1	0	0	12	2	6	20
GARLIC – *Most brands within generic average (0mg).*								
GREEN BEANS (STRING BEANS)								
The Allens Cut Green Beans, NSA	15	0	0	0	3	2	1	10
Butter Kernel Cut Green Beans, NSA	20	0	0	0	4	2	2	10
Del Monte NSA Cut or NSA French Style	20	0	0	0	4	2	2	10
Freshlike NSA French Style or NSA Cu	25	0	0	0	4	2	1	0
Giant NSA French Style or NSA Cut Green Beans	20	0	0	0	4	2	2	15
Great Value Cut Green Beans, NSA	25	0	0	0	4	2	1	0
Our Family Cut, NSA	20	0	0	0	4	2	2	15
Pride Cut Green Beans, NSA	20	0	0	0	4	2	2	10
Safeway Cut, NSA	20	0	0	0	4	2	2	15

	Cal	Fat	Sat	Chol	Carb	Fib	Sug	Sod
Wegmans Foods You Feel Good About								
NSA French Style or NSA Cut Green Beans	20	0	0	0	4	2	2	15
Wylwood Blue Lake Cut, NSA	20	0	0	0	4	2	2	10
REDUCED SODIUM (LESS THAN GENERIC):								
Del Monte Dill Green Beans........................	20	0	0	0	5	1	3	125
Glory Sensibly Seasoned Lower Sodium Beans..	25	0	0	0	5	2	1	160

GREENS – COLLARD, TURNIP AND OTHER GREENS

	Cal	Fat	Sat	Chol	Carb	Fib	Sug	Sod
The Allens Mustard Greens, NSA..................	30	1	0	0	5	3	1	10
Mixed Greens, NSA..................................	30	1	0	0	8	4	1	10
Turnip Greens, NSA.................................	25	1	0	0	3	2	1	15
Collard Greens or Turnip Greens w/Turnips, NSA	30	1	0	0	5	3	1	20
Kale Greens, NSA....................................	30	1	0	0	3	2	1	20
REDUCED SODIUM (LESS THAN GENERIC):								
Glory Sensibly Seasoned Lower Sodium								
Collard Greens, Turnip Greens, or Mixed Greens .	20	0	0	0	4	2	1	240

MIXED VEGETABLES

	Cal	Fat	Sat	Chol	Carb	Fib	Sug	Sod
America's Choice Mixed Veg, NSA	35	0	0	0	7	2	3	25
Del Monte Mixed Vegetables, NSA	40	0	0	0	8	2	3	25
Veg-All Original Mixed Veg, NSA...................	40	0	0	0	8	2	2	25
Wylwood Mixed Vegetables, NSA	45	0	0	0	7	2	2	25
REDUCED SODIUM (LESS THAN GENERIC):								
The Allen's Cut Italian Green Beans w/Potatoes ..	50	0	0	0	10	2	1	160
Glory Sensibly Seasoned								
Lower Sodium Tomatoes & Okra.................	30	0	0	0	6	2	3	170

MUSHROOMS *(also see Asian Vegetables, pg 162)*

	Cal	Fat	Sat	Chol	Carb	Fib	Sug	Sod
Ace of Diamonds Straw Mushrooms.............	30	0	0	0	4	2	1	55
Giorgio Pieces and Stems, NSA	20	0	0	0	3	1	0	20
Pennsylvania Dutchman Stems & Pieces, NSA..	20	0	0	0	3	1	0	20

ONIONS

Cocktail onions – Most brands within generic average (30mg).

	Cal	Fat	Sat	Chol	Carb	Fib	Sug	Sod
Great Value French Fried Onions, 2 tbsp	45	3	2	0	3	0	0	35

PEAS

	Cal	Fat	Sat	Chol	Carb	Fib	Sug	Sod
Del Monte, Fresh Cut, NSA..........................	60	0	0	0	11	4	6	10
Freshlike Tender Garden, NSA	110	1	0	0	19	6	5	10
Giant Sweet Peas, NSA...............................	60	1	0	0	11	4	5	15
Our Family, NSA......................................	60	1	0	0	10	3	5	15
Safeway, NSA	60	1	0	0	10	3	5	15
Wegmans Foods Feel Good NSA Sweet Peas...	60	1	0	0	10	3	5	15
Wylwood Sweet Peas, NSA...........................	60	0	0	0	11	4	6	10

PEPPERS *(see Pickled/Specialty Vegetables, pg 96; Chili Peppers, pg 168)*

POTATOES

	Cal	Fat	Sat	Chol	Carb	Fib	Sug	Sod
Allens Butterfield Shoestring Sticks, 2/3 cup ..	150	9	3	0	16	2	0	90
Giant Whole White, NSA, 2/3 cup	70	0	0	0	15	2	1	15
ShopRite Whole White, NSA, 2/3 cup.............	70	0	0	0	15	2	1	15

PUMPKIN *(see Pastry/Pie Fillings, pg 28)*

SAUERKRAUT

	Cal	Fat	Sat	Chol	Carb	Fib	Sug	Sod
REDUCED SODIUM (LESS THAN GENERIC):								
Bubba's..	15	0	0	0	3	1	0	230
Silver Floss Barrel Cured	20	0	0	0	1	1	0	180

SPINACH

	Cal	Fat	Sat	Chol	Carb	Fib	Sug	Sod
Del Monte Whole Leaf Spinach, NSA	30	0	0	0	4	2	0	85
Popeye Low Salt Spinach	30	0	0	0	4	2	1	35

SQUASH/ZUCCHINI – *Most brands within generic average.*

187

	Cal	Fat	Sat	Chol	Carb	Fib	Sug	Sod

STRING BEANS *(see Green Beans, pg 186)*
SWEET POTATOES AND YAMS – *Most brands within generic average (30–50mg).*
WAX BEANS – *Most brands within generic average (360mg).*

VEGETABLES – DRIED

	Cal	Fat	Sat	Chol	Carb	Fib	Sug	Sod
Mushrooms, shiitake, 4	44	0	0	0	11	2	0	2
Peppers, sweet, red or green, 1/4 cup	5	0	0	0	1	0	0	3

Brands . . .

	Cal	Fat	Sat	Chol	Carb	Fib	Sug	Sod
John Cope's Dried Sweet Corn, 1/4 cup	130	1	0	0	15	1	4	0

VEGETABLES – FRESH

The following vegetables are listed alphabetically.

	Cal	Fat	Sat	Chol	Carb	Fib	Sug	Sod
Artichoke, globe or french, med, 4.6 oz	60	0	0	0	13	7	1	120
Asparagus, 5 spears (5"-7")	16	0	0	0	3	2	2	2
Avocado, 1/2	161	15	2	0	9	7	1	7
Beets, 1/2 cup	29	0	0	0	7	2	5	53
Broccoli, 1/2 cup	15	0	0	0	3	1	1	15
Brussels sprouts, 1/2 cup	19	0	0	0	4	2	1	11
Cabbage, chopped, 1/2 cup	11	0	0	0	3	1	1	8
Carrot, 1 med	25	0	0	0	6	2	3	42
Cauliflower, 1/2 cup	13	0	0	0	3	1	1	15
Celery, 1 med stalk	6	0	0	0	1	1	1	32
Chives, 1 tbsp	1	0	0	0	0	0	0	0
Corn, 1/2 cup	66	1	0	0	15	2	2	12
Cucumber, 1/2 cup	7	0	0	0	1	0	1	1
Eggplant, 1/2 cup	10	0	0	0	2	1	1	1
Fennel bulb, 1/2 cup	13	0	0	0	3	1	0	23
Garlic, 1 clove	4	0	0	0	1	0	0	1
Jerusalem artichoke, 1/2 cup	55	0	0	0	13	1	7	3
Kale, 1/2 cup	17	0	0	0	3	1	0	14
Kohlrabi, 1/2 cup	18	0	0	0	4	2	2	14
Leeks, 1/2 cup	27	0	0	0	6	1	2	9
Lettuce, chopped (avg), 1 cup	8	0	0	0	2	1	1	6
Mushrooms, (avg), 1/2 cup	10	0	0	0	1	0	1	2
Mustard greens, 1/2 cup	7	0	0	0	1	1	0	7
Onion, 1/2 cup chopped	32	0	0	0	7	1	3	3
Parsnips, 1/2 cup	5	0	0	0	12	3	3	7
Peas, green, 1/2 cup	59	0	0	0	10	4	4	4
Pepper, banana, 1 small (4")	9	0	0	0	2	1	1	4
Pepper, jalapeno, 1	4	0	0	0	1	0	0	0
Peppers, sweet, green, 1/2 cup	15	0	0	0	3	1	2	2
Peppers, sweet, red, 1/2 cup	23	0	0	0	4	2	3	3
Potato, russet w/skin, med	168	0	0	0	38	3	1	11
Potato, red w/skin, med	149	0	0	0	34	4	2	13
Pumpkin, 1/2 cup	15	0	0	0	4	0	1	1
Radish, 1 med	1	0	0	0	0	0	0	2
Rutabaga, 1/2 cup	25	0	0	0	6	2	4	14
Shallots, 1 tbsp	7	0	0	0	2	0	0	1
Spinach, 1 cup	7	0	0	0	1	1	0	24
Squash, summer, 1/2 cup	9	0	0	0	2	1	1	1
Squash, winter, 1/2 cup	20	0	0	0	5	1	1	2
Sweet potato, 1/2 cup	57	0	0	0	13	2	3	37
Swiss chard, 1/2 cup	3	0	0	0	1	0	0	38
Tomato, 1 med	22	0	0	0	5	2	3	6

	Cal	Fat	Sat	Chol	Carb	Fib	Sug	Sod
Tomatillo, 1/2 cup	21	1	0	0	4	1	3	1
Turnips, 1/2 cup	18	0	0	0	4	1	2	44
Watercress, 1 cup	4	0	0	0	0	0	0	14
Yam, 1/2 cup	89	0	0	0	21	3	0	7
Zucchini, 1/2 cup	10	0	0	0	2	1	1	6

SALAD – PREPACKAGED

	Cal	Fat	Sat	Chol	Carb	Fib	Sug	Sod
Asian salad kit, 2 1/2 cups w/dressing	120	5	1	0	17	2	8	360
Caesar, 1.5 cups (3.5 oz)	170	14	3	10	8	1	2	380
Lite salad kit	90	6	1	5	8	1	2	340

Brands . . . *(2 cups prep w/dressing unless noted)*

	Cal	Fat	Sat	Chol	Carb	Fib	Sug	Sod
Dole Perfect Harvest Kit, 1.5 cups	160	12	2	0	11	3	7	105
Fresh Express Strawberry Fields Kit, 2.5 cups	200	13	2	0	17	2	12	65
REDUCED SODIUM (LESS THAN GENERIC):								
Et Tu Spinach Kit, 1/6 pkg	90	7	0	5	7	0	3	180
Southwest Ranch Kit, 1/6 pkg	110	10	2	0	5	1	1	190
Fresh Express Coleslaw Kit, 1.5 cups	150	10	2	5	14	2	11	160
Apples & Cheddar Kit, 2.5 cups	150	11	3	10	9	1	7	210

VEGETABLES – FROZEN

(also see Side Dishes, pg 151)

	Cal	Fat	Sat	Chol	Carb	Fib	Sug	Sod
Squash, butternut, 3 oz	48	0	0	0	12	1	2	2
Squash, zucchini, 3 oz	14	0	0	0	3	1	1	2
Corn, 3 oz	74	0	0	0	17	2	2	3
Green beans, 3 oz	33	0	0	0	6	2	2	3
Asparagus, 3 oz	20	0	0	0	3	2	0	7
Brussels sprouts, 3 oz	35	0	0	0	7	3	0	9
Onions, whole, 3 oz	29	0	0	0	7	1	3	9
Greens, turnip, 3 oz	18	0	0	0	3	2	0	10
Collard greens, 3 oz	28	0	0	0	5	3	0	40
Broccoli, 3 oz	22	0	0	0	4	3	1	20
Cauliflower, 3 oz	20	0	0	0	4	2	2	20
Potatoes, whole, 3 oz	66	0	0	0	15	1	1	21
Turnips, mashed, 3 oz	13	0	0	0	2	2	0	21
Mixed vegetables, 3 oz	54	0	0	0	11	3	0	39
Peas and onions, 3 oz	59	0	0	0	11	3	0	51
Peas and carrots, 3 oz	45	0	0	0	9	3	0	66
Artichoke hearts, 3 oz	40	1	0	0	7	1	5	55
Carrots, 3 oz	30	0	0	0	7	3	4	57
Spinach, 3 oz	24	0	0	0	4	2	1	62
Peas, 3 oz	65	0	0	0	11	4	4	91

Brands . . .

Most frozen unprepared vegetables are within the generic average; varieties with added seasonings or sauces may raise sodium content.

	Cal	Fat	Sat	Chol	Carb	Fib	Sug	Sod
Birds Eye Garden or Baby Peas, 2/3 cup	70	0	0	0	12	4	4	0
C&W Early Harvest Petite Peas NSA, 2/3 cup	70	0	0	0	12	4	4	0
Freshlike Green Peas, NSA, 2/3 cup	70	0	0	0	12	4	4	0

VEGETABLES – PICKLED AND SPECIALTY VEGETABLES

(see Asian–Pickled Foods, pg 159; Chili Peppers, pg 168)

VEGETABLES – PREPARED VEGETABLES

(see Pickled/Specialty Vegetables, pg 96; Side Dishes, pg 151; Prepared Salads, pg 153)

MEATS, POULTRY AND MEATLESS ALTERNATIVES

See RESOURCES, page 305, for a partial list of manufacturers and retailers offering low-salt products online or visit **LowSaltFoods.com** *for additional sources.*

MEAT, POULTRY AND MEATLESS ALTERNATIVES

BREAKFAST MEATS

	Cal	Fat	Sat	Chol	Carb	Fib	Sug	Sod
Sausage links, turkey, 1 oz link	66	5	1	45	1	0	0	164
Bacon, pork, fully cooked, 2 slices, 0.6 oz	70	5	2	15	0	0	0	220
Sausage links, smoked, pork, 1 oz link	86	8	3	17	0	0	0	232
Bacon, pork, raw, 2 pan-fried slices, 0.6 oz	80	7	3	15	0	0	1	260
Pancetta, 1 oz	180	16	6	20	0	0	0	320
Sausage patty, pork, patty, 2 oz	170	15	5	40	0	0	0	356
Bacon, Canadian-style, 1 oz slice	45	2	1	15	1	0	0	402
Meatless alternatives:								
Sausage link, meatless, 0.9 oz link	64	5	1	0	2	1	0	222
Bacon, meatless, 2 pan-fried slices, 0.6 oz	50	5	1	0	1	0	0	234
Sausage patty, meatless, 1.4 oz	98	7	1	0	4	1	0	337

NOTE: Some "lower sodium" bacon have 230mg or more sodium per serving.

Brands . . .

BACON *(0.6 oz or 2 slices unless noted)*

	Cal	Fat	Sat	Chol	Carb	Fib	Sug	Sod
Butterball Turkey, Lower Sodium, 0.5 oz slice	25	2	1	10	0	0	0	80
Turkey Bacon, Original, 0.5 oz slice	25	2	1	10	0	0	0	135
Coleman Natural Uncured Hickory Smoked	70	6	2	10	0	0	0	140
Esskay Lower Sodium	60	5	2	10	0	0	0	120
Jennie-O Extra Lean Turkey	20	1	0	10	0	0	0	140
Jimmy Dean Low Sodium Bacon	50	4	2	10	0	0	0	105
Kahn's Lower Sodium	60	5	3	5	0	0	0	105
Shady Brook Farms Turkey, 0.5 oz slice	35	3	1	10	0	0	0	140
Shelton's Turkey Breakfast Strips, 0.5 oz slice	30	2	0	13	0	0	0	115
Wegmans *Food You Feel Good About* Uncured	70	6	2	10	0	0	0	130
Lower Sodium, Less fat, 3 slices	70	5	3	10	0	0	0	135
Food You Feel Good About Uncured Pepper	70	6	2	10	0	0	0	140
Wellshire Farms Black Forest Bacon	80	6	3	15	1	0	0	110

REDUCED SODIUM (LESS THAN GENERIC):

	Cal	Fat	Sat	Chol	Carb	Fib	Sug	Sod
Applegate Farms Organic Uncured Turkey, 1 oz	35	2	0	25	0	0	0	200
Natural Uncured Turkey, 1 oz slice	35	2	0	25	0	0	0	200
Butterball Thin & Crispy Turkey	30	2	1	15	0	0	0	180
Eating Right (Safeway) Turkey, 1 oz slice	40	1	0	25	1	0	0	200
Farmer John Lower Sodium	100	8	3	20	0	0	0	190
Farmland Lower Sodium	80	7	3	15	0	0	0	190
Giant Premium 40% Lower Sodium	80	6	3	15	0	0	0	160
Godshall's Maple Turkey, 1 oz slice	40	1	0	25	2	0	0	190
Turkey, 1 oz slice	40	1	0	25	1	0	0	200
Great Value Lower Sodium Bacon	80	7	3	15	0	0	0	173
Turkey Bacon	35	3	1	10	0	0	0	180
Gwaltney Brown Sugar	70	6	2	20	0	0	0	180
Hatfield Reduced Sodium, 3 slices	70	5	2	5	0	0	0	180
Jennie-O Extra Lean Turkey	35	3	1	13	1	0	0	150
Jimmy Dean Hardwood Smoked Turkey	25	2	1	15	0	0	0	200
Louis Rich Turkey Bacon, 0.5 oz	35	3	1	15	1	0	0	180
Organic Valley Uncured Turkey Bacon, 1 oz sl	40	1	0	25	0	0	0	160
Oscar Mayer Lower Sodium	70	6	3	10	0	0	0	170
Turkey Bacon	35	3	1	15	1	0	0	180
Plumrose Sugar Free Lower Sodium Bacon	80	7	3	15	0	0	0	173
Safeway Select 40% Less Sodium	80	7	3	15	0	0	0	173
Smithfield's Lower Sodium	80	7	3	15	0	0	0	190

191

MEAT, POULTRY AND MEATLESS ALTERNATIVES
Beef, Lamb and Veal – Dried

	Cal	Fat	Sat	Chol	Carb	Fib	Sug	Sod
Thorn Apple Valley								
Lower Sodium Hickory Smoked	80	7	3	15	0	0	0	160
Wellshire Farms Beef Bacon, 2 oz	65	3	1	50	0	0	0	170
Canadian Turkey Bacon, 1 oz	35	1	0	25	0	0	0	180
Classic Sliced or Peppered Turkey Bacon, 1 oz	40	2	0	20	0	0	0	180
BREAKFAST SAUSAGE								
Farmland Pork Patty, Fully Cooked, 1.5 oz	190	18	6	30	0	0	0	75
Pork Links, Fully Cooked, 1.6 oz (2)	200	19	7	30	1	0	0	85
NorthStar Bison Breakfast Sausage, 2 oz	82	2	0	46	0	0	0	32
REDUCED SODIUM (LESS THAN GENERIC):								
Al Fresco All Natural Brkfast Chicken Sausage								
Apple Maple, 1.3 oz	70	3	1	25	4	0	4	170
Wild Blueberry, 1.3 oz	70	3	1	30	5	0	4	170
Applegate Farms Chicken/Apple, 1 oz link	47	3	1	22	1	0	1	150
Chicken & Maple, 1 oz link	50	3	1	22	1	0	1	170
Chicken & Sage, 1 oz link	47	3	1	22	1	0	1	173
Bob Evans Express Fully Cooked Lite Links	80	5	0	15	0	0	0	220
Hans All Natural Chicken Brkfast Links, 1.3 oz	60	3	1	25	0	0	0	250
Jennie-O Turkey Patties, Fully Cooked 1.2 oz	65	4	1	30	0	0	0	250
Jones Dairy Farm								
Golden Brown Patties, 1.4 oz	150	14	5	30	1	0	0	240
All Natural Pork Sausage Patties	130	12	4	30	0	0	0	250
Shelton's Turkey Sausage Patties, 2 oz	160	14	4	40	1	0	0	170
Turkey Breakfast Sausage, 1.6 oz link	150	13	4	35	0	0	0	200
MEATLESS ALTERNATIVES								
CANNED								
REDUCED SODIUM (LESS THAN GENERIC):								
Worthington Saucettes Vegetarian Links	90	6	1	0	1	1	0	200
FROZEN/REFRIGERATED								
SoyBoy Tofu Breakfast Links	65	3	1	0	6	0	1	130
REDUCED SODIUM (LESS THAN GENERIC):								
MorningStar Farms Bacon Strips	60	5	1	0	2	1	0	230
Breakfast Patties, made w/soy, 1.4 oz	80	3	1	0	4	1	1	240
Maple Flavored Sausage Patties, 1.4 oz	80	3	1	0	5	1	2	250
Worthington Stripples Vegetarian Bacon	60	5	1	0	2	1	0	220
Yves Breakfast Patties, 1 oz patty	40	1	0	0	2	1	1	175
Canadian Bacon, 1.5 slices	40	0	0	0	1	0	0	200

BEEF, LAMB AND VEAL – DRIED

	Cal	Fat	Sat	Chol	Carb	Fib	Sug	Sod
Beef, dried, 1 oz	43	1	0	25	1	0	1	1190

Brands . . . *Most brands within generic average.*

BEEF, LAMB AND VEAL – FRESH

(also see Burgers/Patties, pg 193; Canned Meats, pg 194)

	Cal	Fat	Sat	Chol	Carb	Fib	Sug	Sod
Beef, most cuts, trimmed to 1/8" fat, all grades, 4 oz.	265	19	8	75	0	0	0	66
Ground beef, 30% fat, 4 oz	375	34	13	88	0	0	0	76
Lamb, most cuts, trimmed to 1/4" fat, all grades, 4 oz	303	24	11	82	0	0	0	66
Ground, 4 oz	319	26	12	82	0	0	0	67
Liver, 4 oz	151	4	1	308	4	0	0	77
Tongue, 4 oz	253	18	8	98	4	0	0	78
Veal, most cuts, trimmed to 1/4" fat, all grades, 4 oz	127	3	1	94	0	0	0	98
Ground, 4 oz	163	8	3	93	0	0	0	93
Corned beef brisket, 4 oz	226	17	8	61	0	0	0	1380

Brands . . . *Most brands within generic average.*

Cal Fat Sat Chol Carb Fib Sug Sod

BEEF, LAMB AND VEAL – PREPARED ENTREES

(also see Burgers/Patties, pg 193; Dinners/Meals - Frozen, pg 138)

	Cal	Fat	Sat	Chol	Carb	Fib	Sug	Sod
Taco seasoned ground beef, 2 oz	90	5	2	15	5	0	2	360
Corned beef, canned, 2 oz	120	7	3	50	0	0	0	450
Meatballs, 3 oz	290	24	10	50	5	2	1	570
Beef w/gravy, 4 oz	120	6	2	44	4	1	2	610
Meatloaf, 4 oz	192	10	5	44	12	0	6	630
Beef w/BBQ sauce, 4 oz	180	6	2	30	22	2	20	1300

Brands . . . *(3 oz unless noted)*
REDUCED SODIUM (LESS THAN GENERIC):

	Cal	Fat	Sat	Chol	Carb	Fib	Sug	Sod
Chef Express *Smart Selections*								
Beef Tenderloin Steak, Garlic & Herb, 5 oz	250	12	4	90	1	0	1	200
Tyson Beef Shoulder, Steakhouse Blend, 4 oz	140	5	2	55	2	0	0	220
Wegmans Sirloin w/Peppercorn Marinade	130	4	2	65	1	0	1	240

BURGERS AND PATTIES

	Cal	Fat	Sat	Chol	Carb	Fib	Sug	Sod
Chicken patty, uncooked, 4 oz	170	11	4	130	0	0	0	75
Breaded, 2.9 oz	180	9	0	35	9	0	0	480
Seasoned, savory, 4 oz	180	11	4	12	01	0	0	490
Seasoned, char-grilled, 4 oz	190	11	3	115	2	0	0	710
Beef patty, uncooked, 4 oz	319	26	11	89	0	0	0	77
Turkey patty, uncooked, 4 oz	170	9	3	90	0	0	0	85
Char-grilled seasoned, 4 oz	180	10	3	90	0	0	0	660
Breaded, battered, fried, 3.3 oz	266	17	4	58	15	1	0	752
Bison burger, uncooked, 4 oz	380	29	15	75	0	0	0	135
Veggie burger, 2.5 oz	124	4	1	4	10	3	1	398

NOTE: *There is a wide range of sodium in burger patties depending on added ingredients (anywhere from 25mg to more than 700mg). The following have 250mg or less per serving (meatless patties have 300mg or less).*

Brands . . . *(4 oz patty unless noted)*
FROZEN/REFRIGERATED

	Cal	Fat	Sat	Chol	Carb	Fib	Sug	Sod
Applegate Farms Organic Turkey Burgers	190	11	3	75	0	0	0	70
Bubba Burger Sweet Onion	340	26	10	90	2	0	1	80
Philly-Gourmet Homestyle Beef Patties	240	18	7	50	0	0	0	40
Thick & Beefy Homestyle Beef Patties, 6 oz	370	28	12	70	0	0	0	60
Sommers Organic Chicken Burgers	130	5	0	9	5	0	0	65
Turkey Burgers	120	2	0	70	2	0	0	70
Steak-umm Burgers Original, 1/4 lb	240	17	7	75	0	0	0	75
Sweet Onions, 1/3 lb, 5.4 oz	270	18	7	85	3	0	1	80
Original, 1/3 lb, 5.4 oz	320	23	9	105	0	0	0	100

REDUCED SODIUM (LESS THAN GENERIC):

	Cal	Fat	Sat	Chol	Carb	Fib	Sug	Sod
Applegate Farms Chicken Patties	180	9	2	35	12	0	0	210
Health is Wealth Breaded Chicken Patties, 3 oz	130	4	1	35	11	0	0	230

MEATLESS BURGERS AND PATTIES
REDUCED SODIUM (LESS THAN GENERIC):

	Cal	Fat	Sat	Chol	Carb	Fib	Sug	Sod
Boca Burgers Original Vegan	70	1	0	0	6	4	0	280
Bruschetta Tomato Basil Parmesan	70	2	1	5	9	4	0	290
Savory Mushroom Mozzarella	100	3	1	0	11	4	0	300
Grilled Vegetable	80	1	0	0	7	4	1	300
Dr. Praeger's Veggie Burgers Gluten Free Calif	120	6	1	0	13	4	3	180
California, Bombay, Tex Mex, or Italian	110	5	1	0	13	5	2	250
Five-Star Foodies Gourmet Grillers	100	3	1	0	9	1	5	270
Gardenburger Garden Vegan	80	1	0	0	12	4	0	270

193

	Cal	Fat	Sat	Chol	Carb	Fib	Sug	Sod
Gardein The Ultimate Beefless Burger..........	130	5	0	0	6	2	1	280
Sun-Dried Tomato Basil	100	3	1	5	17	4	2	270
Golden Baja Veggie Burgers	100	4	1	10	14	1	2	200
Mon Cuisine Vegan Chicken Patties	100	3	0	0	15	3	1	290
Morningstar Farms Mushroom Lover's........	110	6	1	0	8	1	1	220
Grillers Original	130	6	1	0	5	2	1	260
Tomato & Basil Pizza Burger	120	6	2	10	7	3	2	280
Grillers Vegan...	100	3	0	0	7	4	1	280
Classic Burger made w/soy	150	6	1	0	9	3	2	280
Quorn Turk'y Burger	90	4	1	5	6	2	0	200
Soyboy Okara Courage Burger	130	5	1	0	8	2	1	280
Tofurky SuperBurgers, TexMex	120	2	0	0	14	3	0	250
Wild Wood Organics SprouTofu								
Shiitake Tofu Veggie Burger......................	170	11	2	0	9	2	2	240
Original Veggie Burger..............................	170	12	2	0	7	1	1	300
Worthington FriPats	130	6	1	0	5	3	1	300
Zoglo's Meatless Burgers	131	6	1	0	5	2	0	225
Meatless Chicken Flavor Patties..................	131	6	4	0	5	2	0	225
Mixed Vegetable or Broccoli Patties...........	123	5	4	0	10	2	0	225
Multi-Grain & Vegetable Patties.................	110	2	0	0	20	2	0	225
Tofu Patties...	112	4	1	0	2	2	0	270
MIXES								
Ziyad Falafil Mix, Vegetable Burger, 2 patties..	57	3	0	0	5	0	0	50
REDUCED SODIUM (LESS THAN GENERIC):								
Authentic Foods Falafel, 1/4 cup............	100	1	0	0	17	3	2	240
Sadaf Falafel Mix, 1/4 cup	140	2	0	0	25	2	5	190

CANNED MEATS

	Cal	Fat	Sat	Chol	Carb	Fib	Sug	Sod
Vienna sausage, canned, 2 oz........................	150	12	5	40	1	0	0	260
Turkey, canned, 2 oz....................................	95	4	1	37	1	0	0	262
Chicken, canned, 2 oz..................................	92	4	1	35	0	0	0	282
Chopped ham, canned, 2 oz..........................	136	11	4	28	0	0	0	774

Brands . . . *(2 oz unless noted)*
REDUCED SODIUM (LESS THAN GENERIC):

	Cal	Fat	Sat	Chol	Carb	Fib	Sug	Sod
Hormel Premium White Turkey...................	60	2	1	35	0	0	0	230
Breast of Chicken....................................	60	2	1	40	0	0	0	250
Valley Fresh 100% Natural Premium Turkey.	80	3	1	40	0	0	0	150
100% Natural Premium White Chicken........	80	4	1	50	0	0	0	180
100% Natural White & Dark Chicken..........	80	4	2	50	0	0	0	180

CHICKEN AND TURKEY – FRESH

	Cal	Fat	Sat	Chol	Carb	Fib	Sug	Sod
Turkey, light meat, w/o skin, 4 oz..................	121	1	0	74	0	0	0	58
Dark meat, w/o skin, 4 oz	124	4	1	91	0	0	0	77
Turkey, ground, 4 oz.................................	170	9	3	90	0	0	0	79
Chicken, breast, bone & skin removed, 4 oz.....	123	1	0	65	0	0	0	73
Roasting, skin & meat, 4 oz.......................	242	18	5	82	0	0	0	76
Liver, 4 oz..	130	5	2	386	0	0	0	80
Wing, meat only, 4 oz...............................	141	4	1	64	0	0	0	91
Thigh, meat only, 4 oz	133	4	1	93	0	0	0	96
Drumstick, meat only, 4 oz........................	133	4	1	86	0	0	0	99
Cornish game hen, 1/2	336	24	7	170	0	0	0	102

Brands . . . *Most brands within generic average.*
NOTE: The amount of sodium in packaged poultry varies within brands and cuts of meat. Some may have as much as 190mg sodium per 4-oz serving.

	Cal	Fat	Sat	Chol	Carb	Fib	Sug	Sod

CHICKEN AND TURKEY – PREPARED ENTREES

(also see Entree/Light Meals, pg 143; Entrees – Pasta/Italian Dishes, pg 145; Asian – Entrees/Light Meals, pg 156; Hispanic/Latino – Entrees/Light Meals, pg 163; Mediterranean/Middle Eastern – Meals/Entrees, pg 169)

	Cal	Fat	Sat	Chol	Carb	Fib	Sug	Sod
Taco seasoned ground turkey, 4 oz	250	16	5	75	3	1	1	500
Popcorn chicken, 3 oz	190	9	2	20	18	1	2	510
Turkey roll, light meat, 4 oz	168	8	2	50	0	0	0	560
Italian seasoned ground turkey, 4 oz	160	8	3	80	1	0	0	580
Chicken roll, light meat, 4 oz	176	8	2	58	2	0	0	665
Turkey breast w/gravy, 4 oz	100	2	1	33	3	0	1	735
Chicken breast, oven-roasted, 4 oz	66	0	0	30	2	0	0	915
Turkey, smoked, cooked, light or dark, 4 oz	190	6	0	55	2	0	0	1116

Brands . . . *(4 oz unless noted)*

FRESH

	Cal	Fat	Sat	Chol	Carb	Fib	Sug	Sod
FreeBird Chicken Wings, Barbeque, 2	60	4	1	20	1	0	0	70
Chicken Wings, Buffalo Style, 2	60	4	1	20	1	0	0	115

REDUCED SODIUM (LESS THAN GENERIC):

	Cal	Fat	Sat	Chol	Carb	Fib	Sug	Sod
Foster Farms *Savory Servings*								
Lemon Peppercorn Turkey Tenderloin	110	2	1	50	3	0	1	190
Fire Roasted Chipotle Chicken Tenders	120	2	0	65	2	0	2	200
True BBQ Turkey Tenderloin	110	2	0	45	5	0	3	240

FROZEN

REDUCED SODIUM (LESS THAN GENERIC):

	Cal	Fat	Sat	Chol	Carb	Fib	Sug	Sod
Applegate Farms Organic Chicken Strips	160	7	2	35	11	0	1	180
Chicken Nuggets	180	9	2	35	12	0	0	210
Homestyle Breaded Chicken Breast Tenders	150	5	1	30	14	0	1	230
Barber Foods *Stuffed Chicken Breasts*								
Fit & Flavorful Broccoli & Cheese, 4 oz	190	9	3	35	9	1	1	270
Fully Cooked Asparagus & Cheese, 5 oz	290	16	5	55	15	1	1	320
Foster Farms Turkey Meatballs, Homestyle, 3 oz	160	9	3	30	3	0	0	280
FreeBird Seasoned Grilled Chicken Breasts	120	2	1	55	2	0	0	180
Chickasaurus Rex Breaded Chicken Bites, 3 oz	240	12	4	45	17	1	0	200
Health is Wealth Chicken Nuggets, 3 oz	130	4	1	35	15	0	0	230
Chicken Patties, 3 oz	130	4	1	35	11	0	0	230
Chicken Tenders, 3 oz	130	3	1	35	10	0	0	250
Ian's Chicken Stixs, 3 oz	250	12	2	20	24	0	0	190
Chicken Tenders, Italian Style, 3 oz	220	9	2	50	19	0	2	190
Chicken Nuggets, 3 oz	190	8	2	40	14	0	1	250
Chicken Nuggets, Wheat Free, 3 oz	220	10	1	24	22	0	0	300
Chicken Patties, 3.5 oz	220	9	2	40	16	0	1	300
Chicken Patties, Wheat Free, 3.5 oz	220	10	1	25	22	0	0	300
Shady Brook Farms								
Bacon Ranch Lean Turkey Tenderloins	140	5	0	55	3	0	1	270
Tony Chachere's Tur-Duc-Hen w/Dressing	300	13	4	95	12	0	2	230
Pork Boudin Balls, 2 oz	100	5	2	35	9	0	0	240
Tur-Duc-Hen Stuffed w/Seafood, 5 oz	260	13	4	90	4	0	0	250

GAME MEAT

	Cal	Fat	Sat	Chol	Carb	Fib	Sug	Sod
Rabbit, 3 oz	116	5	1	48	0	0	0	35
Deer, 3 oz	102	2	1	72	0	0	0	43
Buffalo (bison), top round, 3 oz	145	5	2	73	0	0	0	45
Ground, 3 oz	187	13	6	59	0	0	0	55
Elk, 3 oz	94	1	0	47	0	0	0	49

	Cal	Fat	Sat	Chol	Carb	Fib	Sug	Sod
Duck, meat only, 3 oz	111	5	2	65	0	0	0	62
Goose, meat only, 3 oz	135	6	2	71	0	0	0	73

Brands . . . *Most brands are within the generic range.*

HAM AND PORK – CANNED

(see Canned Meats, pg 194)

HAM AND PORK – FRESH

	Cal	Fat	Sat	Chol	Carb	Fib	Sug	Sod
Pork loin roast, boneless, lean, 3 oz	120	4	2	47	0	0	0	38
Pork, whole leg (ham), 3 oz	208	16	6	62	0	0	0	40
Pork, ground, 3 oz	223	18	7	61	0	0	0	47
Pork shoulder, lean, 3 oz	126	6	2	57	0	0	0	65
Ham, cured, 3 oz	137	7	2	48	3	1	0	1095
25% less sodium, 3 oz	140	7	3	49	0	0	0	824
Ham, smoked, 3 oz	140	8	3	50	3	0	3	1150

Brands . . . *(2 oz unless noted)*

REDUCED SODIUM (LESS THAN GENERIC):

	Cal	Fat	Sat	Chol	Carb	Fib	Sug	Sod
Boar's Head Black Forest Smoked Ham	60	1	0	30	2	0	2	440
Deluxe Ham, 42% Lower Sodium	60	1	0	25	2	0	2	460

PREPARED ENTREES

Chef Express Smart Selections

	Cal	Fat	Sat	Chol	Carb	Fib	Sug	Sod
Pork Tenderloin, Chipotle, 4 oz	130	3	1	75	1	0	0	130

REDUCED SODIUM (LESS THAN GENERIC):

Chef Express Smart Selections

	Cal	Fat	Sat	Chol	Carb	Fib	Sug	Sod
Pork Tenderloin, Garlic Peppercorn, 4 oz	150	6	2	60	1	0	0	170

HOT DOGS, FRANKFURTERS AND SAUSAGES

Sausages:

	Cal	Fat	Sat	Chol	Carb	Fib	Sug	Sod
Italian sweet sausage, 2 oz	83	5	2	17	1	0	0	319
Italian sausage, 2 oz	194	18	6	43	0	0	0	409
Vienna sausage, canned, 1.7 oz (3)	110	9	3	42	1	0	0	465
Bratwurst, pork, cooked, 2 oz	166	15	3	44	1	0	0	475
Polish sausage, beef/pork, smoked, 2 oz	169	15	5	4	1	0	0	475
Liverwurst, 2 oz	185	16	6	90	1	0	0	488
Knockwurst, pork/beef, 2 oz	174	16	6	34	2	0	0	527
Braunschweiger, 2 oz	186	16	6	100	2	0	0	658
Kielbasa, turkey/beef, smoked, 2 oz	127	10	3	39	2	0	0	672
Chorizo, 2 oz	258	22	8	50	2	0	0	700
Hot dogs and frankfurters:								
Chicken, 1.6 oz	100	7	2	43	1	0	0	380
Turkey, 1.6 oz	100	8	2	35	2	0	1	485
Corn dog, 2.7 oz	180	10	3	35	15	1	1	490
Beef and pork, 1.6 oz	137	12	5	23	1	0	0	504
Beef, 1.6 oz	149	13	5	24	2	0	2	513

Brands . . . *(1 hot dog/frankfurter unless noted)*

HOT DOGS/FRANKFURTERS

REDUCED SODIUM (LESS THAN GENERIC):

	Cal	Fat	Sat	Chol	Carb	Fib	Sug	Sod
Applegate Farms Uncured Turkey Hot Dogs	40	2	1	25	0	0	0	260
Stadium Organic Uncured Beef	110	8	3	30	0	0	0	330
The Great Organic Uncured Hot Dog	110	8	3	30	0	0	0	330
Boar's Head Lite Beef, Skinless	90	6	3	25	0	0	0	270
Beef, Skinless	120	11	5	20	0	0	0	350
The Buffalo Guys Buffalo Hot Dogs	70	5	1	21	0	0	0	160

	Cal	Fat	Sat	Chol	Carb	Fib	Sug	Sod
Coleman Natural								
All Natural Uncured Franks, Beef & Pork	120	10	4	25	1	0	1	240
Esskay Franks w/Turkey, Pork & Beef	140	12	4	35	3	0	0	220
Franks, Orioles, Jumbo	170	15	4	40	4	0	0	280
Hatfield Reduced Sodium Franks	150	13	6	30	2	0	1	350
Int'l Glatt Kosher Reduced Fat & Sodium Beef	100	8	3	25	0	0	0	200
Beef Frankfurters	160	13	6	30	1	1	0	250
Meal Mart Turkey Franks	100	7	3	45	0	1	0	190
Chicken Franks	100	4	1	35	1	0	0	190
Reduced Fat Beef Franks	110	9	3	30	0	0	0	210
Northstar Bison Buffalo Dogs	81	1	1	47	0	0	0	200
Shelton's Uncured Chicken Franks	80	7	2	35	1	0	0	260
Uncured Turkey Franks	60	5	1	25	1	0	0	260
Wellshire Farms Premium Beef Franks	110	9	4	30	0	0	0	300
Chicken Franks	100	8	2	30	1	0	1	320
Turkey Franks	110	6	2	30	1	0	1	330

CORN DOG
REDUCED SODIUM (LESS THAN GENERIC):

	Cal	Fat	Sat	Chol	Carb	Fib	Sug	Sod
S'Better Beef Corn Dog	180	5	2	30	17	1	5	350

MEATLESS FRANKFURTERS
CANNED

	Cal	Fat	Sat	Chol	Carb	Fib	Sug	Sod
Cedar Lake Deli-Franks	40	0	0	0	1	0	0	110
Tofu Links	35	0	0	0	1	0	0	120

REDUCED SODIUM (LESS THAN GENERIC):

	Cal	Fat	Sat	Chol	Carb	Fib	Sug	Sod
Cedar Lake Tasty Link	70	4	1	0	3	0	0	160
Jumbo Frank	110	5	1	0	3	1	0	180
Vegi-Frank	100	4	1	0	3	0	0	270
Worthington Veja-Links	50	3	1	0	1	0	0	180
LF Veja-Links	45	2	0	0	3	0	0	220
Super Links	110	8	1	0	2	1	0	350
Worthington Loma Linda Linkettes	70	4	1	0	1	1	0	160
Big Franks	110	6	1	0	3	2	0	220
LF Big Franks	80	3	1	0	3	2	0	240
Little Links, 2	90	5	1	0	3	2	0	250

FROZEN/REFRIGERATED
REDUCED SODIUM (LESS THAN GENERIC):

	Cal	Fat	Sat	Chol	Carb	Fib	Sug	Sod
Lightlife Tofu Pups	60	3	1	0	2	1	0	300
Smart Dogs	45	0	0	0	2	1	1	310
Morningstar Farms Veggie Dogs	120	6	1	0	7	1	1	350
SoyBoy Not Dogs	95	3	1	0	10	1	1	240
Tofurky Chipotle Franks	90	3	0	0	5	3	1	270
Veggie Patch Spiced Apple Sausage	110	6	2	0	7	0	5	300
Simply the Best Veggie Dogs	90	5	2	0	3	0	1	310
Sun-Dried Tomato & Artichoke	100	6	2	0	5	1	1	340
Yves Tofu Dogs, 1.4 oz	45	1	0	0	2	0	0	300
Zoglo's Tofu Weiners	69	2	0	0	2	2	0	228

SAUSAGE
FROZEN/REFRIGERATED
REDUCED SODIUM (LESS THAN GENERIC):

	Cal	Fat	Sat	Chol	Carb	Fib	Sug	Sod
Bilinski's All Natural Chicken Sausage								
Peppers & Onions, 2 oz	70	4	2	60	1	0	0	270
Spinach & Garlic, 2 oz	70	4	1	40	1	1	0	270
Sun-Dried Tomato, 2 oz	70	4	2	40	2	0	0	280
Coleman Natural Polish Kielbasa, 2 oz	150	13	5	35	1	0	0	310

	Cal	Fat	Sat	Chol	Carb	Fib	Sug	Sod
D'Artagnan Merguez Sausage, 1.7 oz	160	14	6	35	0	0	0	240
Hans All Natural Chicken Sausage								
Sun-Dried Tomato & Basil, 3 oz	150	9	2	55	3	1	2	300
Shady Brook Farms								
Roasted Garlic Turkey Link	140	8	3	50	2	0	0	240
Chipotle Seasoned Turkey Link, 2.7 oz	130	8	3	50	2	0	0	260
Shelton's Turkey Italian Sausage	170	15	5	40	0	0	0	230
Tony Chachere's Crawfish Boudin, 2 oz	130	5	1	20	17	1	1	210
Pork Boudin, Hot or Smoked Pork Boudin	130	5	2	40	10	0	0	220
Shrimp Boudin, 2 oz	80	5	1	26	15	0	0	230
Andouille, 2 oz	80	3	2	30	2	0	1	300
Smoked or Hot Pork Smoked Sausage, 2 oz	180	12	5	55	1	0	1	300

LUNCHEON/DELI MEATS

	Cal	Fat	Sat	Chol	Carb	Fib	Sug	Sod
Pastrami, 1 oz	27	0	0	13	0	0	0	288
Turkey pastrami, 1 oz	38	2	0	19	1	0	1	280
Bologna, 1 oz	87	8	3	16	1	0	0	302
Turkey bologna, 1 oz	59	4	1	21	1	0	1	351
Salami, 1 oz	74	6	3	20	1	0	0	350
Turkey salami, 1 oz	47	3	1	21	0	0	0	281
Turkey, oven-roasted, 1 oz	29	0	0	12	1	0	1	360
Ham, 1 oz	46	2	1	16	1	0	0	365
Turkey ham, 1 oz	35	1	0	19	0	0	0	291
Beef, 1 oz	50	1	0	12	2	0	0	408
Pepperoni, 1 oz	138	12	4	29	0	0	0	463

Brands . . . *(1 oz serving unless noted)*
NOTE: Some low-sodium brands may be in the deli section of your grocer and are sliced to order.

BEEF

	Cal	Fat	Sat	Chol	Carb	Fib	Sug	Sod
Applegate Farms Roast Beef	40	2	1	15	0	0	0	100
Peppered Eye Round	40	2	1	15	0	0	0	100
Boar's Head NSA Roast Beef	45	2	1	15	0	0	0	20
Deluxe Cap Top Round Roast Beef	40	1	1	15	1	0	0	40
All Natural Roast Beef	40	1	1	18	0	0	0	70
Pepper Seasoned Roast Beef	45	2	1	20	0	0	0	95
Cajun Style Roast Beef	40	1	0	18	0	0	0	130
Dietz & Watson Oven Roasted Angus Roast Beef	35	1	1	15	0	0	0	95
Natural Angus Roast Beef	35	1	1	15	0	0	0	95
London Broil or Italian Roast Beef	35	1	1	15	0	0	0	95
Black Bear Choice Roast Beef	35	1	1	15	0	0	0	95
DiLusso Seasoned Italian Style Roast Beef	40	2	1	18	0	0	0	80
Seasoned Roast Beef	40	2	1	15	0	0	0	105
Wegmans Food You Feel Good About								
Fully Cooked Roast Beef	40	2	0	20	0	0	0	40
Wellshire Farms Sliced Roast Beef	35	2	1	13	0	0	0	115
Sliced Round Cooked Corned Beef	23	1	1	23	1	0	1	125
REDUCED SODIUM (LESS THAN GENERIC):								
Applegate Farms Organic Roast Beef	40	2	1	18	0	0	0	160
Boar's Head Londonport Roast Beef	40	1	1	20	1	0	1	175
Italian Style Roast Beef	40	1	1	20	1	0	0	185
DiLusso Season Cajun Style Roast Beef	40	2	2	15	0	0	0	185
Hatfield Home Style Meat Loaf	70	5	2	15	2	0	1	180
Roast Beef	40	1	0	18	0	0	0	195

	Cal	Fat	Sat	Chol	Carb	Fib	Sug	Sod
FROZEN								
Philly-Gourmet Steaks for Sandwiches, 1.5 oz.	100	9	4	25	0	0	0	20
Steak-umm Sliced Steaks, 1 portion	100	9	4	25	0	0	0	20
BOLOGNA								
Wellshire Farms Sliced Turkey Bologna	30	1	0	10	0	0	0	80
REDUCED SODIUM (LESS THAN GENERIC):								
Applegate Farms Uncured Turkey Bologna ..	45	3	1	15	0	0	0	200
Empire Kosher Chicken Bologna, 0.8 oz sl ...	40	3	1	18	0	0	0	210
Hebrew National Lean Beef Bologna, 2 sl	45	3	1	10	1	0	0	220
Beef Bologna...	80	8	4	15	1	0	0	240
Int'l Glatt Kosher Sliced Beef Bologna	80	7	3	15	1	0	0	220
Shelton's Uncured Turkey Bologna	55	4	1	23	1	0	1	165
CHICKEN AND TURKEY								
Applegate Farms No Salt Turkey	30	0	0	9	0	0	0	15
Butterball Oven Roasted Turkey w/skin	35	1	0	18	0	0	0	130
Oven Roasted Turkey Breast	30	1	0	18	0	0	0	140
Dietz & Watson No Salt Turkey	35	1	0	15	1	0	1	25
Gourmet Lite Turkey Breast..........................	25	1	1	15	1	0	1	120
DiLusso Reduced Sodium Turkey	30	1	0	13	0	0	0	140
Hatfield Black Pepper Turkey Breast	30	1	0	15	0	0	0	117
Meal Mart								
Smoked Turkey or Chicken Breast (avg)	40	2	1	14	0	0	0	95
Turkey Roll..	40	2	1	15	0	0	0	100
REDUCED SODIUM (LESS THAN GENERIC):								
Applegate Farms Smoked Chicken Breast ...	35	1	0	15	1	0	1	155
Oven Roasted Chicken Breast	35	1	0	15	1	0	1	155
Peppered Turkey Breast	25	0	0	15	0	0	0	180
Smoked Chicken Breast	30	1	0	15	1	0	1	180
Oven Roasted or Smoked Turkey Breast......	25	0	0	15	0	0	0	200
Herb Turkey Breast	25	0	0	15	0	0	0	200
Spicy Chipotle Chicken Breast	30	0	0	15	1	0	0	200
Boar's Head All Natural Turkey	30	1	0	15	1	0	0	165
Premium Lower Sodium Turkey Breast..........	30	0	0	10	0	0	0	170
Golden Catering Turkey Breast....................	30	1	0	13	0	0	0	170
All American BBQ Chicken	30	0	0	18	1	0	1	170
Golden Classic Chicken	30	1	0	18	0	0	0	175
Hickory Smoked Chicken Breast.................	30	0	0	13	0	0	0	180
Hickory Smoked Black Forest Turkey..........	30	0	0	13	0	0	0	180
Ovengold Turkey or Lemon Pepper Chicken..	30	1	0	18	1	0	0	180
All Natural Tuscan Turkey Breast	30	1	0	15	0	0	0	190
Blazing Buffalo Chicken..............................	30	1	0	18	0	0	0	195
All Natural Smoked Turkey	30	1	0	13	0	0	0	195
Rotesserie Seasoned Chicken Breast..........	30	1	0	18	0	0	0	200
All Natural French Country Turkey	30	1	0	15	0	0	0	200
Butterball Turkey, Honey Roasted, Thin, 2 sl...	35	1	0	10	3	0	0	195
Turkey Breast, Smoked, Thin, 2 sl	30	1	0	10	2	0	1	195
Turkey Breast, Honey Roasted or Smoked ...	30	1	0	10	3	0	0	200
Turkey, Oven Roasted, Thin, 2 sl	30	1	0	10	2	0	0	210
Turkey Breast, Honey Roasted, Tub, 4 sl......	34	1	0	11	3	0	0	211
Turkey Breast, Oven Roasted	30	1	0	10	2	0	0	220
Turkey Breast, Rotisserie, Tub, 4 sl.............	34	1	0	11	2	0	0	223
Chicken, Oven Roasted, Thin, 2 sl	25	1	0	10	2	0	0	225
Turkey, Oven Roasted, Tub, 4 sl	34	1	0	11	2	0	0	228
Dietz & Watson Banquet Breast of Turkey ...	25	1	0	15	0	0	0	160

199

MEAT, POULTRY AND MEATLESS ALTERNATIVES
Luncheon/Deli Meats

	Cal	Fat	Sat	Chol	Carb	Fib	Sug	Sod
Smoked Peppercorn Turkey Breast	25	1	0	15	0	0	0	160
Pepper & Garlic Turkey	30	1	0	15	0	0	0	200
Gourmet Breast of Chicken	35	1	1	15	1	0	1	200
Black Forest Turkey	25	1	0	15	0	0	0	200
Oven Classic Turkey Breast	30	1	0	15	1	0	1	200
Maple & Honey Cured Turkey Breast	30	1	0	15	1	0	1	200
DiLusso Oven Roasted Chicken	25	1	0	10	0	0	0	210
Mesquite Style Chicken	30	1	0	15	0	0	0	225
Empire Kosher Turkey Breast, Oven Prep	25	0	0	15	1	0	0	150
Foster Farms Smoked Turkey	30	1	0	10	1	0	0	210
Turkey Breast, Oven Roasted	30	0	0	10	0	0	0	220
Deli Tub, Turkey, Oven Roasted, 2 sl	30	1	0	8	1	0	0	220
Hatfield Premium Turkey Breast	30	0	0	18	0	0	0	177
Hod Golan Mexican Smoked Turkey Breast	25	1	0	10	1	0	0	170
Smoked Turkey Breast	25	1	0	10	1	0	0	170
Turkey Delight	39	1	1	15	1	0	0	185
Hormel *Natural Choice* Smoked Deli Turkey	25	1	0	13	1	0	1	225
Oscar Mayer / Louis Rich								
Deli Fresh Turkey Breast, Mesquite, 0.9 oz	25	1	0	10	1	0	0	185
Deli Fresh Turkey Breast, Oven Roasted	23	0	0	10	1	0	0	230
Turkey, White, Oven Roasted	30	2	0	10	1	0	0	220
Shady Brook Farms								
Oven Roasted Turkey Breast	30	0	0	15	1	0	1	205
Hickory Smoked Honey Turkey Breast	30	0	0	15	2	0	2	215

HAM AND PORK

	Cal	Fat	Sat	Chol	Carb	Fib	Sug	Sod
Wellshire Farms Sliced Turkey Ham	30	1	0	10	0	0	0	80
Sliced Virginia Brand Deli Ham	30	1	1	13	1	0	0	90
Sliced Tavern Ham	100	1	1	13	1	0	0	90

REDUCED SODIUM (LESS THAN GENERIC):

	Cal	Fat	Sat	Chol	Carb	Fib	Sug	Sod
Applegate Farms Black Forest Ham	30	1	1	15	0	0	0	160
Honey Ham	35	1	0	15	2	0	2	225
Boar's Head Season Cooked Fresh Ham	40	2	1	18	0	0	0	155
All Natural Smoked Uncured Ham	30	1	0	18	1	0	1	160
All Natural Uncured Ham	35	1	0	18	1	0	1	170
Dietz & Watson Roast Sirloin of Pork	30	1	1	15	0	0	0	175
Barbecue or Italian Style Roast of Pork	30	1	1	15	0	0	0	195
Esskay FF Lower Sodium Ham	20	0	0	15	0	0	0	165
FF Lower Sodium Virginia or Honey Ham	20	0	0	13	1	0	1	165
Farmer John Mission Loaf or Ham Roll	30	1	1	13	1	0	1	225
Hatfield Roast Pork	30	1	0	10	0	0	0	160
Original Loaf	65	5	2	10	2	0	2	200
Pickle & Pimiento Loaf	60	4	2	8	3	0	3	205
Imported Brand Cooked Ham	30	1	0	5	1	0	1	205
Reduced Sodium Ham (tub), 3 slices	35	1	0	10	1	0	1	225
Plumrose Lower Sodium Ham	30	1	0	10	0	0	0	160
Russer Cooked Ham, Reduced Sodium	30	1	0	10	1	0	0	230
Wellshire Farms Black Forest Deli Ham	50	1	1	23	2	0	0	175

PASTRAMI

	Cal	Fat	Sat	Chol	Carb	Fib	Sug	Sod
Wellshire Farms Sliced Beef Pastrami Round	23	1	1	23	1	0	1	125

REDUCED SODIUM (LESS THAN GENERIC):

	Cal	Fat	Sat	Chol	Carb	Fib	Sug	Sod
Applegate Farms Turkey Pastrami	25	0	0	15	0	0	0	180
Hod Golan Dark Turkey Pastrami	35	2	1	20	1	0	0	170
Hod Lavan Smoked Turkey Pastrami	38	2	1	15	2	0	0	220

	Cal	Fat	Sat	Chol	Carb	Fib	Sug	Sod
PEPPERONI AND SALAMI								
REDUCED SODIUM (LESS THAN GENERIC):								
Applegate Farms Uncured Turkey Salami	35	1	1	15	0	0	0	180
Hebrew National Beef Salami, 1.5 slices	75	7	3	18	0	0	0	210
Int'l *Glatt Kosher* Beef Salami or Garlic Stick.	80	7	3	15	1	0	0	220
MEATLESS ALTERNATIVES								
REDUCED SODIUM (LESS THAN GENERIC):								
Field Roast Lentil Sage, 2 slices.................	73	2	0	0	6	2	1	180
Wild Mushroom, 2 slices	67	2	0	0	4	1	0	180
Lightlife *Smart Deli* Baked Ham Style, 2 sl ...	35	1	0	0	2	1	1	195
Tofurky Oven Roasted or Peppered, 3 slices .	60	2	0	0	3	2	1	180
Hickory Smoked, 3 slices	60	2	0	0	3	2	1	180
Italian Deli, 3 slices...................................	66	3	0	0	4	3	1	216
Cranberry & Stuffing, 3 slices	60	2	0	0	5	2	1	222
"Philly-Style" Steak, 3 slices	60	2	0	0	4	2	0	222
Yves Deli Turkey, 2 slices...........................	50	1	0	0	3	0	0	170
Roast w/o the Beef, 2 slices.......................	55	1	0	0	2	1	1	180
Meatless Canadian Bacon, 1.5 slices..........	40	0	0	0	1	0	0	200
Deli Bologna or Meatless Ham, 2 slices (avg)	45	1	0	0	2	0	0	225

PATÉ

	Cal	Fat	Sat	Chol	Carb	Fib	Sug	Sod
Chicken liver paté, 1 oz..................................	57	4	1	111	2	0	0	109
Goose liver paté, smoked, 1 oz	131	12	4	43	1	0	0	198

Brands . . . *Most brands within generic average.*

SANDWICH SPREADS

(also see Vegetable Spreads, pg 95; Dips/Spreads, pg 220)

	Cal	Fat	Sat	Chol	Carb	Fib	Sug	Sod
Chicken spread, 1 oz..................................	44	5	1	16	1	0	0	202
Roast beef, 1 oz.......................................	65	5	2	20	1	0	0	205
Deviled ham, 1 oz	75	6	2	18	0	0	0	230
Deviled ham, canned, 1 oz	90	8	3	18	1	0	0	240
Ham salad, 1 oz..	61	4	1	11	3	0	0	259
Pork and beef, 1 oz..................................	67	5	2	11	3	0	0	287
Ham and cheese, 1 oz...............................	69	5	2	17	1	0	0	339
Minced pork & ham, 1 oz	90	8	3	20	1	0	0	395
25% lower sodium, 1 oz	90	8	3	20	1	0	0	295

Brands . . .
	Cal	Fat	Sat	Chol	Carb	Fib	Sug	Sod
Dixie Carb Counters Chicken (Not!) Salad Mix..	95	1	0	0	8	5	0	119
REDUCED SODIUM (LESS THAN GENERIC):								
Dixie Carb Counters Tuna (Not!) Salad Mix ..	80	2	0	0	8	3	0	204

SAUSAGE

(see Breakfast Meats, pg 191; Sausages, pg 197)

VEGETARIAN MEAT AND POULTRY – PREPARED ENTREES

	Cal	Fat	Sat	Chol	Carb	Fib	Sug	Sod
Vegetarian meatloaf, 2 oz.............................	110	5	1	0	4	3	1	308
Vegetarian fillet, 3 oz..................................	247	15	2	0	8	5	1	417

Brands . . . *(3 oz serving unless noted)*
FROZEN/REFRIGERATED
	Cal	Fat	Sat	Chol	Carb	Fib	Sug	Sod
Mon Cuisine Vegan Chicken Nuggets, 9 oz........	35	1	0	0	5	1	0	95
REDUCED SODIUM (LESS THAN GENERIC):								
Al Safa Halal Falafel, 3 oz (3)....................	282	15	2	3	27	3	6	162
Veggie Samosa, 2 oz (2)	110	4	0	0	17	1	0	240
Gardein 7 Grain Crispy Tenders, 2 pcs	100	4	0	0	8	1	0	250

201

MEAT, POULTRY AND MEATLESS ALTERNATIVES
Vegetarian Meat and Poultry Substitutes

	Cal	Fat	Sat	Chol	Carb	Fib	Sug	Sod
Mandarin Orange Crispy Chick'n, 3.3 oz	165	5	0	0	10	0	2	290
Michael Angelo's Eggplant Cutlets, 5.4 oz	250	15	2	0	23	3	1	150
Mon Cuisine Vegan Italian Shell Pasta	250	3	0	0	43	11	5	210
Vegetarian Stuffed Cabbage in Tomato Sauce	220	5	0	0	36	5	8	260
Vegan Breaded Chicken Cutlet, 10 oz	300	7	1	0	44	7	3	270
Vegan Chicken Patties, 10 oz	100	3	0	0	15	3	1	290
MorningStar Farms								
Veggie Cakes Ginger Teriyaki	110	2	1	0	19	2	2	320
Southwestern Style, 2.4 oz cake	130	3	1	0	21	2	0	340
Grillers Chik'n, 2.4 oz	80	3	0	0	7	5	0	350
Nate's Meatless Meatballs								
Savory Mushrrom, 1.5 oz	100	5	0	0	6	2	1	230
Classic Flavor, 1.5 oz	190	5	0	0	5	2	1	270
Zesty Italian, 1.5 oz	90	5	0	0	4	2	1	340

(VEGETARIAN MEAT AND POULTRY SUBSTITUTES)

	Cal	Fat	Sat	Chol	Carb	Fib	Sug	Sod
Tofu:								
Plain, soft, 3 oz	45	3	0	0	2	0	0	0
Plain, firm, 3 oz	50	3	0	0	2	0	0	30
Plain, extra firm, 3 oz	45	2	0	0	2	0	0	55
Plain lite, firm, 3 oz	30	1	0	0	1	0	0	70
Seasoned, 3 oz	90	5	1	0	3	1	1	220
Tempeh, plain, 3 oz	160	9	1	0	8	4	1	7
Ground beef, meatless, 2 oz	60	1	0	0	6	3	0	350
Beef strips, meatless, 3 oz	120	1	0	0	4	1	1	370
Textured vegetable protein (TVP), 1/4 cup	80	0	0	0	7	4	3	594

Brands . . . *(2 oz unless noted)*

MEAT AND POULTRY

CANNED/SHELF-STABLE

	Cal	Fat	Sat	Chol	Carb	Fib	Sug	Sod
Dixie Diner Carver's Choice Cuts, 1/2 cup	100	2	0	0	7	4	2	0
Meat Not, 1/3 cup	100	2	0	0	7	4	2	0
Beef (Not!) Chunks or Strips, 1.8 oz	140	2	1	0	15	9	4	5
Chicken (Not!) Chunks or Strips, 1.8 oz	140	2	1	0	15	9	4	5
Turkey (Not!) Ground, 1.8 oz	140	2	1	0	15	9	4	5
Worthington Loma Linda								
Vege-Burger, 1/4 cup	60	1	0	0	2	2	0	130

REDUCED SODIUM (LESS THAN GENERIC):

	Cal	Fat	Sat	Chol	Carb	Fib	Sug	Sod
Cedar Lake Nuti-Loaf, 2.3 oz	140	10	0	0	8	2	1	160
Hostess Cuts, 4 oz	100	0	0	0	9	0	0	290
Beef Strips, 2.1 oz	90	1	0	0	4	0	0	300
Dixie Diner Soysage Pattie Mix, Sausage	118	2	0	0	12	5	2	303
Beef (Not!) Crumbles, 3.1 oz	118	2	0	0	12	5	2	343
Soysage Crumblers - Sausage, 3.1 oz	118	2	0	0	12	5	2	343
Worthington Diced Chik, 1/4 cup	50	0	0	0	2	1	0	220
Meatless Chicken Style Roll, 2 oz	90	5	1	0	2	1	0	240
Vegetarian Burger, 1/4 cup	70	2	0	0	3	1	0	250
Multigrain Cutlets, 2 slices (3.4 oz)	100	1	1	0	5	3	0	290
LF Vegetable Steaks, 2 slices (2.6 oz)	80	1	1	0	3	2	0	300
Worthington Loma Linda Tender Rounds	120	5	1	0	6	1	1	340
Zoglo's *Vegetarian Choice* Tofu Cutlets, 2.6 oz	139	7	1	0	8	2	0	250
Tofu/Corn or Tofu/Mix Veg Cutlets, 2.9 oz	152	7	1	0	13	2	0	250
Tofu Patties, 3.1 oz	112	4	1	0	2	2	0	270

FROZEN/REFRIGERATED

	Cal	Fat	Sat	Chol	Carb	Fib	Sug	Sod
Clawson Paneer, 1 oz	100	8	5	10	1	0	1	0

	Cal	Fat	Sat	Chol	Carb	Fib	Sug	Sod
REDUCED SODIUM (LESS THAN GENERIC):								
Field Roast								
Quarter Loaf Smoked Tomato, 2 oz	90	2	0	0	7	3	2	290
Quarter Loaf Wild Mushroom, 2 oz	110	2	0	0	9	2	2	300
Quarter Loaf Lentil Sage, 2 oz	110	2	0	0	9	3	1	310
Lightlife *Smart Ground* Mexican Style, 1/3 c	70	0	0	0	7	3	1	220
Morningstar Farms *Meal Starters*								
Grillers Recipe Crumbles, 2/3 cup	80	3	0	0	5	3	1	230
Quorn Grounds	90	2	1	0	9	5	1	170
Yves Meatless Ground, 1/3 cup	60	1	0	0	5	2	1	270
Meatless Taco Stuffers, 1/3 cup	90	3	0	0	5	2	1	300
Meatless Ground Turkey, 1/3 cup	60	1	0	0	4	2	0	330
Lettuce Wraps (Asian meatless ground round)	60	1	0	0	8	2	4	350
MIXES								
Harvest Direct Veggie Ribs Mix, 2 tbsp	160	0	0	0	7	2	1	40
Seitan Quick Mix, 1/3 cup	160	1	0	0	11	2	0	60
Soy BBQ	60	0	0	0	8	3	2	120
Soy Chicken Breast, 0.6 oz pc	52	0	0	0	3	3	0	120
Soy Taco Mix	60	0	0	0	8	3	1	135
REDUCED SODIUM (LESS THAN GENERIC):								
Authentic Foods Falafel Mix, 1/4 cup	100	1	0	0	17	3	2	240
Harvest Direct Soy Chicken Chunk or Strip	41	0	0	0	2	2	0	275
TEMPEH								
FROZEN/REFRIGERATED								
Plain tempeh – *Most brands of plain tempeh within generic average (0mg).*								
Lightlife Garden Veggie Tempeh, 4 oz	240	10	2	0	17	10	1	10
Tofurky *Tempeh* Spicy Veggie, 3 oz	145	5	1	0	20	7	0	25
REDUCED SODIUM (LESS THAN GENERIC):								
Tofurky *Tempeh* Coconut Curry Strips, 5 sl	120	3	2	0	12	5	0	280
Sesame Garlic Strips, 5 slices (3 oz)	90	4	1	0	13	5	2	340
TOFU								
PLAIN TOFU – *Most brands of plain tofu within generic average (0mg–70mg).*								
BAKED/FLAVORED								
REDUCED SODIUM (LESS THAN GENERIC):								
More Than Tofu Pesto, 1/4 pkg	90	5	1	0	3	1	1	160
Peanut & Ginger or Spicy Thai, 1/4 pkg	90	5	1	0	3	1	1	160
Indian Marsala or Spinach Jalapeno, 1/4 pkg	80	4	1	0	3	2	1	160
Garlic Shiitake or Savory Portabella, 1/4 pkg	80	4	1	0	3	2	1	160
Italian Herb, 1/4 pkg	80	4	1	0	3	2	1	160

NOODLES, PASTA, RICE AND GRAINS

See RESOURCES, page 305, for a partial list of manufacturers and retailers offering low-salt products online or visit **LowSaltFoods.com** *for additional sources.*

NOODLES, PASTA, RICE AND GRAINS

GRAINS

(also see Side Dishes, pg 151; Rice, pg 209)

	Cal	Fat	Sat	Chol	Carb	Fib	Sug	Sod
Wheat bran, uncooked, 1/2 cup	63	1	0	0	19	12	0	1
Oat bran, uncooked, 1/2 cup	116	3	1	0	31	7	1	2
Millet, uncooked, 1/2 cup	378	4	1	0	73	9	-	5
Couscous, uncooked, 1/2 cup	325	1	0	0	67	4	1	9
Barley, pearl, uncooked, 1/2 cup	352	1	0	0	78	16	1	9
Buckwheat groats, roasted, 1/2 cup	284	2	0	0	62	8	-	9
Bulgur, uncooked, 1/2 cup	239	1	0	0	53	13	0	12
Quinoa, uncooked, 1/2 cup	318	5	1	0	59	5	0	18

Brands . . . *Most brands within generic average.*

GRAINS – SIDE DISHES

	Cal	Fat	Sat	Chol	Carb	Fib	Sug	Sod
Tabouli, mix, 2/3 cup prep	95	0	0	0	22	4	1	340
Couscous, parmesan, mix, 1 cup prep	200	2	1	5	39	2	3	580
Falafel, mix, 1/4 cup	120	2	0	0	20	4	3	610

Brands . . . *(1 cup unless noted)*

	Cal	Fat	Sat	Chol	Carb	Fib	Sug	Sod
Bountiful Pantry Couscous w/Cranberries	150	0	0	0	33	2	6	0
Couscous & Lentil Salad w/Cranberries	200	1	0	0	40	7	9	15
Ziyad Falafil Mix, Vegetable Burger, 2 patties	57	3	0	0	5	0	0	50

REDUCED SODIUM (LESS THAN GENERIC):

	Cal	Fat	Sat	Chol	Carb	Fib	Sug	Sod
Sadaf Falafel Mix, 1/4 cup	140	2	0	0	25	2	5	190

PASTA AND NOODLES

(also see Entrees–Pasta/Italian Dishes, pg 145; Side Dishes, pg 151)

	Cal	Fat	Sat	Chol	Carb	Fib	Sug	Sod
Lasagne, dry, 2 oz	210	1	0	0	40	2	0	0
Farfel, matzo, 1 oz	105	0	0	0	21	-	-	0
Macaroni and spaghetti, dry, 2 oz	211	1	0	0	43	2	1	3
Macaroni and spaghetti, whole wheat, dry, 2 oz	198	1	0	0	43	5	0	5
Noodles, egg, dry, 2 oz	219	3	1	48	41	2	1	12
Pasta, fresh-refrigerated, 4.5 oz	369	3	0	93	70	-	-	33

Brands . . . *Most brands within generic average.*

PASTA AND NOODLES – SIDE DISHES

	Cal	Fat	Sat	Chol	Carb	Fib	Sug	Sod
Noodles w/parmesan sauce, mix, 1/2 pkg	220	5	3	10	37	1	2	680
Pasta salad, mix 1/4 pkg	170	1	0	0	36	0	3	800
Pasta w/alfredo sauce, mix, 1/2 pkg	250	5	3	50	41	1	4	980

Brands . . .

SHELF-STABLE MIXES

Frontier Soups Salad! Pasta Salad Mix

	Cal	Fat	Sat	Chol	Carb	Fib	Sug	Sod
Pesto Italian	160	4	0	0	27	2	2	0
Mediterranean or Country French (avg)	135	1	0	0	28	2	1	10

REDUCED SODIUM (LESS THAN GENERIC)

Betty Crocker Suddenly Salad

	Cal	Fat	Sat	Chol	Carb	Fib	Sug	Sod
Creamy Parmesan	160	1	1	0	33	1	2	270
Ranch & Bacon or Chipotle Ranch (avg)	160	1	0	0	34	2	4	295
Leonard Mountain Pasta Salad, all, 1/6	220	1	0	0	43	0	0	175

PASTA FIXINGS – PASTA SAUCE

	Cal	Fat	Sat	Chol	Carb	Fib	Sug	Sod
Red clam sauce, 1/2 cup	60	1	0	10	8	1	4	350

NOODLES, PASTA, RICE AND GRAINS
Pasta Fixings – Pasta Sauce

	Cal	Fat	Sat	Chol	Carb	Fib	Sug	Sod
Alfredo sauce, ready-to-use, 1/4 cup	110	10	5	35	3	0	1	420
Mix, 2 tbsp...	80	4	0	10	9	0	3	690
White clam sauce, 1/2 cup................................	140	10	2	15	5	0	1	510
Marinara/spaghetti, ready-to-use, 1/2 cup	111	3	0	0	18	3	11	580
Pesto, 1/4 cup	110	8	2	5	8	2	4	720

Brands . . . *(1/2 cup serving unless noted)*
PESTO
FROZEN/REFRIGERATED

	Cal	Fat	Sat	Chol	Carb	Fib	Sug	Sod
Armanino Tomato & Garlic Pesto, 1/4 cup	210	20	0	5	5	1	3	130
Scarpetto Pesto Sauce, 1/4 cup	108	9	2	3	1	0	0	100
REDUCED SODIUM (LESS THAN GENERIC):								
Ciba Naturals Cilantro Lime Pesto, 1/4 c ...	270	29	3	5	2	1	1	160
Sun-Dried Tomato Pesto, 1/4 cup.............	260	23	2	0	11	3	3	170
Artichoke Lemon Pesto, 1/4 cup.............	210	21	3	5	3	0	1	260
Basil, made w/Almonds Pesto, 1/4 cup	280	28	4	5	3	1	0	230
Monterey Pasta Pesto Cream Sauce, 1/4 c ..	120	10	6	40	4	0	1	220
Rising Sun Farms								
Organic Basil/Dried Tomato	220	22	3	0	6	2	2	260
Organic Garlic Galore Pesto	240	24	3	0	4	2	0	280
Organic Basil & Garlic Pesto	240	26	4	0	4	2	0	300
MIXES								
REDUCED SODIUM (LESS THAN GENERIC):								
Simply Organic Sweet Basil.....................	10	0	0	0	2	1	0	210
SHELF-STABLE								
Bella Sun Luci Tomato Pesto	270	27	3	5	8	1	5	70
Bella Terra Traditional Basil Pesto, 3 tbsp.....	100	10	0	0	0	0	0	110
REDUCED SODIUM (LESS THAN GENERIC):								
DaVinci Pesto Genovese	400	40	6	0	8	2	0	250
Meditalia Basil Pesto	46	1	0	0	15	0	0	160
Melissa's Basil Pesto	340	34	6	10	3	0	1	230
Robt Rothschild Farm Artichoke Pesto, 2 tbsp ..	45	4	1	0	2	0	0	170
Stonewall Kitchen Basil Pesto, 2 tbsp.......	110	11	2	5	2	1	0	150
Sun-Dried Tomato Pesto, 2 tbsp.............	70	6	1	0	4	1	2	200
Turtledove Savory Basil Pesto	44	6	2	4	2	0	0	208
Lemon Artichoke Heart	100	8	2	20	4	0	0	300

RED PASTA SAUCE
FROZEN/REFRIGERATED

	Cal	Fat	Sat	Chol	Carb	Fib	Sug	Sod
REDUCED SODIUM (LESS THAN GENERIC):								
Scarpetta Tuscan Vodka Sauce	120	11	6	35	5	1	3	240
Arrabbiata Sauce	40	2	0	0	5	1	3	250
Barely Bolognese	45	2	1	0	6	2	4	290
Marinara Sauce	45	2	1	0	7	2	3	300
MIXES								
Bernard LS Spaghetti Sauce Mix	55	0	0	0	14	0	4	140
REDUCED SODIUM (LESS THAN GENERIC):								
Simply Organic Garlic Pasta	15	0	0	0	4	1	0	170
READY-TO-USE								
Anjon's Gourmet Marinara	70	6	1	0	5	1	3	120
Casa Visco FF Sauce	30	0	0	0	6	1	3	110
Dave's Gourmet Roasted Garlic/Sweet Basil	45	2	0	0	7	2	4	125
Eden Organic Spaghetti, NSA....................	70	3	0	0	9	5	4	10
Fanny's Meat Sauce for Pasta	230	7	0	15	35	0	2	80
Francesco Rinaldi NSA	70	3	0	0	12	2	6	40
Furmano's Spaghetti Sauce	50	1	0	0	10	2	6	90

Pasta Fixings – Pasta Sauce

	Cal	Fat	Sat	Chol	Carb	Fib	Sug	Sod
Lucini Italia Sicilian Eggplant & Olive Sauce.	70	5	1	0	6	1	1	110
Med-Diet Spaghetti	20	0	0	0	3	0	0	100
Mother Teresa's Pasta Sauces, all	40	1	0	0	7	1	3	20
Palmieri Meat (Flavored) Sauce	35	3	1	0	1	0	1	115
Robt Rothschild Farm Artichoke Pasta	80	5	0	0	8	0	7	90
LE Roselli's LS Spaghetti	45	1	0	0	9	2	3	35
Victoria LS Marinara Sauce	70	4	1	0	8	1	5	120
Walnut Acres Tomato & Basil, LS	40	0	0	0	9	1	7	20
REDUCED SODIUM (LESS THAN GENERIC):								
Alessio's Homemade Spaghetti Sauce	80	4	1	0	10	3	8	179
Amy's *Light in Sodium* Family Marinara	80	5	1	0	9	2	5	290
Light in Sodium Tomato Basil Pasta	90	5	1	0	11	2	6	290
Bove's Marinara or Basil Pasta Sauce	80	4	1	0	7	1	2	240
Mushroom & Wine or Roasted Garlic (avg)	75	5	1	0	7	1	2	265
Sweet Red Pepper	110	3	1	5	7	2	6	290
Casa Visco Homestyle	90	3	1	0	12	3	0	150
Peppers & Onion	40	3	0	0	6	1	3	260
Tomato Basil, Fra Diavolo	80	3	1	0	13	3	1	260
Filetto di Pomodoro	80	3	1	0	13	3	1	260
Catanzaro's Pasta Sauce	160	10	1	0	14	4	6	210
Chef's Meat Flavored Pasta Sauce	120	4	2	20	19	4	19	160
Plain Pasta Sauce	90	3	1	0	12	4	7	160
Classico Spicy Red Pepper	60	3	1	0	8	2	5	300
Colavita Marinara	70	3	0	0	9	2	6	220
Classic Hot	80	3	0	0	12	3	6	250
Garden Style	60	3	0	0	12	3	0	290
Dave's Gourmet Wild Mushroom	60	3	0	0	7	1	2	270
Red Heirloom or Spicy Heirloom Marinara	45	2	0	0	7	2	4	280
Dean & Deluca Marinara Sauce	80	5	1	0	8	1	1	290
Arrabbiata Sauce	110	8	1	0	9	1	1	300
Dei Fratelli Spaghetti Sauce	60	1	0	0	9	3	7	220
Tomato Basil	60	2	0	0	9	2	7	260
Arrabbiata	50	2	0	0	8	2	5	300
Delallo Imported Roasted Garlic	90	7	1	0	7	2	0	300
Delicae' Gourmet Artichoke Pasta Sauce	50	0	0	0	12	3	8	190
Vokda Pink Peppercorn	50	0	0	0	11	2	8	200
Romesco	130	10	1	0	9	3	4	210
Fra Diablo	50	9	9	9	12	3	7	220
Sun-Dried Tomato & Basil	60	0	0	0	14	3	8	260
Dell'Amore Original Recipe or Spicy	80	4	0	0	10	2	6	250
Don Brunno Marinara or Arrabbiata Sauce	70	5	0	0	7	1	4	290
Eden Organic Spaghetti	70	3	0	0	9	5	4	300
Enrico's Traditional Pasta Sauce, NSA	60	2	0	0	12	0	11	25
Francesco Rinaldi Premium Vodka Sauce	60	4	2	10	4	0	4	290
Premium Sun-Dried Tomato Alfredo	60	4	2	10	5	0	4	290
Frank's Vodka Sauce	153	14	7	35	5	1	2	231
Frescorti Garden Vegetable	60	2	0	0	10	1	8	270
Gia Russa Artichoke	90	7	1	0	6	2	3	200
Lucini Italia Rustic Tomato Vodka Sauce	70	3	1	10	10	2	2	230
Hearty Artichoke Tomato Sauce	50	2	0	0	7	3	1	230
Sicilian Olive & Wild Caper Sauce	50	2	0	0	8	2	2	290
Mom's Puttanesca or Martini Sauce	120	8	4	20	6	1	3	250
Paesana Fra Diavolo	70	4	0	0	7	2	3	280
Sicilian Gravy	110	7	1	0	9	2	5	300
Palmieri Marinara or Spaghetti Sauce, 2/3 c	90	3	0	0	13	4	11	170

	Cal	Fat	Sat	Chol	Carb	Fib	Sug	Sod
Roasted Garlic or Tomato Basil, 2/3 cup	90	3	0	0	13	4	11	170
Primavera or Puttanaesca Sauce (avg)	60	4	1	0	6	1	3	240
Portobello Mushroom or Roasted Eggplant	70	4	1	0	8	1	3	250
Fra Diavolo	60	4	0	0	5	1	3	250
Paul Sorvino Italian Vodka Sauce	90	7	4	15	6	1	4	150
Puttanesca	60	4	1	0	6	1	4	220
Arrabbiata	60	4	1	0	6	1	4	250
Marinara	60	4	1	0	6	1	4	260
Rao's *Homemade* Puttanesca	80	5	1	0	6	2	3	250
Rising Moon Organics Garlic & Basil	35	0	0	0	8	2	4	190
Garlic & Merlot	40	0	0	0	8	2	4	190
Port & Asiago	45	1	0	0	8	2	4	200
Garlic & Chanterelle Mushroom	40	0	0	0	9	2	4	250
Olive & Asiago	45	2	1	0	8	2	3	260
Robert Rothschild Farm								
Vodka Pasta Sauce	140	9	3	10	10	2	9	270
Sal & Judy's *Heart Smart*, all varieties	35	1	0	0	6	4	2	250
Sclafani Homestyle Spaghetti	45	2	1	0	7	3	1	300
Seeds of Change Arrabiatta di Roma	80	6	1	0	6	2	0	300
Serafina Arrabbiata	80	6	1	0	5	1	3	280
ShopRite *Organic* Tomato Basil	60	1	0	0	10	2	6	300
The Silver Palate Tuscan Marinara	60	7	1	5	13	1	3	270
Testo's Marinara	60	5	1	0	4	1	1	290
Veroli Foods Classic or Chunky Marinara	60	4	1	0	6	1	3	300
Vincent's Marinara	80	5	0	0	8	2	4	210
Vodka Sauce	190	15	7	25	13	2	6	240
Vito Marcello's Tomato Basil Marinara	90	3	0	0	13	4	11	170
Puttanesca Sauce	50	4	1	0	4	1	3	240
Fra Diavolo Sauce	60	4	0	0	5	1	11	250
Walnut Acres								
Garlic-Garlic or Roasted Garlic (avg)	55	1	0	0	11	1	7	280
Sweet Pepper & Onion	50	1	0	0	9	1	6	280

ALFREDO AND WHITE SAUCES
MIXES

	Cal	Fat	Sat	Chol	Carb	Fib	Sug	Sod
Chef Creations Alfredo Sauce, 1/4 cup	120	12	8	45	2	0	2	140
REDUCED SODIUM (LESS THAN GENERIC):								
Road's End Organics Alfredo Sauce, 1/4 c	35	1	0	0	6	3	0	200
Tony Chachere's Cream Sauce Mix, 1/4 c	15	0	0	0	0	0	0	190

READY-TO-USE
Walden Farms

	Cal	Fat	Sat	Chol	Carb	Fib	Sug	Sod
Scampi, 2 tbsp	0	0	0	0	0	0	0	130
REDUCED SODIUM (LESS THAN GENERIC):								
Classico Mushroom Alfredo	70	5	3	35	3	2	0	300
Francesco Rinaldi Dried Tomato Alfredo	60	4	2	10	5	0	4	290

(POLENTA)

	Cal	Fat	Sat	Chol	Carb	Fib	Sug	Sod
Polenta, instant, 1/4 cup	140	0	0	0	32	4	0	0
Ready-to-eat, 4 oz	88	0	0	0	20	1	0	376
Mix, prep, 3/8 cup	260	5	2	5	48	4	3	550

Brands . . .
MIXES
Instant – *Most brands within generic average (0mg).*

	Cal	Fat	Sat	Chol	Carb	Fib	Sug	Sod
Bob's Red Mill Polenta Corn Grits, 1/4 cup	130	0	0	0	27	2	0	0

	Cal	Fat	Sat	Chol	Carb	Fib	Sug	Sod

READY-TO-USE

REDUCED SODIUM (LESS THAN GENERIC):

	Cal	Fat	Sat	Chol	Carb	Fib	Sug	Sod
Ferrara Pronto Polenta, 2 oz	60	0	0	0	19	1	1	200
Monterey Pasta Co Polenta, Original	80	0	0	0	16	2	0	198

RICE

	Cal	Fat	Sat	Chol	Carb	Fib	Sug	Sod
White rice, uncooked, 1/2 cup	351	1	0	0	77	1	0	1
Brown rice, uncooked, 1/4 cup	344	3	1	0	72	3	0	4
Wild rice, uncooked, 1/4 cup	286	1	0	0	60	5	2	6
Instant rice, 1/2 cup	190	1	0	0	43	1	0	15

Brands . . . *Most brands within generic average.*

RICE – SIDE DISHES

(also see Asian–Entrees/Light Meals, pg 156; Mediterranean/Middle Eastern–Meals/Entrees, pg 169)

	Cal	Fat	Sat	Chol	Carb	Fib	Sug	Sod
Risotto, mix, 1/4 cup	150	0	0	0	34	0	0	420
Rice w/vegetables, frozen, 1 cup	180	4	2	10	31	2	2	480
Rice and beans, mix, 1/4 cup	160	0	0	0	35	3	1	490
Rice pilaf, mix, prep, 1 cup	210	5	1	0	41	1	0	710
Spanish rice, canned, 1/4 cup	90	3	0	0	15	1	1	770
Mix, prep, 1 cup	300	2	1	0	65	2	2	1000
Long grain and wild rice, mix, prep, 1 cup	220	5	1	0	42	2	0	800
Flavored rice, mix, prep, 1 cup	320	2	0	0	51	2	2	1070
1/3 less salt, prep, 1 cup	280	1	0	0	53	1	2	640
Fried rice, mix, prep, 1 cup	260	1	0	0	47	1	3	1095

Brands . . .

MIXES

	Cal	Fat	Sat	Chol	Carb	Fib	Sug	Sod
Bountiful Pantry Mushroom Herb Risotto	170	0	0	0	38	1	0	0
Wild Rice Pilaf w/Mushrooms	170	2	0	0	35	2	0	0
Pumpkin Risotto w/Cranberries	190	1	0	0	45	2	6	0
Risotto w/Garden Vegetables	170	1	0	0	40	2	1	10
Wild Rice Pilaf w/Cranberries	200	2	0	0	44	3	7	15
Neera's Northern Indian Biryani	132	1	0	0	29	0	0	4
Indian Dal w/Chaunk	140	1	0	0	23	0	0	4
Indian Urad & Channa Dal	104	1	0	0	18	0	0	4
Jamaican-Style Dirty Rice	175	6	0	0	28	0	0	5
Indian Shahi Pilau	286	8	0	0	48	0	0	6
Stonewall Kitchen Veg Risotto Mix, 1/2 cup	30	1	0	0	33	3	3	20
REDUCED SODIUM (LESS THAN GENERIC):								
Goya Mexican Rice	160	0	0	0	37	0	1	325
Sadaf Basmati Rice Mix Sweet Harmony, 2 oz	210	2	0	0	43	3	4	250
Wild West Favorite, 2 oz mix	200	2	0	0	43	3	1	310
Herb Rice, 2 oz mix	200	2	0	0	43	2	1	320
Sweet Delight, 2 oz mix	210	3	0	0	43	4	8	320
Seeds of Change Tapovan White Basmati Rice	190	3	0	0	38	1	0	160
Rishikesh Brown Basmati, 1 cup	190	4	0	0	37	2	1	170
Tigris A Mixture of 7 Whole Grains, 1 cup	260	4	1	0	50	5	1	220
Stonewall Kitchen Mushroom Risotto Mix	40	2	1	5	31	2	1	180
Taste Adventure Lentil/Rice Bombay Curry	150	1	0	0	32	3	1	250
Tasty Bite Thai Lime Rice, 1/2 pkg	210	5	2	0	38	1	2	300
Zatarain's Jambalaya Mix, Reduced Sodium	130	0	0	0	29	1	0	360
SEASONING MIXES FOR RICE								
Perez *Mix for Rice* Dried Veg, Raisins & Spice	129	8	0	0	12	0	0	140
Pine Nuts, Raisins, Blueberries, 2 tbsp	145	10	3	0	12	0	0	140

SNACK FOODS

See RESOURCES, page 305, for a partial list of manufacturers and retailers offering low-salt products online or visit **LowSaltFoods.com** *for additional sources.*

SNACK FOODS

CHIPS AND NIBBLERS

	Cal	Fat	Sat	Chol	Carb	Fib	Sug	Sod
Banana chips, 1 oz	147	10	8	0	17	2	10	2
Apple chips, 1 oz	140	7	1	0	20	2	11	15
Taro chips, 1 oz	141	7	2	0	19	2	1	97
Tortilla chips, 1 oz	139	6	1	0	19	1	0	110
Baked, low fat, 1 oz	118	2	1	1	23	2	0	119
Ranch flavor, 1 oz	142	7	1	0	18	1	1	147
Nacho cheese flavor, 1 oz	146	7	1	0	18	1	1	174
Oriental mix, rice based, 1 oz	143	7	1	0	15	4	1	117
Potato chips, 1 oz	155	11	3	0	14	1	0	149
Reduced fat, 1 oz	134	6	1	0	19	2	0	139
Sour cream & onion flavor, 1 oz	151	10	3	2	15	2	0	177
Barbecue flavor, 1 oz	139	9	2	0	15	1	0	213
Cheese flavor, 1 oz	141	8	2	1	16	2	0	225
Corn nuts, regular, 1 oz	125	4	1	0	21	2	0	157
Nacho, 1 oz	124	4	1	0	20	2	0	180
Barbecue, 1 oz	124	4	1	0	20	2	0	277
Corn chips, 1 oz	160	10	2	0	15	1	1	170
Barbecue flavor, 1 oz	150	10	2	0	15	1	1	280
Chex mix, 1 oz	120	5	2	0	18	2	–	288
Cheese puffs, 1 oz	158	10	2	0	15	1	1	298
Sesame sticks, 1 oz	153	10	2	0	13	1	0	422
Pork skins, plain, 1 oz	155	9	3	27	0	0	0	521
Barbecue flavor, 1 oz	153	9	3	33	1	0	0	756

Brands . . . *(1 oz unless noted)*

CORN AND TORTILLA CHIPS

There are many low sodium chips, the following have 120mg or less per serving.

	Cal	Fat	Sat	Chol	Carb	Fib	Sug	Sod
Bachman's Restaurant Style Tortilla Chips	140	6	1	0	19	2	0	50
Sweet Potato Tortilla Chips	130	5	1	0	20	3	2	70
Tortilla Dipping Strips	140	6	1	0	20	2	0	85
Multigrain Tortilla Chips	140	6	1	0	19	5	0	95
Bearito's Blue, White, or Yellow, NSA	140	6	1	0	19	2	0	5
Blue Corn Chips	150	7	1	0	19	2	0	65
Blue, White, or Yellow Tortilla Chips	140	6	1	0	19	2	0	65
Chi-Chi's Fiesta Authentic or Rounds	140	7	1	0	18	1	0	120
Corazonas Lightly Salted Tortilla Chips	140	7	1	0	18	3	0	75
Doritos Toasted Corn	140	7	1	0	18	1	0	120
Eatsmart Naturals Whole Grain Tortilla Chips	150	7	1	0	19	3	2	80
Food Should Taste Good Cinn or Choc (avg)	140	7	1	0	18	4	4	80
Sweet Potato, Lime or Multigrain (avg)	140	6	1	0	18	3	2	80
Yellow Corn	140	7	1	0	19	3	0	85
Frontera Blue Corn, Thick/Crunchy or Thin/Crispy	130	5	1	0	20	2	0	75
Lime & Sea Salt	140	6	1	0	18	2	0	75
Fritos Lightly Salted Corn Chips	160	10	2	0	16	1	0	80
Scoops! Corn Chips	160	10	2	0	16	1	0	110
Garden of Eatin' Blue Chips NSA	140	7	1	0	18	2	0	10
Blue Chips or Mini Yellow Rounds	140	7	1	0	18	2	0	60
Mini White Rounds or Mini White Strips	140	6	1	0	19	2	0	60
Black Bean Chips or White Chips (avg)	140	7	1	0	18	3	0	70
Red Chips, Yellow Chips, or Little Soy Blues	140	7	1	0	18	2	0	70

211

SNACK FOODS
Chips and Nibblers

	Cal	Fat	Sat	Chol	Carb	Fib	Sug	Sod
Sunny Blues	150	8	1	0	17	2	0	70
Key Lime Jalapeno or Maui Onion (avg)	140	7	1	0	18	2	0	80
Sesame Blues	150	8	1	0	16	2	0	90
Multi Grain Blues, Sea Salt	130	7	1	0	16	2	1	110
Baked Blue or Yellow Chips (avg)	120	3	1	0	20	3	0	120
Veggie Chips, Beet & Garlic or Veg Medly	140	6	1	0	19	2	1	120
Focaccia Tortilla Chips	140	6	1	0	19	1	0	120
Grande Restaurant Style Tortilla Chips	130	5	1	0	20	1	0	95
Original Lightly Salted	140	6	1	0	20	2	0	95
Multigrain Lightly Salted	140	5	1	0	20	2	0	100
Guiltless Gourmet Unsalted Yellow Corn	120	2	0	0	22	2	1	26
Kettle Brand Tias! Toasted Corn Tortilla Chips	150	8	1	0	17	1	0	120
Laurel Hill Chips, all varieties	140	6	1	0	19	2	1	80
Lundberg Rice Chips Sesame & Seaweed	140	7	1	0	18	1	0	90
Sante Fe Barbecue or Sea Salt	140	7	1	0	18	1	0	110
Maine Coast Sea Chips	146	7	0	0	17	4	0	65
Nature's Promise (Giant Foods)								
Natural Blue or Natural Yellow (avg)	140	6	1	0	18	1	0	65
Old Dutch Restaurante Style Fiesta	150	7	1	0	19	1	0	30
Restaurante Style Multigrain	150	7	1	0	20	3	1	70
Restaurante Style Dip Strips	140	7	1	0	18	1	0	80
Restaurante Style Original	150	7	1	0	19	2	0	95
Restaurante Style Bite Size	150	8	1	0	18	1	0	105
Que Pasa, all varieties	135	6	1	0	19	2	0	42
Robert Rothschild Farm Tortilla Chips	140	6	1	30	19	1	0	30
Santitas Yellow Tortilla Triangles	140	6	1	0	19	2	0	110
White Tortilla Triangles	140	6	1	0	19	2	0	115
Yellow Tortilla Rounds or Strips	140	6	1	0	20	1	0	120
Snyder's of Hanover Restaurant Tortilla Chips	130	5	0	0	20	4	0	120
SunChips Original	140	6	1	0	19	3	2	120
Tostitos Natural Blue Corn	140	6	1	0	19	1	0	80
Artisan Roasted Garlic & Black Bean	140	7	1	0	18	2	0	90
Artisan Fire-Roasted Chipotle	140	7	1	0	18	2	1	90
Natural Yellow Corn	140	6	1	0	19	1	0	100
Bite Size Whole Grains or Multigrain Scoops (avg)	140	7	1	0	18	2	1	110
Multigrain	150	7	1	0	19	2	1	110
Dipping Strips! or Restaurant Style	140	7	1	0	19	2	0	115
Crispy Rounds or Scoops!	140	7	1	0	18	2	0	120
Wild Harvest Organic Yellow Corn Tortilla Chips	140	6	1	0	18	1	0	65
Black Bean Tortilla Chips	140	7	1	0	18	4	0	70
Blue Corn Tortilla Chips	140	6	1	0	18	2	0	100
Xochitl Corn Chips, NS	135	6	1	0	19	2	0	0

FRUIT CHIPS – *Most fruit chips within generic average (2-15mg).*

PITA AND BAGEL CHIPS *(see Crackers, pg 214)*

POTATO AND VEGETABLE CHIPS *(1 oz unless noted)*
There are many low sodium chips, the following have 130mg or less per serving.

	Cal	Fat	Sat	Chol	Carb	Fib	Sug	Sod
Boulder Canyon No Salt Natural Potato Chips	140	7	1	0	17	2	1	0
Reduced Sodium Potato (avg)	140	7	1	0	17	2	1	70
Olive Oil Natural Potato Chips	140	7	1	0	16	0	0	120
Corazonas Slightly Salted Potato Chips	130	6	1	0	18	2	0	90
Spicy Rio Habanero Potato Chips	130	6	1	0	18	2	1	120
Dirty Potato Chips, Unsalted	150	8	2	0	17	1	0	10
Potato Chips, Sea Salted	150	8	2	0	16	1	0	85
Sea Salted Sweet Potato Chips	150	9	1	0	15	2	5	90

	Cal	Fat	Sat	Chol	Carb	Fib	Sug	Sod
Dutch Gourmet Thick Cut Sea Salt Potato	160	11	1	0	14	1	0	50
Thick Cut Honey Dijon Potato Chips	160	10	1	0	15	1	1	65
Thick Cut Szechwan or Slow Cooked Ribs	160	10	1	0	15	1	1	70
Good Health Natural Foods								
Glories Sea Salt Sweet Potato Chips	160	10	1	0	14	2	4	45
Olive Oil Potato Chips Sea Salt	150	8	1	0	16	0	0	65
Olive Oil Potato Chips Garlic	130	6	1	0	17	2	0	70
Olive Oil Potato Chips Cracked Pepper	140	8	1	0	16	1	0	90
Avocado Oil Potato Chips Sea Salt	140	8	2	0	17	1	0	100
Avocado Oil Potato Chips Chilean Lime	140	7	1	0	17	0	0	115
Avocado Oil Potato Chips Barcelona BBQ	140	7	1	0	17	1	1	130
Hawaiian Original, Maui Onion or Luau BBQ (avg)	140	9	3	0	15	1	1	120
Herr's Lightly Salted Potato Chips	140	8	3	0	16	1	0	90
Kettle Brand Unsalted Potato Chips	150	9	1	0	16	2	0	5
Baked Salt & Pepper Potato	120	3	1	0	21	2	0	110
Sea Salt, Krinkle Cut or Organic Sea Salt	150	9	1	0	16	1	0	115
Krunchers! Sweet Hawaiian Onion	140	7	1	0	17	1	2	95
Original	140	7	1	0	17	1	1	105
Lay's Honey Mustard Potato Chips	160	10	1	0	16	1	2	80
Lightly Salted Potato Chips	160	10	1	0	16	1	1	85
Kettle Cooked Original Potato Chips	160	9	1	0	16	1	1	90
Honey Barbecue Potato Chips	160	10	1	0	16	1	2	105
Kettle Cooked Sea Salt & Cracked Pepper	150	9	1	0	16	1	1	110
Kettle Cooked Maui Onion Potato Chips	150	9	1	0	17	1	1	115
Wavy Ranch Potato Chips	160	10	1	0	15	1	1	120
Kettle Cooked Sharp Cheddar or Jalapeno	150	9	1	0	16	1	1	130
Kettle Cooked Spice Rubbed BBQ Potato	140	8	1	0	17	1	2	130
Maui Style Maui Onion Potato Chips	150	9	1	0	17	1	1	115
Michael Season's Thin/Crispy Unsalted Potato	140	7	1	0	17	1	0	10
Ripple, Lightly Salted	140	7	1	0	17	1	0	130
Lightly Salted Thin & Crispy or Mediterranean	140	7	1	0	17	1	0	130
Old Dutch Dutch Crunch Rip-L LS Kettle Chips	150	8	1	0	16	1	0	50
Rip-L LS Potato Chips	150	8	1	0	17	1	0	60
Original Potato Chips	160	10	1	0	15	1	0	130
Dutch Crunch Parmesan/Garlic Kettle Chips	150	9	1	0	15	1	1	130
Pringles 100 Calorie Original	100	6	2	0	13	1	0	110
Ruffles Baked! Original	120	3	0	0	22	2	1	125
Seneca Cinnamon Sweet Potato Chips	150	7	1	0	18	4	8	30
Terra AuNatural Unsalted Potato Chips	120	9	1	0	15	2	0	0
Hickory BBQ Unsalted Potato or Sweets & Beets	150	9	1	0	15	1	0	5
Lemon Pepper Unsalted Potato Chips	150	10	1	0	15	1	0	5
Sweet Potato, NSA	160	11	1	0	15	3	3	10
Crinkles Candied Sweet Potato Chips	160	11	1	0	15	3	3	10
Sweets & Carrots	150	9	1	0	15	5	7	20
Exotic Harvest Sweet Onion	140	6	1	0	18	3	5	40
Original	150	9	1	0	16	3	3	50
Yukon Gold Onion & Garlic	130	5	1	0	19	1	1	65
Red Bliss Olive Oil & Fine Herbs	140	7	1	0	18	3	1	70
Yukon Gold Original	130	5	1	0	19	0	0	80
Red Bliss Sun-Dried Tomato & Vinegar	140	7	1	0	18	3	1	85
Sweet Potato Krinkle Cut Sea Salt	160	11	1	0	15	3	3	90
Kettles Sea Salt	140	7	1	0	18	1	0	100
Stripes & Blues Sea Salt	140	8	1	0	16	2	5	110
Yukon Gold Salt & Vinegar	130	5	1	0	20	2	1	110
Potpourri Potato Chips or Taro Chips (avg)	140	7	1	0	18	4	2	110

SNACK FOODS
Crackers

	Cal	Fat	Sat	Chol	Carb	Fib	Sug	Sod
Red Bliss Made w/Olive Oil	140	7	1	0	18	2	0	110
Terra Stix Original	150	9	1	0	16	3	3	110
Tim's Unsalted Potato Chips	130	6	2	0	18	1	1	0
Original Lightly Salted Potato Chips	140	9	2	0	15	1	0	110
All Natural Sea Salt Potato Chips	130	6	2	0	18	1	1	110
Jalapeno Potato Chips	140	9	2	0	15	1	0	130
Utz NSA or NSA Barbeque Potato Chips	150	9	2	0	14	1	0	5
Kettle Classics Sweet Potato Chips	150	9	2	0	16	2	3	65
Kettle Classics Reduced Fat Potato Chips	130	6	1	0	18	1	0	75
Natural 40% Reduced Fat Potato Chips	130	6	1	0	18	1	0	75
Wavy or Ripple Potato Chips	150	9	2	0	14	1	0	95
Wood Stock Farms Veggie Chips	130	5	0	0	18	2	5	70

OTHER CRUNCHIES AND NIBBLERS *(also see Nuts/Seeds, pg 224)*

	Cal	Fat	Sat	Chol	Carb	Fib	Sug	Sod
A&Js Lasagna Chips Sea Salt	128	5	1	0	17	1	0	62
Lasagna Chips Garlic & Oregano	130	5	1	0	19	1	0	62
Lasagna Chips Barbecue	130	5	1	0	18	1	0	98
Lasagna Chips Tomato Basil	130	5	1	0	18	1	0	139
Barbara's Bakery Cheese Puffs	150	10	2	0	16	0	0	130
Beanfield's Bean & Rice Chips, Naturally Salted	140	6	0	0	18	4	0	5
Bean & Rice Chips Sea Salt	140	6	0	0	18	4	0	140
Burns & Ricker Garlic Bagel Chips	110	0	0	0	22	1	2	30
Party Mix	107	0	0	0	23	1	2	38
Eatsmart Naturals Garden Veggie Sticks	140	6	1	0	20	1	0	120
Genisoy Soy Crisps Apple Cinnamon	120	4	0	0	15	2	3	55
Sweet Crisps Cinnamon Streusel or Choc Mint	90	4	3	0	12	1	6	70
Good Health Natural Foods Humbles								
Baked Hummus Chips, Sesame Garlic	120	4	0	0	17	1	1	135
Lundberg Rice Chips Sesame & Seaweed	140	7	1	0	18	1	0	90
Rice Chips Santa Fe Barbecue or Sea Salt	140	7	1	0	18	1	0	110
New York Style Bagel Chips, Plain	140	6	3	0	17	1	1	70
Bagel Chips, Cinnamon Raisin	130	6	3	0	17	1	7	80
Pita Chips, Maple Cinnamon	130	5	3	0	18	1	2	90
Mini Bagel Chips, Cinnamon Raisin	130	6	3	0	17	1	1	115
Original Tings Crunchy Corn Sticks	150	8	1	0	18	0	0	140
Pirate's Booty Choc Rice & Corn Puffs	140	8	1	0	17	1	5	40
Veggie Rice & Corn Puffs	130	5	1	0	17	1	1	90
NY Pizza Rice & Corn Puffs	130	5	1	0	18	1	1	120
Barrrrrbeque Rice & Corn Puffs	130	5	1	0	19	1	2	135
Aged White Cheddar Rice & Corn Puffs	130	5	1	0	19	0	0	140
Sour Cream & Onion Rice & Corn Puffs	130	5	1	0	18	1	1	140
Shibolim Rice Chips Whole Grain Choc Coated, 2	36	1	1	0	5	0	2	8
Rice Chips Whole Grain, Carob, 2	39	2	1	0	5	0	2	10
Woodstock Farms Sesame Sticks, No Salt	160	11	2	0	13	1	0	0
Rice Cracker Mix	110	0	0	0	24	1	1	120

CRACKERS

	Cal	Fat	Sat	Chol	Carb	Fib	Sug	Sod
Rice crackers, unsalted, 0.5 oz	55	1	0	0	11	1	0	0
Salted, 0.5 oz	55	1	0	0	11	1	0	10
Crispbread, rye, 0.5 oz	52	0	0	0	12	2	0	37
Norweigan flatbread, 0.5 oz	53	0	0	0	12	2	0	38
Melba toast, plain, 0.5 oz	55	0	0	0	11	1	0	118
Whole wheat, 0.5 oz	53	0	0	0	11	1	0	119
Rye, 0.5 oz	55	0	0	0	11	1	0	128
Cheese crackers, 0.5 oz	71	4	1	2	8	0	0	141
Wheat crackers, 0.5 oz	71	3	1	0	10	1	2	142

214

	Cal	Fat	Sat	Chol	Carb	Fib	Sug	Sod
Saltines, 0.5 oz	63	1	0	0	11	0	0	167
Unsalted tops, 0.5 oz	63	1	0	0	11	0	0	109
Oyster crackers, 0.5 oz	63	1	0	0	11	0	0	167
Sandwich w/peanut butter filling, 1 pkg	138	7	1	0	16	1	3	201
w/cheese filling, 1 pkg	134	6	2	1	17	1	1	392

Brands . . . *(0.5 oz unless noted)*
There are many low-sodium crackers, the following have 125mg or less per serving.

	Cal	Fat	Sat	Chol	Carb	Fib	Sug	Sod
Andre's Carbo Save Crackerbread, all, 1 oz	140	8	1	0	8	4	2	120
Aunt Gussie's Cracker Flats								
Spelt Cinnamon Raisin, 0.9 oz	100	2	0	0	19	1	5	40
Spelt Sesame or *Spelt* Garlic, 0.9 oz	60	2	0	0	12	2	0	80
Spelt Everything, 0.9 oz	60	1	0	0	2	1	0	110
Back to Nature Multigrain Flax Flatbread Crackers	130	4	0	0	20	2	2	120
Blue Diamond Nut-Thins Almond, Hint of Salt, 1 oz	130	3	0	0	24	1	0	80
Nut-Thins Almond or Hazelnut, 1 oz	130	3	0	0	23	1	0	115
Bremner LS Wafers	70	2	0	0	12	0	0	10
Original Wafers or Sesame Wafers	70	2	0	0	11	1	0	120
Bisca Organic Water Crackers, Sesame	60	2	0	0	10	0	0	75
Organic Water Crackers, Cracked Pepper	60	1	0	0	11	0	0	80
Organic Water Crackers, Garlic & Herb	60	1	0	0	12	0	0	85
Organic Water Crackers, Original, 0.6 oz	70	1	0	0	13	0	0	95
CaPeachio's Sesame Crackers	70	2	0	0	11	0	0	70
Original or Peppercorn & Poppy Crackers	60	1	0	0	12	0	0	75
Garlic & Herb Crackers	60	1	0	0	12	0	0	110
Carr's Water Crackers, Toasted Sesame, 0.6 oz	70	2	1	0	12	1	0	100
Water Crackers, Plain or Cracked Pepper	70	2	1	0	13	1	0	100
Water Crackers, Whole Wheat, 0.6 oz	80	4	2	0	11	1	3	100
Entertainment Collection, 0.6 oz	80	3	2	0	12	1	1	110
Water Crackers, Roasted Garlic/Herbs, 0.6 oz	70	2	1	0	13	1	0	120
Dare All Natural Water Crackers, Cracked Pepper	60	1	0	0	12	0	0	45
All Natural Water Crackers, Toasted Sesame	70	2	0	0	11	0	0	45
All Natural Water Crackers, Original	60	1	0	0	12	0	0	50
Cabaret Crackers	70	4	1	0	9	0	1	65
Breton Minis, Garden Vegetable	80	4	1	0	10	1	1	100
Bremner Wafers	70	2	0	0	11	0	0	105
Breton Original or Sesame Crackers (avg)	65	4	2	0	8	1	2	110
Vinta Original Crackers or Squares	70	3	1	0	8	1	0	120
Vivant Crackers	60	3	2	0	9	0	2	120
Deli-catessen Rosemary Snack Sticks	70	1	0	0	10	1	2	110
Sweet Peppers w/Basil Crackers	70	3	1	0	10	1	1	115
Wheat Extraordinaire Crackers	70	3	1	0	10	1	1	120
Eating Right Whole Grain Water Crackers, 1.3 oz	60	1	0	0	12	1	0	85
Multigrain & Flax Water Crackers, 0.9 oz	60	1	0	0	12	1	0	85
Ener-G Cinnamon Crackers, 1 oz	70	5	0	0	12	5	3	85
Foods Alive Maple & Cinnamon Flax, 1 oz	150	8	1	0	12	8	4	15
Foods Alive Hemp Flax Crackers, 1 oz	150	9	1	0	10	8	2	65
Kashi Heart to Heart Roasted Garlic, 1 oz	120	4	0	0	22	4	0	75
Heart to Heart Whole Wheat, 1 oz	120	4	0	0	22	4	0	85
Kedem Whole Wheat Crackers, Garlic & Dill	52	2	0	0	9	1	0	70
Sesame Seed	56	2	0	0	8	2	0	70
Whole Wheat Crackers, Plain	60	2	1	0	10	1	0	80
Mariner Biscuit, all crackers except Cheddar	60	2	0	0	10	0	0	45
Medford Farms Stone Ground Less Salt	60	2	0	0	11	1	0	75
Milton's Crispy Sea Salt	70	3	2	0	10	0	0	90

215

SNACK FOODS
Crackers

	Cal	Fat	Sat	Chol	Carb	Fib	Sug	Sod
Everything Multi-Grain	70	0	0	0	10	1	1	100
Roasted Garlic or Whole Wheat Multi-Grain	70	0	0	0	10	1	1	100
Original Multi-Grain	70	3	0	0	10	0	1	105
Nabisco Ritz Crackers, Hint of Salt	80	4	1	0	10	0	1	35
Ritz Brown Sugar	80	4	1	0	11	0	2	65
Triscuits Hint of Salt, 1 oz	130	5	1	0	19	3	0	50
Wheat Thins Hint of Salt, 1 oz	150	5	1	0	23	2	4	60
Ritz Whole Wheat, 0.5 oz	70	3	1	0	11	1	1	120
Triscuits Garden Herb	120	4	1	0	20	3	0	125
Wheat Thins Flatbread Garlic & Parsley	60	2	0	0	12	1	2	125
Wheat Thins Flatbread Tuscan Herb	60	2	0	0	12	1	2	125
Nejaimes Lavasch Flatbread Cracker, all	60	2	0	0	10	1	1	65
Partners Parmesan & Herb	60	2	1	0	8	0	1	95
Olive Oil & Sea Salt	50	2	0	0	8	0	1	110
Roasted Garlic & Rosemary	60	1	0	0	10	0	2	110
Asiago & Black Pepper	50	2	0	0	8	0	1	115
All Natural Sweet Onion	120	4	2	10	16	1	3	120
Sun-Dried Tomato & Herb	70	3	2	5	11	1	2	125
Pepperidge Farm Entertaining Quartet, 4	70	3	1	5	10	1	1	95
Golden Butter, 4	70	3	1	5	11	0	1	100
Entertaining Trio, 4	70	3	1	5	11	1	1	110
Harvest Wheat, 3	80	4	1	0	11	1	2	125
Red Oval Farms								
Stoned Wheat Thins Lower Sodium	60	2	1	0	10	1	0	70
Roland Cracked Pepper Water Crackers	60	2	0	0	10	0	0	65
Toasted Sesame or Garlic/Herb Water Crackers	60	1	0	0	11	0	0	65
Whole Wheat Water Crackers	60	2	0	0	9	1	0	105
Country Style Natural Butter Water Crackers	70	2	0	0	9	0	1	110
Shibolim *Crisp Snax* Spelt Original	80	1	0	0	11	2	0	55
Knockers Spelt or Whole Wheat, Unsalted	53	1	0	0	11	2	0	7
Knockers Whole Wheat Sesame	54	2	0	0	10	2	0	45
Crisp Snax Spelt Sesame	60	1	0	0	11	2	0	55
Crisp Snax Wh Wheat Onion, or Garlic	50	0	0	0	11	2	0	55
Crisp Cracker Spelt or Wheat	90	0	0	0	19	2	0	115
Venus Cracked Pepper or Garden Vegetable	60	0	0	0	12	0	1	80
Garlic & Herb	60	0	0	0	12	0	1	90
Multi Grain	60	0	0	0	12	0	1	100
Wegmans Water Crackers, Toasted Sesame	60	2	0	0	12	1	0	75
Water Crackers, Classic	60	1	0	0	12	1	0	80
Water Crackers, Cracked Pepper/Poppy Seed	60	1	0	0	12	1	0	80
Stone Ground Wheat, Reduced Sodium	60	1	0	0	11	1	0	80
Classic Entertainment Crackers	70	3	1	0	10	0	1	90
Vegetable Crackers	70	3	0	0	10	1	1	100
Wheat Entertainment Crackers	70	3	1	0	10	1	1	120
Wellington Toasted Sesame Water Crackers	60	2	0	0	12	0	0	40
Plain or Cracked Pepper Water Crackers	60	1	0	0	12	0	0	40
Garlic & Herb	60	1	0	0	12	0	0	110
Wild Harvest Organic Pepper Water Crackers	70	1	0	0	14	1	0	80
Original Water Crackers	70	0	0	0	14	1	0	85

BAGEL AND PITA CHIPS

	Cal	Fat	Sat	Chol	Carb	Fib	Sug	Sod
New York Style *Bagel Crisps* Plain, 1 oz	140	6	3	0	17	1	1	70
Bagel Crisps Cinnamon Raisin, 1 oz	130	5	3	0	19	0	7	85
Sami's Bakery Millet & Flax, 1 oz	66	2	0	0	11	8	0	90
Millet & Flax, Cinnamon, 1 oz	87	3	0	0	12	8	1	90
Stacy's Pita Chips, Cinnamon Sugar	140	5	1	0	20	1	6	115

216

	Cal	Fat	Sat	Chol	Carb	Fib	Sug	Sod

GRAHAM CRACKERS *(see Graham/Other Sweet Crackers, pg 223)*

MATZOS *(see Matzos, pg 224)*

MELBA AND CRISP TOAST

	Cal	Fat	Sat	Chol	Carb	Fib	Sug	Sod
Alessi Crispy Sliced Toasts, Whole Wheat	70	0	0	0	13	1	1	70
Crispy Sliced Toasts, Regular	50	0	0	0	8	0	1	70
Devonsheer Unsalted Melba Toast	60	0	0	0	13	1	0	0
Melba Rounds, Onion	50	0	0	0	11	1	0	95
Melba Toast, Rye or Whole Wheat	60	0	0	0	13	1	0	100
Melba Toast, Plain	60	0	0	0	13	1	0	115
Melba Rounds, Sesame	60	2	1	0	10	1	0	125
Grille' Toast No Sodium	70	1	0	0	14	1	1	4
Plain or Whole Wheat	70	1	0	0	14	1	1	90
Kavli 5 Grain	40	0	0	0	9	2	0	30
Crispy Thin	50	0	0	0	11	2	1	45
Hearty Thick	70	1	0	0	15	3	0	55
Golden Rye	60	1	0	0	12	7	1	70
Garlic	50	1	0	0	10	2	1	115
New York Style *Panetini* Original	70	4	2	0	9	1	0	75
Old London *Melba Toast* Unsalted Whole Grain	60	0	0	0	12	2	0	0
Melba Toast Sourdough	60	0	0	0	12	1	0	105
Melba Toast Classic or *Melba Snacks* Classic	60	0	0	0	13	1	0	110
Melba Toast Rosemary & Olive Oil or Rye	60	1	0	0	12	1	0	110
Ry-Krisp FF Natural or Light Rye	50	0	0	0	11	3	0	65
Sesame	60	2	0	0	10	3	0	80
FF Seasoned	60	2	0	0	10	3	0	90
Shibolim Crisp Bread, Spelt or Whole Wheat (avg)	95	1	0	0	19	4	0	0
Wasa Sourdough	35	0	0	0	9	2	0	45
Whole Grain	40	0	0	0	10	2	0	50
Fiber	35	1	0	0	8	2	0	60
Whole Wheat, Light Rye, or Hearty (avg)	50	0	0	0	11	2	1	70
Multi Grain	45	0	0	0	10	2	0	80
Sesame	60	2	0	0	9	1	0	85
Crisp'n Light, 7 Grain	60	0	0	0	13	2	1	95
Crisp'n Light, Mild Rye	80	0	0	0	16	2	1	120

RICE CRACKERS AND OTHER THINS

Unsalted rice crackers – *Most brands within generic average (0mg).*

Salted rice crackers – *Most brands within generic average (10mg), however, some brands have up to 200mg sodium.*

	Cal	Fat	Sat	Chol	Carb	Fib	Sug	Sod
Blue Diamond *Nut-Thins* Almond or Hazelnut	130	3	0	0	23	1	0	115
New York Style *Risotto Chips* Sea Salt, 1 oz	140	7	1	0	19	2	1	110
Risotto Chips Parmesan/Roasted Garlic, 1 oz	140	7	1	0	19	2	1	120

SALTINES, OYSTER AND SOUP CRACKERS

	Cal	Fat	Sat	Chol	Carb	Fib	Sug	Sod
Barbara's Bakery Wheatines Original	60	1	0	0	11	1	1	80
Bremner Soup & Chili Crackers	60	2	0	0	11	0	0	110
Jacob's Cream Crackers	70	2	0	0	11	1	0	80
Nabisco *Premium* Saltines Hint of Salt	70	2	0	0	11	0	0	30
Premium Saltines Unsalted Tops	70	2	0	0	13	0	0	75
Wegmans Saltines Unsalted Tops	70	2	1	0	11	0	0	125

SANDWICH CRACKERS – *Most brands within generic average (201-392mg).*

DIET, ENERGY AND SNACK BARS

(also see Granola/Cereal/Breakfast Bars, pg 69)

	Cal	Fat	Sat	Chol	Carb	Fib	Sug	Sod
Diet meal bar, milk choc peanut, 2 oz	212	5	3	4	33	3	14	140
Power/energy bar, 2 oz	212	6	3	2	28	4	16	215

SNACK FOODS
Diet, Energy and Snack Bars

	Cal	Fat	Sat	Chol	Carb	Fib	Sug	Sod
Brands . . .								
There are many low-sodium brands, the following have 110mg or less per serving.								
Atkins *Advantage*								
Dark Choc Almond Coconut Crunch,1.4 oz	190	15	7	0	16	8	1	35
Endulge Peanut Caramel Cluster, 1.2 oz	140	9	3	5	12	5	1	50
Endulge Caramel Nut Chew, 1.2 oz	130	8	4	5	17	6	1	70
Endulge Choc Coconut, 1.4 oz	170	12	10	0	19	9	1	65
Endulge Choc Caramel, 1.2 oz	120	5	4	0	23	9	1	85
Endulge Nutty Fudge Brownie, 1.4 oz	170	12	6	0	18	6	0	90
Advantage Coconut Almond Delight, 1.6 oz	200	16	11	0	18	6	1	90
Day Break Choc Hazelnut, 1.4 oz	180	14	4	0	18	7	1	95
Day Break Cranberry Almond, 1.2 oz	140	5	3	0	16	5	1	100
Endulge Peanut Butter Cups, 1.2 oz	160	13	7	5	18	5	0	105
Day Break Cinnamon Bun, 1.4 oz	160	8	5	0	18	5	1	105
Day Break Cherry Pecan, 1.2 oz	160	11	2	0	15	4	3	110
Day Break Choc Oatmeal, 1.4 oz	130	5	2	0	24	10	1	110
Attune *Probiotic Wellness Bar* Dark Choc, 0.7 oz	80	6	4	0	11	3	6	0
Mint Choc or Almond Milk Choc, 0.7 oz (avg)	100	7	4	0	12	3	8	10
Probiotic Wellness Bar Choc Crisp, 0.7 oz	90	6	4	0	12	3	8	20
Candice Foods Protein Bars, all, 2 oz (avg)	225	10	2	0	30	5	12	15
Clif Blueberry or Cherry Pomegranate, 1.4 oz	130	5	0	0	26	4	17	10
Apple or Raspberry, 1.4 oz	130	5	0	0	25	4	17	15
Crunch Choc Chip, 1.5 oz	180	8	1	0	27	3	11	100
Crunch Blueberry Crisp, 1.5 oz	180	9	2	0	26	3	11	105
Crunch Honey Oat, 1.5 oz	180	8	1	0	28	3	11	110
Divine Foods *Boomi Bar* Almond Protein Plus	270	7	1	15	20	4	15	12
Boomi Bar Cashew Protein Plus, 1.7 oz	250	15	3	15	20	2	16	20
Boomi Bar Walnut Date, 1.7 oz	200	9	1	0	27	2	18	20
Boomi Bar Macadamia Paradise, 1.7 oz	240	12	3	0	25	3	12	25
Boomi Bar Maple Pecan, 1.7 oz	200	11	1	0	28	3	20	30
Boomi Bar Healthy Hazel, 1.7 oz	230	13	1	0	23	1	4	40
Boomi Bar Perfect Pumpkin, 1.7 oz	230	9	2	0	23	1	3	45
Boomi Bar Cranberry Apple, 1.7 oz	210	9	1	0	28	4	18	50
Boomi Bar Pistachio Pineapple, 1.7 oz	200	9	2	0	28	3	17	50
Boomi Bar Cashew Almond, 1.7 oz	260	14	2	0	23	1	3	55
Boomi Bar Fruit & Nut, 1.7 oz	210	9	1	0	27	3	13	55
Boomi Bar Pineapple Ginger, 1.7 oz	200	8	1	0	29	3	16	70
Boomi Bar Apricot Cashew, 1.7 oz	190	7	1	0	28	3	13	75
Dixie Diner *Soy Rocks* Crunchy Choc, 1.1 oz	113	4	2	0	13	4	3	3
Soy Rocks Crunchy Apple, 1.1 oz	90	3	1	0	15	12	3	3
Soy Rocks Caramel Choc, 1.1 oz	104	5	3	1	12	8	2	42
Sticky Bar, Banana/Pecan/Flax, 1.1 oz	149	13	3	1	11	7	1	45
Ener-G Choc Chip Snack Bars, 1.5 oz	160	6	4	0	31	4	14	15
Fi-Bar, 1.2 oz (avg)	120	2	1	0	26	3	12	25
Glucerna *Mini Snack Bars* Oatmeal Raisin, 0.7 oz	70	2	1	0	12	1	5	30
Mini Snack Bars Choc Peanut, 0.7 oz	80	3	1	0	12	1	4	60
Meal Bars Choc Chunk, 2 oz	210	6	5	0	34	4	10	85
Kind Almond Cashew w/Flax + Omega-3, 1.4 oz	180	10	2	0	20	4	13	0
Almond & Coconut, 1.4 oz	210	13	6	0	19	4	10	10
Fruit & Nut Delight or Almond & Apricot (avg)	185	11	4	0	21	5	12	15
Cranberry Almond + Antioxidants, 1.4 oz	190	13	2	0	20	3	12	20
Dark Choc Cherry Cashew + Antioxidants	180	9	3	0	22	3	14	20
Pomegranate Blueberry Pistachio + Antioxidants	170	8	1	0	24	4	13	25
Blueberry Pecan + Fiber, 1.4 oz	180	10	1	0	23	5	12	25
Apple Cinnamon & Pecan, 1.4 oz	180	10	1	0	23	3	13	25

	Cal	Fat	Sat	Chol	Carb	Fib	Sug	Sod
Peanut Butter & Strawberry, 1.4 oz	190	11	2	0	18	4	10	30
Peanut Butter Dark Choc + Protein	200	13	4	0	17	3	10	50
Almond Walnut Macadamia + Protein	190	12	2	0	15	3	8	75
Ian's Go Bars Cinnamon Bun, 1 oz	100	2	1	0	21	1	7	45
Go Bars Apple Pie, 1 oz	100	2	1	0	19	1	9	60
Larabar Tropical Fruit Tart, 1.6 oz	210	12	7	0	25	5	19	0
Cinnamon Roll or Choc Coconut Chew (avg)	240	13	2	0	30	5	23	0
Cherry Pie, 1.7 oz	200	8	1	0	30	5	23	0
Cashew Cookie or Banana Bread, 1.7 oz (avg)	230	12	3	0	26	5	19	0
Pecan Pie, 1.6 oz	220	14	1	0	24	4	18	0
Lemon Bar or Key Lime Pie, 1.8 oz (avg)	220	11	3	0	30	4	23	0
Ginger Snap, 1.8 oz	240	14	1	0	27	6	20	0
Coconut Cream Pie, 1.8 oz	220	11	7	0	31	6	24	5
Jocalat Choc Hazelnut or Choc, 1.7 oz	200	10	2	0	27	5	21	0
Jocalat Choc Mint, 1.7 oz	190	9	2	0	26	5	20	0
Jocalat Choc Coffee, 1.7 oz	210	11	2	0	27	5	21	0
Apple Pie, 1.6 oz	190	10	1	0	24	5	18	10
Peanut Butter Cookie, 1.7 oz	220	12	2	0	23	4	18	45
Peanut Butter & Jelly, 1.7 oz	210	10	2	0	27	4	19	60
Luna Caramel Nut Brownie, 1.7 oz	180	6	3	0	27	3	12	110
Nature's Path Optimum Energy Bar								
Blueberry, Flax & Soy, 2 oz	200	3	0	0	38	5	20	100
Orange Choc, 2 oz	220	6	2	0	37	4	19	120
Nature Valley Nut Clusters Nut Lovers	150	9	1	0	14	1	6	100
Nut Clusters Nut Lovers	140	7	1	0	16	2	7	125
New England Naturals Organic								
Antioxidant Bar or Choc Omega Bar	140	4	0	0	25	2	11	0
Maple Nut Bar	120	2	0	0	27	6	8	5
Nutiva Flax-Raisin, 1.4 oz	200	15	2	0	15	4	8	0
Flax-Choc, 1.4 oz	200	12	2	0	19	5	10	5
Hempseed, 1.4 oz	210	14	2	0	11	5	5	5
Odwalla Chewy Nut Sweet/Salty Almond, 1.6 oz	220	11	1	0	22	6	8	65
Original Choco-wallo, 2 oz	210	5	2	0	39	5	16	75
Original Super Food, 2 oz	200	4	2	0	39	3	18	85
Original Mocha-walla, 2 oz	210	4	2	0	38	3	15	90
Chewy Nut Choc Chip Trail Mix, 1.6 oz	200	7	2	0	28	2	15	90
Original Strawberry Pomegranate, 2 oz	200	2	0	0	42	3	18	95
Original Banana Nut, 2 oz	220	5	1	0	39	5	17	105
Omega Smart most, 2.3 oz (avg)	220	9	0	0	33	6	25	0
Power Bar Iron Girl Strawberry & Cranberry	160	3	2	0	29	2	10	50
Pria French Vanilla Crisp	110	3	3	0	17	1	9	80
Pria Choc Peanut Crunch	110	4	2	0	16	1	10	85
Iron Girl Cocoa Crunch	160	4	2	0	28	2	8	85
Pure & Simple Energy Cranberry Oatmeal Cookie	130	3	1	0	23	2	10	90
Pure & Simple Energy Roasted Peanut Butter	140	4	1	0	22	2	10	90
Pria Mint Choc Chip	110	4	3	0	15	1	9	90
Pria Double Choc Cookie	110	3	3	0	16	1	10	100
PrānaBar Apricot Goji or Cashew Almond (avg)	220	14	2	0	24	3	15	30
Apricot Pumpkin, 1.7 oz	190	11	2	0	23	2	16	30
Pear Ginseng, 1.7 oz	220	15	2	0	21	4	12	30
Coconut Acai, 1.7 oz	220	13	2	0	26	3	18	35
Supercharger Blueberry Coconut, 1.7 oz	210	11	6	0	26	4	18	70
Supercharger Goldenberry Goji, 1.7 oz	180	7	3	0	29	3	22	75
Supercharger Raspberry Pomegranate, 1.7 oz	200	9	4	0	29	5	21	75
Apple Pie, 1.7 oz	230	12	1	0	28	4	11	85

219

SNACK FOODS
Dips and Spreads

	Cal	Fat	Sat	Chol	Carb	Fib	Sug	Sod
Supercharger Mango Maca, 1.7 oz	230	15	6	0	23	3	17	90
Pure Protein Choc Deluxe	180	5	3	15	17	2	2	115
Raw Indulgence								
Raw Revolution 100 Calorie bars, all (avg)	100	6	1	0	10	1	6	3
Raw Revolution 1.6 oz bar, all (avg)	170	7	2	0	25	4	18	5
Raw Revolution 2.2 oz bar, all (avg)	280	16	3	0	30	4	19	5
Slim Fast Choc Nougat Gone Nuts, 0.8 oz	100	5	3	0	14	1	7	55
Choc Mint, 0.8 oz	100	4	3	0	16	3	7	65
Chocolatey Vanilla Blitz, 0.9 oz	100	3	2	0	17	1	6	70
Peanut Butter Crunch Time, 0.8 oz	100	4	2	0	16	0	13	70
Double-Dutch Choc, 0.8 oz	100	4	3	0	16	2	7	80
Choc Cookie Doug, 1.9 oz	200	4	3	5	32	5	13	110
Choc Fudge Brownie, 1.9 oz	200	4	3	5	32	5	13	110
SoyJoy Pineapple, 1 oz	140	6	3	20	17	3	12	40
Mango Coconut, 1 oz	140	6	4	20	16	3	11	45
Strawberry or Blueberry, 1 oz (avg)	135	6	3	20	17	4	12	45
Apple Walnut or Banana, 1 oz (avg)	140	6	3	20	16	3	10	50
Berry, 1 oz	130	5	2	15	17	3	12	50
Supreme Protein Cookies 'n Cream 1.6 oz	180	7	5	5	15	1	4	70
Rocky Road Brownie, 1.8 oz	210	9	6	5	16	1	3	70
Peanut Butter & Jelly, 1.8 oz	200	8	5	8	18	1	5	95
Peanut Butter Pretzel Twist, 1.8 oz	210	9	6	5	17	1	3	100
Tigers Milk Protein Rich, 1.3 oz	140	5	3	0	18	1	13	60
Peanut Butter Crunch, 1.3 oz	150	6	2	0	19	1	13	75
Peanut Butter or Peanut Butter & Honey, 1.3 oz	150	6	2	0	18	1	13	80

(DIPS AND SPREADS)

(also see Chutney/Relish/Other Accompaniments, pg 75; Vegetable Spreads, pg 95; Sauces/Toppings/Fruit Dips, pg 133; Salsa/Taco Sauce, pg 164)

	Cal	Fat	Sat	Chol	Carb	Fib	Sug	Sod
Guacamole, 2 tbsp	60	5	1	0	3	0	2	140
Hummus, 2 tbsp	70	4	0	0	6	2	1	150
Bean, 2 tbsp	40	1	0	0	5	1	0	170
French onion dip, refrigerated, 2 tbsp	60	5	3	20	2	0	1	180
Creamy herbal, refrigerated, 2 tbsp	100	9	2	5	2	1	1	190
Spinach dip, refrigerated, 2 tbsp	60	5	2	5	3	0	1	240
Ranch dip, mix, 1 tsp	5	0	0	0	1	0	0	210
Cheese, 2 tbsp	60	4	2	5	3	0	0	330
Onion soup and dip, mix, 1 tsp	200	0	0	0	4	0	0	700

Brands . . . *(2 tbsp unless noted)*

REFRIGERATED

	Cal	Fat	Sat	Chol	Carb	Fib	Sug	Sod
Arriba! 3 Bean Dip	30	0	0	0	5	0	0	100
Chipotle con Queso Dip	30	2	0	0	3	0	0	135
Salsa con Queso Dip	15	0	0	0	3	0	0	135
Bison Creamy Dill Dip	50	5	3	15	2	0	1	130
Cabot Dip Salsa Grande Sour Cream Dips	50	5	3	15	1	0	0	130
Dip Ranch or Garden Veggie	50	5	3	15	1	0	1	140
Cedarlane 5 Layer Mexican Dip	60	3	2	10	4	1	2	100
De LA Casa 5 Layer Dip	45	3	2	0	4	1	1	110
Don Loco Spicy Guacamole Dip	60	5	1	0	3	2	0	75
Guacamole Dip	60	5	1	0	3	2	0	80
Emerald Valley 3 Bean Dip	35	0	0	0	6	2	1	140
Marie's Creamy Dill Dip	100	10	3	15	2	0	1	140
Guacamole	40	3	2	5	3	1	1	140
Opaa! Cucumber Yogurt Sauce	35	3	2	10	1	0	1	50

220

	Cal	Fat	Sat	Chol	Carb	Fib	Sug	Sod
Sabra Caponata	55	5	1	0	2	1	0	65
Vegetarian Liver	70	6	0	30	2	0	1	70
Ratatouille	35	3	0	0	2	0	1	80
Classic Babaganoush	80	8	1	5	3	2	0	135
TGI Friday's Spinach, Cheese/Artichoke Dip	45	4	2	10	2	0	0	115
Wild Garden Hummus Dip, Red Pepper	35	2	0	0	4	1	1	70

MIXES

Many mixes require additional ingredients which may raise sodium content.

	Cal	Fat	Sat	Chol	Carb	Fib	Sug	Sod
Cook in the Kitchen Boursen Cheese Dip	0	0	0	0	1	0	0	0
Horseradish Dip	0	0	0	0	0	0	0	35
Cheesy Garlic Dip	0	0	0	0	0	0	0	50
Sweet Onion Dip	0	0	0	0	0	0	0	75
Goodman's Onion Soup & Dip Mix LS	30	1	0	0	6	1	3	115
Julia's Pantry *Sassy Dip & Seasoning*								
Sweet Onion or Roasted Garlic (avg)	7	0	0	0	2	0	1	41
Sweet & Spicy, Havanero, or Jalapeno	6	0	0	0	2	0	1	72
Chipotle, Original, or Ghost Pepper	6	0	0	0	2	0	1	72
Laurie's Kitchen Sesame Garlic Dip Mix	10	0	0	0	1	0	0	35
Roasted Pepper Dip Mix	5	0	0	0	1	0	0	40
Chipotle Chile Dip Mix	5	0	0	0	1	0	0	45
Bacon Cheddar Dip Mix	5	0	0	0	1	0	0	55
White Cheddar Merlot Dip Mix	10	0	0	0	1	0	0	110
Sundried Tomato Pesto Dip Mix	5	0	0	0	1	0	0	125
Spinach Artichoke Dip Mix	5	0	0	0	1	0	1	130
Lays *Dip Creations* Onion or Country Ranch	5	0	0	0	1	0	0	140
McCormick Vegetable Dip Mix	5	0	0	0	1	0	0	130
French Onion Dip Mix	5	0	0	0	1	0	0	140
Pantry Blends Dip Mix Chipotle Bacon or BLT	5	0	0	0	1	0	0	10
Cool Ranch Salsa	5	0	0	0	1	0	0	45
Crab Dip	5	0	0	0	1	0	0	55
Country Spinach	5	0	0	0	1	0	0	70
Rabbit Creek Roasted Garlic Red Pepper	0	0	0	0	0	0	0	0
Sweet Bell Peppers w/a Hint of Jalapeno	10	0	0	0	3	0	2	0
Buffalo Wing or Git Up & Go Garlic	0	0	0	0	1	0	0	0
Bleu Cheese, Blood Mary, Crab, or Lobster	3	0	0	0	1	0	0	0
Caramelized Onion w/Horseradish	5	0	0	0	1	0	1	0
Guacamole, Garlic Onion, or Mexican Dip	2	0	0	0	1	0	0	2
Country Herb or Fiery Smoked Chipotle (avg)	4	0	0	0	1	0	0	18
Smokin' Pig	5	0	0	0	1	1	0	30
Bacon! Bacon! Who's Got the Bacon?	5	0	0	0	1	0	1	35
Creamy Spinach w/Roasted Garlic or Spinach	5	0	0	0	1	0	0	45
Dilly Cucumber or Dilly Ranch	1	0	0	0	0	0	0	46
Cheesy Onion Veg or BLT (avg)	4	0	0	0	1	0	1	48
Pigs in the Spinach Patch	10	0	0	0	1	0	1	50
Sun Dried Tomato w/Herb	0	0	0	0	0	0	0	50
Cheesy Bacon	6	0	0	0	1	0	0	54
Jalapeno Bacon Cheddar or Parmesan Dill (avg)	5	0	0	0	1	0	0	55
Zesty Bacon w/Cheese	10	0	0	0	1	1	0	55
Smoky Horseradish	7	0	0	0	1	1	0	65
Blooming Onion or Cheesy Country Veg	5	0	0	0	1	0	0	90
Cracked Pepper Ranch or Spicy Ranch	0	0	0	0	1	0	0	90
Garlicky Veg	9	0	0	0	1	0	0	104
This Little Piggy Loves Garlic Veg Dip	5	0	0	0	1	1	0	130
Garden Fest Dip Mix	10	0	0	0	1	0	1	130
Simply Organic Creamy Dill or Guacamole	5	0	0	0	1	0	0	95

SNACK FOODS
Dips and Spreads

	Cal	Fat	Sat	Chol	Carb	Fib	Sug	Sod
French Onion	5	0	0	0	2	0	1	130
Stonewall Kitchen Artichoke Spinach Dip Mix	5	0	0	0	1	0	0	120
Curry Dip Mix	5	0	0	0	1	0	0	125
Vegetable Dip Mix	5	0	0	0	1	0	0	140
Tostitos *Dip Creations* Guacamole Seasoning	5	0	0	0	1	0	0	120
Wise Green Onion Dip Mix	5	0	0	0	1	0	1	140
SHELF-STABLE								
Desert Pepper Tuscan White Bean	30	1	0	0	5	1	1	45
El Paso Chili Co. Bean Dips (avg)	25	0	0	0	5	2	1	20
Guiltless Gourmet Mild or Spicy Black Bean	40	0	0	0	7	2	0	125
Island Grove Oriental Sweet Heat	25	0	0	0	5	0	5	95
Key Lime Honey Ginger	125	10	1	0	9	0	8	90
Florida Keys' Key Lime Pepper	50	3	0	0	8	0	8	130
Florida Orange Poppy	55	3	0	0	7	0	6	132
Key Lime Honey Mustard	150	10	2	10	7	0	7	140
Roads End Organics Nacho Cheese, Mild or Spicy	20	0	0	0	3	1	0	110
Robert Rothschild Farm								
Roasted Pineapple & Habanero Dip	60	0	0	0	14	0	14	0
Spice Maple Pumpkin Dip, 2 tbsp	40	0	0	0	10	1	7	0
Roasted Red Pepper & Onion Dip, 1 tbsp	20	0	0	0	5	0	5	15
Red Pepper Dip	80	7	4	20	5	0	5	85
Mediterranean Dip	70	7	3	5	2	0	1	110
Blue Cheese & Chive Dip	70	7	4	5	1	0	0	135
Stonewall Kitchen Honey Mustard Dip, 1 tsp	15	0	0	0	3	0	3	25
Maple Mustard Dip, 1 tsp	20	1	0	0	3	0	3	25
Orange Ginger Mustard Dip, 1 tsp	15	0	0	0	3	0	2	35
Black Bean Dip	35	2	0	0	4	1	0	105
White Bean Dip	40	2	0	0	5	2	0	140

HUMMUS

Most brands are low sodium, the following have 120mg or less sodium per serving.

	Cal	Fat	Sat	Chol	Carb	Fib	Sug	Sod
FROZEN/REFRIGERATED								
Eat Well Enjoy Life Edamame Hummus	80	7	1	0	2	1	0	85
Emerald Valley Roasted Red Pepper Hummus	60	4	0	0	4	0	0	100
Traditional Hummus	60	4	0	0	5	0	0	110
Marzetti Hummus, Original or Roasted Garlic	70	6	1	0	4	1	0	110
Roasted Garlic Hummus	70	6	1	0	4	1	0	110
Nasoya Super Hummus, Original or Spinach	50	3	0	0	2	1	1	120
Sabra Classic or Roasted Garlic Hummus	70	6	1	0	4	1	0	120
Roasted Red Pepper or Luscious Lemon	70	6	1	0	3	1	0	120
Sun Dried Tomato or Spinach & Artichoke	70	9	2	0	4	2	0	120
Tahini Hummus	80	6	1	0	4	4	0	120
Sonny & Joe's Tehini Dip	60	5	1	0	3	1	0	85
Turkish Dip	25	2	0	0	3	1	1	95
Hummus	80	5	1	0	6	1	1	100
Garlic Addition Hummus	70	5	1	0	5	1	0	100
Hummus Pinoli or Just Hummus	80	6	1	0	4	1	0	115
Hot Enough Hummus?	70	6	1	0	4	1	1	120
Summer Fresh Roasted Garlic Hummus	60	4	0	0	6	2	0	115
Wildwood *Probiotic Hummus* Red Pepper	60	5	0	0	3	1	1	80
Probiotic Hummus LF Classic	45	3	0	0	4	1	1	85
Probiotic Hummus Classic or Spicy Cayenne	70	5	1	0	3	1	1	95
SHELF-STABLE								
Al Wadi Hommos Tahina	40	2	1	0	4	1	0	90
Robt Rothschild Farm Roasted Garlic	60	4	0	0	5	1	1	60
Jalapeno Hummus	50	4	0	0	5	1	0	90

	Cal	Fat	Sat	Chol	Carb	Fib	Sug	Sod
Roasted Eggplant & Pepper Hummus	50	2	0	0	6	1	0	110
Wild Garden Hummus Dip, all	35	2	0	0	4	1	0	70

BREAD DIP SEASONINGS

	Cal	Fat	Sat	Chol	Carb	Fib	Sug	Sod
Rabbit Creek Gourmet Pesto	5	0	0	0	3	0	0	1
Cheesy Roasted Tomato	26	1	1	5	0	1	0	6
Cheesy Pesto	31	1	1	5	2	1	0	50
Sun-Dried Tomato	21	0	0	0	5	0	0	50

CHEESE BALL SEASONINGS

	Cal	Fat	Sat	Chol	Carb	Fib	Sug	Sod
Cedar Hill Seasonings Mexican	70	1	0	0	17	0	4	30
Cravings Hors D'oeuvre Mix								
Wine & Cheese Cheeseball	28	0	0	1	6	0	3	22
Bacon & Scallion Cheeseball	18	1	0	0	3	0	2	35
Hors D'oeuvre Mix Spinach Artichoke	19	0	0	0	4	0	1	69
Rabbit Creek Gourmet Toffee Crunch	16	0	0	0	4	0	4	0
Cinnamon Apple or Luscious Raspberry	10	0	0	0	3	0	3	0
Raspberries & Red Zinfandel	10	0	0	0	3	0	3	0
Crab Rangoon	3	0	0	0	1	0	0	0
Cranberry Pecan	19	1	0	0	4	1	3	0
Sweet Pepper	120	0	0	0	3	0	5	0
White Choc Raspberry	30	1	1	0	7	0	5	3
Fall Harvest or Pumpkin Pie Spice	23	1	0	0	5	0	3	4
Key Lime	26	0	0	0	6	0	5	4
White Choc & Raspberries Wine	310	1	0	0	7	0	5	5
Herbs w/Chardonnay Wine	5	0	0	0	1	0	0	24
Menage A Trois of Berries	10	0	0	0	2	1	1	30
Bacon Onion	3	0	0	0	0	0	0	33
Savory Herb	4	0	0	0	1	0	2	35
Spinach Delight	6	0	0	0	0	0	0	43
Dill of a Ranch	2	0	0	0	0	0	0	46

GRAHAM AND OTHER SWEET CRACKERS

	Cal	Fat	Sat	Chol	Carb	Fib	Sug	Sod
Graham crackers, 1 oz	120	3	0	0	22	1	9	172
Chocolate graham crackers, 1 oz	137	7	4	0	19	1	12	82
Brands . . . *(1 oz unless noted)*								
Annie's Homegrown Choc Bunny Grahams	130	5	0	0	21	2	9	75
Choc Chip Bunny Grahams	130	5	0	0	21	1	7	95
Bunny Graham Friends	130	5	0	0	22	2	7	105
Health Valley Rice Bran Graham Crackers	110	3	0	0	19	3	4	70
Amaranth or Oat Brand Grahams (avg)	120	3	0	0	22	3	3	80
Keebler Cinnamon Grahams, 0.7 oz	100	3	1	0	16	0	4	90
New Morning Cinnamon Grahams	130	3	0	0	24	1	7	85
Honey Grahams	130	3	0	0	24	1	6	95
Pepperidge Farm Goldfish Grahams Choc	130	4	1	0	22	2	0	125
Goldfish Grahams Cinnamon or Vanilla	140	5	1	0	22	1	0	135
Goldfish S'mores Adventure	130	4	2	0	24	1	11	140
Safeway Cinnamon Grahams	130	3	2	0	25	1	10	105
Honey Grahams	140	3	2	0	24	1	7	120

GRANOLA, CEREAL AND SNACK BARS

(see Granola/Cereal/Breakfast Bars, pg 69; Diet/Energy/Snack Bars, pg 217)

JERKY AND MEAT SNACKS

	Cal	Fat	Sat	Chol	Carb	Fib	Sug	Sod
Beef sticks, smoked, 1 oz	156	14	6	38	2	0	0	420
Beef jerky, chopped & formed, 1 oz	116	7	3	14	3	1	0	627

	Cal	Fat	Sat	Chol	Carb	Fib	Sug	Sod
Brands . . . *(1 oz unless noted)*								
Shelton's Turkey, Original or Hot & Spicy, 0.5 .	50	1	0	25	1	0	0	125
Snatch Beef Jerky Whiskey Row, 1 oz...........	50	1	0	20	2	0	2	50
Peppered Ale, 1 oz	50	2	0	20	1	0	1	85
Original Peppered, 1 oz...............................	50	1	0	20	1	0	1	105
REDUCED SODIUM (LESS THAN GENERIC):								
JuJu Jerky Turkey or Beef Jerky, 1 oz	70	1	0	30	3	1	2	170

MATZOS

	Cal	Fat	Sat	Chol	Carb	Fib	Sug	Sod
Matzo, plain, 1 oz..	112	0	0	0	24	1	0	1
Whole wheat, 1 oz	100	0	0	0	22	3	0	1
Egg, 1 oz	111	1	0	24	22	1	0	6
Egg and onion, 1 oz....................................	111	1	0	13	22	1	0	81

Brands . . . *Most brands within generic average.*

NUTS AND SEEDS

	Cal	Fat	Sat	Chol	Carb	Fib	Sug	Sod
Unsalted nuts:								
Almonds, dry roasted, unsalted, 1 oz............	169	15	1	0	5	3	1	0
Hazelnuts, dry roasted, unsalted, 1 oz	183	18	1	0	5	3	1	0
Pecans, dry roasted, unsalted, 1 oz	201	21	2	0	4	3	1	0
Macadamia nuts, dry roasted, unsalted,1 oz......	204	22	3	0	4	2	1	1
Pine nuts, unsalted, 1 oz............................	191	19	1	0	4	1	1	1
Walnuts, unsalted, 1 oz................................	185	18	2	0	4	2	1	1
Mixed nuts, dry roasted, unsalted, 1 oz.........	168	15	2	0	7	3	1	3
Pistachios, unsalted, 1 oz	162	13	2	0	8	3	2	3
Cashews, dry roasted, unsalted, 1 oz............	163	13	3	0	9	1	1	5
Salted/flavored nuts:								
Macadamia nuts, dry roasted, salted, 1 oz	203	22	3	0	4	2	1	75
Peanuts, choc covered, 1 oz	210	15	5	0	18	2	15	80
Almonds, dry roasted, salted, 1 oz	169	15	1	0	5	3	1	96
Pecans, dry roasted, salted, 1 oz.................	201	21	2	0	4	3	1	109
Peanuts, honey roasted, 1 oz......................	170	13	3	0	7	1	4	110
Pistachios, salted, 1 oz...............................	161	13	2	0	8	3	1	115
Cashews, dry roasted, salted, 1 oz	163	13	3	0	9	1	0	181
Mixed nuts, dry roasted, salted, 1 oz	168	15	2	0	7	3	1	190
Lightly salted, 1 oz.................................	168	15	2	0	7	3	1	95
Almonds, chili-flavored, 1 oz........................	170	15	1	0	5	3	1	210
Mixed nuts and seed snacks:								
Tropical mix, 1 oz......................................	115	5	2	0	12	1	7	35
Trail mix, regular, 1 oz	131	8	2	0	14	2	5	65
Peanut bar, 1.6 oz bar................................	235	15	2	0	21	2	19	70
Seeds:								
Sunflower seeds, salted, 1 oz	165	14	*3*	0	7	3	1	116
Unsalted, 1 oz	165	14	*3*	0	7	3	1	0
Pumpkin seeds, salted, 1 oz	190	15	4	0	4	3	1	130
Unsalted, 1 oz	180	14	4	0	4	3	1	5
Sesame sticks, 1 oz....................................	153	10	2	0	13	1	0	422

Brands . . . *(1 oz unless noted)*

NUTS

Unsalted nuts – *Most brands within generic average (0-4mg).*

	Cal	Fat	Sat	Chol	Carb	Fib	Sug	Sod
Dave's Gourmet Dave's Lucky Nuts	160	14	2	0	5	2	1	65
Dave's Smokin' BBQ'd Nuts	160	14	2	0	5	2	1	130
Dave's Burning Nuts	200	17	8	0	7	3	1	135

	Cal	Fat	Sat	Chol	Carb	Fib	Sug	Sod
Eden Organic Pistachios	160	12	2	0	7	3	1	60
Organic Tamari Almonds	160	11	1	0	8	4	0	65
Planters Cocktail Peanuts, Lightly Salted	170	14	2	0	5	2	1	55
Sahale Snacks Glazed Nuts, Valdosta Pecans	130	11	1	0	9	2	7	50
Soledad Almonds, 1/4 cup	130	9	1	0	10	3	7	60
KSAR Pistachios, 1/4 cup	150	11	2	0	11	3	3	65
Pomegranate Cashews, 1/4 cup	150	10	2	0	11	1	6	90
Sing Buri Cashews, 1/4 cup	130	9	2	0	10	1	6	100
Almond Peanut Butter & Jelly, 1/4 cup	160	12	1	0	7	3	6	100

NUT BARS *(see Diet/Energy/Snack Bars, pg 217)*

TRAIL MIX AND OTHER SNACK MIXES

	Cal	Fat	Sat	Chol	Carb	Fib	Sug	Sod
Back to Nature Bar Harbor Blend Trail Mix	130	7	2	0	17	2	14	0
Harvest Blend Trail Mix	150	10	1	0	12	3	7	5
Monterey Blend Trail Mix	140	6	1	0	19	3	14	5
Sonoma Blend Trail Mix	130	1	0	0	32	2	28	5
Nantucket Blend Trail Mix	130	7	1	0	15	3	11	25
Pacific Heights Blend Trail Mix	160	11	3	0	13	3	9	40
Eden Organic Wild Berry Mix	150	8	1	0	13	4	1	10
All Mixed Up Too	140	11	2	0	10	4	3	15
All Mixed Up	160	12	2	0	7	4	2	70
Emerald Breakfast on the Go Trail Mix								
Breakfast Blend, 1 oz	120	4	52	0	19	2	14	45
Great Value Choc Nut Antioxidant, 1.2 oz	150	5	1	0	24	2	6	0
Good Health Energy, 1 oz	150	8	1	0	12	3	7	0
Grizzlie's Granolas All Organic Trail Mix	110	7	5	0	14	2	10	0
7th Heaven Organic Trail Mix	140	9	3	0	13	2	10	0
Organic Nectarine Nut Mix	130	8	5	0	13	2	8	0
Applenut Mix	140	10	1	0	12	2	8	5
Oregon Trail Mix or Organic	140	10	2	0	12	2	8	20
Cherub Almond Trail Mix	130	7	2	0	15	2	11	25
Curry Cashew Trail Mix or Organic	150	10	2	0	13	2	5	35
Woodstock Farms Organic Trail Mix	140	6	1	0	10	2	7	0
California Supreme Mix	150	9	1	0	12	2	7	0
Cape Cod Cranberry or Gourmet (avg)	120	4	1	0	19	2	16	6
Cascade or Enchanted Trail Mix (avg)	120	3	1	0	23	2	17	9
Tropical Mix	90	0	0	0	22	2	15	10

SEEDS

	Cal	Fat	Sat	Chol	Carb	Fib	Sug	Sod
David Pumpkin Seeds	160	12	3	0	4	1	0	10
Reduced Sodium Sunflower Seeds	190	14	2	0	7	3	1	75
Eden Organic Spicy Pumpkin, 1/4 cup	200	16	3	0	5	5	0	75
Organic Pumpkin Seeds, 1/4 cup	200	16	3	0	5	5	0	100
Woodstock Farms Sesame Sticks, No Salt	160	11	2	0	13	1	0	0
Sunflower Seeds Hulled Roasted No Salt	180	15	2	0	5	3	0	0

POPCORN AND PUFFED CORN/RICE SNACKS

	Cal	Fat	Sat	Chol	Carb	Fib	Sug	Sod
Popcorn, air-popped, 1 oz	110	1	0	0	22	4	0	2
Popcorn, caramel-coated w/o peanuts, 1 oz	122	4	1	1	22	2	15	58
w/peanuts, 1 oz	113	2	0	0	23	1	13	84
Popcorn, cheese-flavor, 1 oz	149	9	2	3	15	3	1	252
Popcorn, butter-flavor, ready-to-eat, 1 oz	160	11	2	0	14	1	0	300
Popcorn, microwave, 1 oz	160	12	3	0	17	4	0	390

Brands . . . *(1 oz or about 2 1/2 cups unless noted)*

POPCORN – MICROWAVE

	Cal	Fat	Sat	Chol	Carb	Fib	Sug	Sod
Bearitos Organic, NS, 10 cups	110	2	0	0	23	5	0	0

	Cal	Fat	Sat	Chol	Carb	Fib	Sug	Sod
Garden of Eatin' No Oil Added	55	1	0	0	12	2	0	45
Natural Butter	75	3	2	0	11	2	0	90
Orville Redenbacher's Caramel	170	8	2	0	24	1	12	35
Popcorn Indiana Cocoa Kettle	140	6	0	0	22	2	10	20
Smart Balance Smart 'n Healthy	120	2	0	0	24	5	0	85
REDUCED SODIUM (LESS THAN GENERIC):								
Newman's Own Light Butter	1204	2	0	0	19	4	0	170

POPCORN – READY-TO-EAT

	Cal	Fat	Sat	Chol	Carb	Fib	Sug	Sod
Caramel-coated popcorn – *Most brands within generic average (58-84mg).*								
Bachman's Lite Popcorn	110	2	0	0	22	4	0	110
Bearitos Organic, Lite, NS, 4 cups	120	2	0	0	24	1	0	100
Erin's All Natural Low Saturated Fat, LS	130	6	1	0	18	4	0	135
Good Health Natural Foods								
Half-Naked Popcorn	120	3	0	0	21	4	4	140
Herr's Popcorn Light	120	4	1	0	19	3	1	80
Northern Lites FF Caramel Corn	110	0	0	0	26	1	17	80
Pirate's Booty Chocolate	140	8	1	0	17	1	5	40
Veggie	130	5	1	0	17	1	1	90
New York Pizza	120	5	1	0	18	1	1	120
Barrrrrbeque	130	5	1	0	19	1	2	135
Sour Cream & Onion	130	5	1	0	18	1	1	140
Aged White Cheddar	130	5	1	0	19	0	0	140
Popcorn Indiana Cinnamon Sugar	130	5	0	0	21	2	7	115
Original Kettlecorn	130	5	0	0	21	2	6	130
Poppycock Choc Lovers Popcorn Snack	160	7	3	5	22	1	14	100
Pecan Delight or Cashew Lovers	150	7	2	5	20	1	13	105
Smartfood Popcorn Clusters, Cranberry Almond	120	2	0	0	24	5	10	75
Vic's Gourmet White Lite, 1 cup	40	2	0	0	6	0	0	45
Gourmet White, 1 cup	60	4	0	0	6	0	0	85
Ya Ya's Herb & Garden Veg Popcorn	160	10	1	0	15	2	0	110
Light Popcorn	130	3	1	0	21	1	0	140

POPCORN SEASONING

	Cal	Fat	Sat	Chol	Carb	Fib	Sug	Sod
Kernal Season's Apple Cinnamon, 1/4 tsp	4	0	0	0	1	0	1	0
Kettle Corn or Caramel, 1/4 tsp	5	0	0	0	1	0	1	0
Choc Marshmallow, 1/4 tsp	3	0	0	0	1	0	0	1
BBQ, 1/4 tsp	3	0	0	0	1	0	1	5
Sour Cream & Onion, 1/4 tsp	2	0	0	0	0	0	0	35

PRETZELS

	Cal	Fat	Sat	Chol	Carb	Fib	Sug	Sod
Unsalted pretzel, 1 oz	108	1	0	0	22	1	1	82
Choc coated pretzel, 1 oz	130	5	2	0	20	1	10	161
Pretzel, plain, 1 oz	108	1	0	0	23	1	1	385
Soft pretzel, 1 oz	95	1	0	0	19	1	0	393
Brands . . . *(1 oz unless noted)*								
Bachman's LS Mini Pretzels	110	0	0	0	25	1	0	50
Funky Chunky Choc Pretzels	140	6	5	0	19	1	10	90
Good Health Natural Foods								
Peanut Butter Filled Pretzels, Unsalted	140	6	1	0	15	3	2	80
Snyder's of Hanover Unsalted Mini Pretzels	110	0	0	0	25	1	1	75
Nibblers Honey Mustard & Onion	130	3	2	0	23	1	1	95
Pretzel Dips Hershey's Milk Choc	130	6	4	5	18	1	10	100
Pretzel Dips Hershey's White Choc	140	6	3	5	19	0	11	110
Olde Tyme Pretzels	120	1	0	0	24	1	1	120
Pretzel Dips Hershey's Special Dark	140	5	3	5	22	2	8	130

	Cal	Fat	Sat	Chol	Carb	Fib	Sug	Sod
Unique Pretzels Unsalted Cheese Splits.........	110	2	1	5	21	1	0	103
Unsalted Multigrain Splits.............................	115	2	0	0	22	1	0	105

FROZEN/REFRIGERATED

	Cal	Fat	Sat	Chol	Carb	Fib	Sug	Sod
Hanover Soft Baked Pretzel	160	0	0	0	33	1	2	130
SuperPretzel Soft Pretzel Bites, 1.9 oz	150	1	0	0	32	1	1	115
Soft Pretzel, 2.3 oz....................................	180	1	0	0	36	2	1	140

RICE CAKES AND SNACKS

	Cal	Fat	Sat	Chol	Carb	Fib	Sug	Sod
Rice cakes, 1 oz	70	0	0	0	14	0	0	60
Unsalted, 1 oz	70	0	0	0	14	0	0	0
Rice cakes, caramel, 1 oz	100	0	0	0	22	0	6	60
Mini cakes, 1 oz	110	1	0	0	26	1	9	310
Rice cakes, cheese flavored, 1 oz	140	5	1	0	21	1	1	400

Brands . . . *(1 oz unless noted)*

  Unsalted rice cakes – Most brands within generic average (0mg).
  Plain rice cakes – Most brands within generic average (60mg).

	Cal	Fat	Sat	Chol	Carb	Fib	Sug	Sod
EnviroKidz Crispy Rice Peanut Choco Drizzle...	120	5	1	0	18	1	8	50
Crispy Rice Fruity Burst..............................	110	3	1	0	21	1	8	65
Crispy Rice Peanut Butter...........................	110	3	0	0	20	1	7	65
Crispy Rice Berry Blast or Choc (avg)............	110	3	0	0	21	1	7	70
Kellogg's Rice Krispies Treats								
Strawberry, 0.8 oz.....................................	90	2	1	0	16	0	8	95
Chocolatey Drizzle, 0.8 oz	100	3	2	0	17	0	8	95
Original, 0.8 oz...	90	3	1	0	17	0	7	105
Lundberg Green Tea w/Lemon Rice Cakes	80	0	0	0	17	1	2	0
Apple Cinnamon or Buttery Caramel Rice Cakes	70	1	0	0	16	1	2	0
Cinnamon Toast Rice Cakes	80	1	0	0	18	1	3	0
Honey Nut Rice Cakes.................................	80	1	0	0	18	1	2	5
Rice w/Popcorn or Mochi Sweet Rice Cakes....	60	1	0	0	14	1	0	35
Caramel Corn Rice Cakes	80	1	0	0	18	1	2	40
Mother's Salted Butter Rice Cakes.................	70	0	0	0	16	0	0	90
Paskesz Multigrain Squares, SF, 3 cakes........	57	0	0	0	12	2	0	0
Spelt or Whole Wheat Squares, SF, 3 cakes ...	63	0	0	0	13	2	0	0
Ultra-thin Rice Cake Minis, SF, 10 cakes	76	0	0	0	17	1	0	0
Quaker Rice Cakes Apple Cinnamon...............	100	0	0	0	22	0	6	0
Rice Cakes Lightly Salted	70	0	0	0	14	0	0	30
Rice Cakes Caramel Corn	100	0	0	0	22	0	6	60
Rice Cakes Choc Crunch.............................	120	2	0	0	22	0	6	60
Mini Delights Chocolatey Drizzle, 0.7 oz	90	4	4	0	14	1	6	65
Mini Delights Chocolatey Mint, 0.7 oz............	90	4	3	0	14	1	7	70
Mini Delights Cinnamon Streusel, 0.7 oz	90	4	3	0	14	1	6	95
Mini Delights Caramel Drizzle, 0.7 oz	90	4	3	0	15	1	8	75
Quakes Choc or Apple Cinnamon (avg)	120	2	0	0	27	1	8	100

SNACK BARS

(see Granola/Cereal/Breakfast Bars, pg 69; Diet/Energy/Nutritional Bars, pg 217)

SOUPS AND CHILI

See **RESOURCES**, *page 305, for partial list of manufacturers and retailers offering low-salt products online or visit* **LowSaltFoods.com** *for additional sources.*

Cal Fat Sat Chol Carb Fib Sug Sod

SOUPS AND CHILI

BOUILLON, STOCKS AND BROTHS

	Cal	Fat	Sat	Chol	Carb	Fib	Sug	Sod
Stock, seafood, 1 cup	10	0	0	0	0	0	0	420
Broth, vegetable, 1 cup	15	0	0	0	3	0	1	570
Bouillon, beef, 1 cube	9	0	0	0	1	0	1	611
Bouillon, chicken, 1 cube	11	1	0	0	1	0	1	743
Broth, beef, 1 cup	17	1	0	0	0	0	01	782
Lower sodium, 1 cup	10	1	0	0	1	0	1	440
Broth, chicken, 1 cup	17	0	0	5	1	0	1	980
Lower sodium, 1 cup	10	1	0	5	1	0	1	570

Brands . . . *(1 cup unless noted)*

CANNED/READY-TO-USE

	Cal	Fat	Sat	Chol	Carb	Fib	Sug	Sod
Campbell's Chicken Broth, LS, 1 can	25	1	1	5	1	0	1	140
Das Dutchman Essenhaus Chicken Broth	30	0	0	0	0	0	0	65
Health Valley Beef Broth, FF, NSA	10	0	0	0	0	0	0	120
Chicken Broth, NSA	35	2	1	0	0	0	0	130
Imagine Organic Chicken Broth, LS	20	1	0	5	1	0	0	95
Beef Broth, LS	20	1	0	5	1	0	0	140
Vegetable Broth, LS	20	1	0	0	3	1	1	140
Chicken Cooking Stock, LS	15	1	0	0	1	–	–	140
Beef Flavored Cooking Stock, LS	10	0	0	0	1	–	–	140
More Than Gourmet Cullinary Veg Stock	15	0	0	0	2	0	1	75
Nature's Promise Chicken, LS	50	0	0	0	0	0	0	140
O Organics Organic Chicken Broth, LS	5	0	0	0	1	0	1	140
Pacific Natural LS Chicken or LS Veg Broth	15	0	0	0	3	1	2	140
Shelton's Chicken Broth, FF, LS	10	0	0	0	0	0	0	60
Organic Chicken Broth, FF, LS	20	0	0	0	0	0	0	100

REDUCED SODIUM (LESS THAN GENERIC):

	Cal	Fat	Sat	Chol	Carb	Fib	Sug	Sod
Kitchen Basics Unsalted Chicken Stock	24	0	0	0	1	0	0	150

CUBE, POWDER AND GLACÉ CONCENTRATE *(1 tsp or cube unless noted)*

	Cal	Fat	Sat	Chol	Carb	Fib	Sug	Sod
Bernard Soup/Gravy Base, Beef or Chicken	20	1	0	0	3	0	1	10
Celibr Gluten-Free Bouillon, all flavors	5	0	0	0	1	0	0	123
Croyden House LS Instant, Chicken	15	0	0	0	0	0	0	5
Edward & Sons LS Veggie, 1/2 cube	20	2	1	0	1	0	0	135
Frontier LS Veg Broth, 2 tbsp	50	0	0	0	12	2	0	50
Goya Beef or Chicken Bouillon, 1/4 tsp	5	0	0	0	1	0	1	130
Harvest Sun Organic LS Veg Bouillon, 1/2 cube	20	0	0	0	3	0	0	89
Herb-Ox Beef or Chicken Bouillon, LS	10	0	0	0	2	0	1	5
Home Again SF Beef or Chicken Base	20	1	0	0	3	0	0	0
L.B. Jamison's Chicken Soup Base, LS	25	2	0	0	3	0	2	55
Med-Diet Cream Soup Base	92	5	0	0	11	0	0	65
Beef-like Clear Broth	10	0	0	0	2	0	0	105
Clear Chicken Broth	12	0	0	0	2	0	0	120
Vegetable Broth	12	0	0	0	3	0	0	138
Miller's Chicken Base, LS	25	1	0	0	3	0	0	10
Beef Base, LS, 1 tsp	25	1	0	0	3	0	0	60
Minor's LS Chicken, Turkey, or Roasted Chicken	15	1	0	5	1	0	0	135
LS Beef, Ham, or Veg Base (avg)	15	1	0	0	3	0	0	140
More Than Gourmet Veggie Glace Gold, 2 tsp	15	0	0	0	3	0	1	60
Veggie Stock Gold, 2 tsp	10	0	0	0	2	0	1	80
Orrington Farms Chicken Base, LS	25	1	0	0	3	0	0	15
Beef Base, LS, 1 tsp	25	1	0	0	3	0	0	60
Rapunzel NSA Veg Bouillon, 1/2 cube	24	2	1	0	1	0	0	101

229

SOUPS AND CHILI
Chili

	Cal	Fat	Sat	Chol	Carb	Fib	Sug	Sod
RC Fine Foods Beef or Chicken Base, Very LS	10	0	0	0	2	0	0	30
Supreme Turkey, LS	10	1	0	0	1	0	0	135
Supreme Chicken, Beef, or Ham Base, LS	10	1	0	0	1	0	0	140
Supreme Vegetable Base, LS	10	0	0	0	2	0	1	140
Advantage Chicken, Beef, or Veg	10	1	0	0	1	0	0	140
Vogue Cuisine Onion Base, 1 tsp	15	0	0	0	2	0	0	136
VegeBase, 1 tsp	15	0	0	0	2	0	0	140
Wyler's Chicken or Beef Bouillon SF	10	0	0	0	2	0	0	0

FROZEN/REFRIGERATED

Knorr *Ultimate Low Sodium*

	Cal	Fat	Sat	Chol	Carb	Fib	Sug	Sod
Vegetarian Vegetable Base, 3/4 tsp	10	0	0	0	2	0	0	95
Roasted Beef Base, 1 tsp	20	1	0	0	2	0	0	125
Roasted Chicken Base, 1 tsp	25	1	0	5	2	0	0	130

CHILI

	Cal	Fat	Sat	Chol	Carb	Fib	Sug	Sod
Chili mix, 1/6 pkg	60	2	0	0	10	0	0	980
Chili w/o beans, 1 cup	302	18	6	54	16	3	3	996
Less sodium chili w/o beans, 1 cup	220	9	4	40	18	3	3	710
Chili w/beans, 1 cup	287	14	6	44	30	11	3	1336
Less sodium chili w/beans, 1 cup	260	7	3	30	33	7	5	880

Brands . . . *(1 cup unless noted)*

CANNED

	Cal	Fat	Sat	Chol	Carb	Fib	Sug	Sod
Health Valley Tame Tomato Chili, NSA	210	3	0	0	41	8	11	70
REDUCED SODIUM (LESS THAN GENERIC):								
Amy's Light in Sodium Spicy or Med Chili	280	9	1	0	35	7	5	340
Dixie Diner Carb Counters Cup o'Chili	109	1	0	0	10	5	1	369

FROZEN/REFRIGERATED

REDUCED SODIUM (LESS THAN GENERIC):

	Cal	Fat	Sat	Chol	Carb	Fib	Sug	Sod
Tabatchnick Organic or Vegetarian Chili	180	4	0	0	28	8	3	360

MIXES

NOTE: Several chili mixes have a separate salt packet. If the packet is not added, the sodium per serving is significantly less.

	Cal	Fat	Sat	Chol	Carb	Fib	Sug	Sod
Ass Kickin' Chili Fixin's	180	1	0	0	33	0	0	75
Green Chili & Corn Stew	80	1	0	0	18	0	0	110
Bountiful Pantry Lentil Chili (dry mix only)	180	1	0	0	31	14	3	5
White Bean Chili	190	1	0	0	36	13	5	10
5 Bean Chili	200	0	0	0	36	15	4	20
Quinoa & Corn Chili (dry mix only)	120	3	0	0	22	7	4	25
Delicaé Pantry Slow Cooker SW Roadhouse	120	0	0	0	17	3	4	45
Dixie Diner Dusty Roads Chili Mix	157	2	0	0	23	9	4	124
Frontier Soups Ski Country Chili	140	1	0	0	25	8	0	15
White Bean Chili	90	0	0	0	22	10	1	25
Cinncinati Chili Mix	80	3	2	0	12	4	1	50
Hurst HamBeens Chili Beans	120	1	0	0	20	9	1	70
Leonard Mt Boot Scootin' Chili Red or Green	90	1	0	0	19	2	1	101
Slow Cooker Gourmet Chili Mix	140	1	0	0	26	9	5	15
Texas Roadhouse Chili	120	0	0	0	17	3	4	45
REDUCED SODIUM (LESS THAN GENERIC):								
Canterbury Naturals White Lightning Chicken	120	1	0	0	23	7	3	220

CHILI SEASONING

	Cal	Fat	Sat	Chol	Carb	Fib	Sug	Sod
Chili seasoning, 1/4 pkg	30	1	0	0	5	2	1	310
30% less sodium, 1/4 pkg	30	5	0	0	5	1	0	210

	Cal	Fat	Sat	Chol	Carb	Fib	Sug	Sod
Brands . . .								
Harvest Direct Soy Chili Mix, 1 oz mix...........	60	0	0	0	8	3	2	1
New Traditions Chili Mix, 1 tsp mix	15	0	0	0	3	0	0	0
WhoopAss Chili Mix, 1 oz mix......................	60	1	0	0	12	0	0	40
Williams								
Chili Seasoning Chipotle or Onion.................	15	1	0	0	2	1	1	0
Original or Tex-Mex Style, 1/8 pkg...............	10	0	0	0	2	1	1	0
Chicken, 1/5 pkg...	20	0	0	0	5	0	0	20

SOUPS

	Cal	Fat	Sat	Chol	Carb	Fib	Sug	Sod
Clam chowder, manhattan, 1 cup....................	77	2	0	3	12	2	3	576
New england, 1 cup............................	91	3	1	8	13	1	0	881
Tomato, 1 cup..	73	1	0	0	16	2	10	667
Chicken noodle, 1 cup.....................................	66	2	1	14	8	0	1	678
Mix, prep, 1 cup......................................	56	1	0	10	9	0	1	561
Gazpacho, 1 cup..	46	0	0	0	4	1	1	739
Cream of mushroom, 1 cup	103	7	2	0	8	0	2	780
Chicken w/rice, 1 cup.....................................	58	2	0	6	7	1	0	791
Vegetable beef, 1 cup....................................	79	2	1	5	10	2	1	795
Cream of potato, 1 cup	74	2	1	6	12	1	2	803
Cream of chicken, 1 cup.................................	113	7	2	10	9	0	1	825
Vegetable, 1 cup..	73	2	0	0	12	1	4	827
Split pea w/ham, 1 cup	193	4	2	8	28	2	1	851
Cream of celery, 1 cup	91	6	1	14	9	1	2	863
Chicken gumbo, 1 cup....................................	57	1	0	4	8	2	2	873
Onion, 1 cup..	57	2	0	0	8	1	3	900
Mix, prep, 1 cup......................................	28	0	0	0	6	1	2	796
Oyster stew, 1 cup	59	4	3	14	4	0	0	910
Minestrone, 1 cup..	84	3	1	1	11	1	2	915
Matzo ball soup, 1 cup	40	1	0	0	9	1	2	1040
Reduced sodium, 1 cup............................	50	1	0	0	10	1	2	640
Black bean, 1 cup	114	2	0	0	19	8	3	1203
Brands . . . *(1 cup unless noted)*								
CANNED/SHELF-STABLE								
Campbell's Split Pea, LS, 1 can.................	240	4	2	5	38	6	6	30
Chunky Veg Beef, LS, 1 can....................	170	5	2	30	18	6	7	50
Cream Of Mushroom, LS, 1 can.................	160	8	3	10	19	3	6	60
Tomato w/Tomato Pieces, LS, 1 can..............	150	4	2	10	25	4	16	90
Chicken w/Noodles, LS, 1 can	160	5	2	30	17	2	4	140
Gold's Borscht, Unsalted, 6 oz................	50	0	0	0	13	1	11	30
Health Valley Lentil, NSA	140	2	0	0	27	8	5	30
Black Bean, NSA	140	2	0	0	29	6	4	30
Potato Leek, NSA	100	2	0	0	20	3	2	30
Minestrone, NSA	90	2	0	0	16	3	5	50
Vegetable, NSA.......................................	100	3	0	0	18	4	4	50
Tomato, NSA	100	3	1	5	19	3	13	60
Mushroom Barley, NSA.............................	90	3	0	0	15	3	3	60
Split Pea, NSA	140	3	1	0	26	8	4	85
Rice Primavera, NSA................................	110	3	0	0	17	3	3	135
Chicken Noodle, NSA................................	80	3	0	15	12	3	1	135
Imagine Light in Sodium Sweet Potato...........	110	1	0	0	23	3	7	140
REDUCED SODIUM (LESS THAN GENERIC):								
Amy's Light in Sodium Minestrone	90	2	0	0	17	3	5	290
Light in Sodium Butternut Squash	100	3	0	0	20	2	4	290

SOUPS AND CHILI
Soups

	Cal	Fat	Sat	Chol	Carb	Fib	Sug	Sod
Light in Sodium Lentil	150	5	1	0	20	5	3	290
Light in Sodium Lentil Veg	150	4	1	0	23	6	5	340
Light in Sodium Cream of Tomato	100	2	2	10	17	3	11	340
Imagine *Organic*								
Light in Sodium Creamy Garden Broccoli	70	2	0	0	12	2	1	200
Light in Sodium Creamy Red Bliss Potato	100	3	0	0	18	2	2	220
Light in Sodium Creamy Harvest Corn	110	3	0	0	20	3	4	220
Light in Sodium Creamy Garden Tomato	80	1	0	0	16	2	2	300
Manischewitz								
Chicken Noodle, Reduced Sodium	180	2	1	70	20	1	2	260
Borscht, Reduced Sodium, 6 oz	64	0	0	0	16	0	16	274
Meal Mart *Amazing Meals*								
Chicken Soup w/Matzoh Balls, 12 oz	160	4	1	55	9	0	0	220
Pacific Natural Foods								
Creamy Butternut Squash, Light Sodium	90	2	0	0	17	3	4	280
Pritikin Ready-to-eat, all (avg)	90	0	0	0	18	3	2	290
ShariAnn's French Green Lentil	130	0	0	0	22	1	0	320
Streit's Hearty Vegetarian Vegetable	130	3	0	0	24	3	9	300
FROZEN/REFRIGERATED								
Tabachinack Barley & Mushroom, LS	80	1	0	0	17	4	1	40
Vegetable, LS	90	2	0	0	17	4	3	45
Pea, LS	140	0	0	0	34	14	0	50
REDUCED SODIUM (LESS THAN GENERIC):								
Blount Spiced Pumpkin Bisque	230	16	10	50	20	2	8	190
Moosewood Tibetan Curried Lentil	130	4	0	0	19	7	5	320
Tabachinack Cabbage	90	1	0	0	21	1	11	160
Wilderness Wild Rice	80	1	0	0	16	1	1	220
Cream of Mushroom	100	5	3	15	11	1	3	260
Balsamic Tomato & Rice	110	4	0	0	18	3	10	260
Minestrone	100	2	0	0	18	4	3	320
Old Fashioned Potato	100	2	0	0	21	2	2	330
Yankee Bean	180	2	0	0	33	10	2	340
Vegetable	90	2	0	0	17	4	3	350
MIXES								
Some mixes require additional ingredients which may raise sodium content.								
Ass Kickin' Green Chili & Corn Stew	80	1	0	0	18	3	3	110
Bean Cuisine Louisiana Cajun Bean	90	0	0	0	17	4	0	0
Mediterranean Ministrone	90	0	0	0	18	0	1	0
13 Bean Bouillabaise or Lots of Lentil	100	0	0	0	17	5	1	0
Island Black Bean or White Bean Provencial	100	0	0	0	17	6	2	0
Split Pea or Utima Pasta Fagioli (avg)	100	0	0	0	18	4	2	5
Bob's Red Mill 13 Bean	270	1	0	0	49	15	4	15
Vegi Soup Mix	350	2	0	0	63	19	6	30
Bountiful Pantry Hearty Lentil & Vegetable	180	0	0	0	34	6	4	10
Moroccan Lentil Soup	150	1	0	0	30	6	3	10
Pasta e Fagioli or Italian Bean Soup (avg)	190	1	0	0	37	12	4	15
Jambalaya	190	1	0	0	41	2	1	15
Hearty Fisherman Stew	150	1	0	0	28	10	3	15
Heritage Bean Soup	200	1	0	0	36	12	1	15
Black Bean Soup or Split Pea & Herbs (avg)	190	1	0	0	35	14	7	20
Pumpkin Chowder	150	0	0	0	34	6	13	25
Quinoa & Red Lentil Chowder	170	2	0	0	33	6	2	25
Farmhouse Chowder	220	2	0	0	42	9	5	25
Roasted Tomato & Pasta Soup	100	1	0	0	21	4	3	25
Quinoa Vegetable Soup	110	2	0	0	22	3	5	30

	Cal	Fat	Sat	Chol	Carb	Fib	Sug	Sod
Butternut Squash & Apple	120	1	0	0	27	3	10	30
Wild Rice & Veggie Chowder	120	1	0	0	24	3	3	30
Country or Southwestern Corn Chowder	110	1	0	0	24	3	4	35
Garden Veggie & Pasta	100	1	0	0	20	3	5	35
Golden Pea & Vegetable	180	2	0	0	33	13	4	45
Curried Potato & Carrot Soup	100	1	0	0	23	5	5	50
Bean & Potato Soup	200	1	0	0	39	12	4	55
Thai Sweet Potato Bisque	70	0	0	0	31	3	11	70
Tuscan Minestrone Soup	120	1	0	0	24	4	6	75
Vegetable Cheddar Chowder	130	1	0	0	27	5	4	75
Canterbury Naturals Black Bean & Pasta	110	1	0	0	20	4	0	80
Delicaé Pantry Slow Cooker Caribbean Black Bean	180	0	0	0	34	5	6	5
Farmer's Hearty Split Pea	90	0	0	0	34	6	5	5
Country Harvest Corn Chowder	80	0	0	0	18	2	1	25
Potato Leek or New England Clam Chowder	80	0	0	0	19	1	1	25
Grandpa's Favorite Beef Barley	110	0	0	0	22	6	2	25
Southern Italian Pasta e Fagioli	120	1	0	0	24	5	3	25
Thai Curry Lentil	180	0	0	0	35	6	6	35
Manhattan Clam Chowder	80	0	0	0	17	3	4	35
Slow Cooker Soup U.S. Senate Bean	190	1	0	0	38	8	5	40
Mexican Fiesta Tortilla Soup	110	1	0	0	23	7	5	65
Mother's Comfort Chicken Noodle Soup	50	0	0	0	12	2	2	80
Dixie Diner Creme of Mushroom & Gravy	39	1	0	0	6	1	0	133
Frontier Soups French Onion Soup	90	0	0	0	11	2	2	0
Asparagus Almond Soup	77	0	0	0	11	1	1	0
Squash & Lentil Soup	80	0	0	0	16	2	1	0
Internat'l Collection Hungarian Goulash	80	0	0	0	19	6	1	5
Beef Goulash or Minestrone Soup (avg)	80	0	0	0	18	6	0	5
Sausage Lentil Soup	60	0	0	0	15	6	0	5
Mushroom Barley or Broccoli Cheddar (avg)	73	0	0	0	16	3	1	7
Wild Rice Soup or Tortilla Soup (avg)	61	1	0	0	12	3	0	8
Corn Chowder	55	0	0	0	13	1	0	8
Beef Barley Bean Stew or 11 Bean Soup (avg)	65	0	0	0	17	8	2	10
Chicken Stew	70	0	0	0	15	4	2	10
Fisherman's Stew	44	0	0	0	9	2	0	11
Split Pea Soup	93	0	0	0	18	5	0	14
Black Bean Soup	150	1	0	0	29	11	2	15
Spicy Fiesta Soup	70	2	0	0	18	7	1	15
Chicken Noodle Soup	70	1	0	10	15	1	2	20
Wild Rice & Mushroom Soup	45	0	0	0	10	1	1	20
Red Bean Gumbo	80	0	0	0	22	7	1	20
Red Pepper Corn Chowder	120	0	0	0	25	1	1	25
Potato Leek or Vegetable Soup (avg)	75	0	0	0	16	2	1	25
Garden Gazpacho	22	0	0	0	5	1	0	27
Jambalaya	72	1	0	0	16	1	1	28
Wedding Soup	80	0	0	0	16	1	1	30
Golden Peanut Soup	70	1	0	0	24	2	3	35
Internat'l Collection Italian Wedding	80	1	0	0	12	1	1	35
Cranberry Bean Soup	110	0	0	0	22	9	1	36
Far East Ginger Beef Bowl	160	3	0	0	31	3	2	55
Goodman's Noodleman Noodle LS	50	1	0	10	9	1	2	95
Onion Soup & Dip, LS	30	1	0	0	6	1	3	115
Goya 16 Bean	90	0	0	0	26	15	1	85
Hurst's HamBeens 15 Bean	120	1	0	0	20	9	1	70
Cajun 15 Bean	120	1	0	0	20	9	1	100

SOUPS AND CHILI
Soups

	Cal	Fat	Sat	Chol	Carb	Fib	Sug	Sod
Just Delicious Foods Minestrone..............	30	0	0	0	11	2	1	0
Seafood or Golden Corn Chowder (avg).........	45	1	0	0	10	1	0	0
Albondigas...	58	0	0	0	22	2	0	0
Chicken Rice & Curry Spice......................	60	0	0	0	10	5	1	1
Red Lentil..	110	0	0	0	16	12	2	4
Barley Beef..	100	0	0	0	19	2	0	5
Navy Bean..	120	1	0	0	21	0	0	7
Split Pea...	150	1	0	0	21	14	5	10
Chicken Vegetable..................................	120	0	0	0	21	12	0	10
Black Beans & Rice.................................	60	1	0	0	31	20	0	20
Tortilla	60	1	1	0	21	19	0	32
Kedem Vegetable Soup Mix....................	110	0	0	0	21	6	3	30
Leonard Mountain Country Harvest Lentil	101	1	1	0	20	1	0	70
Manischewitz Veg w/Mushrooms..................	120	0	0	0	22	3	1	70
Rabbit Creek Gourmet Tortilla Soup.............	15	0	0	0	4	1	0	16
Country Bean..	95	2	0	0	27	14	1	20
Stonewall Kitchen French Onion..................	90	0	0	0	11	1	0	0
New England Corn Chowder.......................	55	0	0	0	13	1	0	8
Potato Leek..	93	0	0	0	18	5	0	14
Italian Wedding Soup..............................	80	1	0	0	16	1	1	35
Farmers Market Veg	143	1	0	0	31	6	0	49
REDUCED SODIUM (LESS THAN GENERIC):								
Ass Kickin' Black Bean or Tortilla & Bean	150	4	0	0	23	6	3	290
Cook in the Kitchen Pasta Primavera Soup...	120	0	0	0	24	1	1	260
Dixie Diner Cheese (Not!) Chicken Enchilada ..	122	1	0	0	19	6	2	304
Goodman's *Noodleman* Reduced Sodium Matzo..	24	0	0	0	1	0	0	150
Hurst's HamBeens Chili 15 Bean Soup........	120	1	0	0	20	9	1	170
Chicken 15 Bean Soup.............................	120	1	0	0	20	9	1	250
Beef 15 Bean Soup.................................	120	1	0	0	20	9	1	310
Legumes Plus Cajun/Brown Rice Lentil........	190	1	0	0	-	-	-	170
Zesty Tomato Lentil Soup.........................	180	1	0	0	-	-	-	250
Leonard Mountain Sailor Soup	157	1	1	0	34	3	0	150
Hunky Chunky Veggie Stew.......................	101	1	1	0	20	2	0	150
Spuds 'N Chives Potato Soup	90	5	1	0	22	2	0	172
4 Amigos Tortilla or 2 Amigos Green Chili	75	3	0	0	10	1	0	190
3 Amigos Enchilada Stew or Peppadew Stew..	75	3	0	0	10	1	0	190
Mama Leone Tuscany Veg or Italian Wedding ..	125	0	0	0	36	2	1	170
Pasta e Fagioli Italian or Minestrone............	125	1	0	0	25	2	1	245
Rabbit Creek Gourmet								
Cheesy Potato w/Bacon	100	2	0	5	18	1	4	300
Taste Adventure Minestrone......................	160	1	0	0	30	9	4	250
Williams								
Country Store 50% Less Sodium Tortilla......	90	2	0	0	20	2	1	330

SOUP CUPS *(1 soup cup unless noted)*

	Cal	Fat	Sat	Chol	Carb	Fib	Sug	Sod
REDUCED SODIUM (LESS THAN GENERIC):								
Dr. McDougalls *Light Sodium* Soup Cups								
Lentil Couscous	190	1	0	0	37	9	3	330
Edward & Sons Miso-Cup Reduced Sodium ..	25	1	0	0	3	1	1	270
Health Valley Zesty Black Bean w/Rice........	100	0	0	0	22	4	2	320
OrGran Garden Veg Soup Cup..................	47	0	0	0	3	0	0	200
Tomato Soup Cup	126	0	0	0	7	0	4	200

SOUP SEASONING MIX

	Cal	Fat	Sat	Chol	Carb	Fib	Sug	Sod
Bob's Red Mill Bean Soup Seasoning, 1 tsp....	4	0	0	0	0	0	0	56

PART 2

FAST FOOD
AND
CASUAL DINING
RESTAURANTS

FAST FOOD AND CASUAL DINING RESTAURANTS

237

NOTE: All sodium amounts listed in the following section are in milligrams (mg).

FAST FOOD AND CASUAL DINING RESTAURANTS

A & W

BURGERS/SANDWICHES/ENTREES 520–1,570
Corn Dog Nuggets, 5 pc [520] • Hot Dog, plain [740]
Crunchy Shrimp [820] • Grilled Chicken Sandwich [820] • Hamburger [860]

SIDES 290–2,440
French Fries, small [290]

CONDIMENTS 100–250
Ketchup [100] • Sweet & Sour Sauce [120] • Marinara Dipping Sauce [125]

SWEETS/SMOOTHIES 85–570
SMOOTHIES: Strawberry or Strawberry Banana, 16 oz/20 oz [85–100] •
Pineapple Banana, 16 oz/20 oz [100–110]
Root Beer or Diet Root Beer Float, sm/med [100–105]
Choc Fudge Blendrrr: 16 oz [100] • 20 oz [125]
ORANGE FLOAT: sm [115] • med [120]
Vanilla Cone, reg [115] • Strawberry Sundae [140] • Hot Fudge Sundae [140]

APPLEBEE'S

APPETIZERS *(1/4 serving)* 133–1,518
TRIOS CLASSIC WINGS: So BBQ [133] • Honey BBQ [168] • Sweet & Spicy [210]
Chips & Spicy Chipotle Lime Salsa [203] • Trios Spinach Artichoke Dip [223]

ENTREES *(w/o sides)* 410–6,620
Kid's Sirloin Steak, 4 oz [410] • Loaded Baked Potato [500]
Kid's Fried Shrimp [540] • New York Strip, 12 oz [550]
   TOPPERS 180–1,120
   Sauteed Garlic Mushrooms [180] • Grilled Onions [280]

SALADS *(w/o dressing unless noted)* 125–3,420
Caesar (w/dressing), side [125] • House Salad (w/dressing), side [380]
Grilled Chicken Caesar, half [450] • Oriental Chicken Salad, half [480]
Grilled Steak Caesar, half [540] • Oriental Chicken Salad (w/dressing) [600]
   DRESSINGS 250–490
   Bleu Cheese [250] • Buttermilk Ranch [310]

SOUPS 980–1,690

BURGERS/SANDWICHES 440–3,740
Kid's Corn Dog [440] • Kid's Mini Hamburger [490]
Kid's Grilled Chicken Sandwich [560] • Kid's Mini Cheeseburger [610]

SIDES 0–1,660
Fresh Fruit [0] • Applesauce [0] • Kid's Steamed Broccoli [25]
Guacamole [150] • Baked Potato [170] • Cole Slaw [190]

DESSERTS 65–980
KID'S SUNDAE: Vanilla [65] • Strawberry [65] • Oreo Cookie [170]
  ADD: Hershey's Syrup [25]
Hot Fudge Sundae Shooter [125] • Brownie Bite [200]

ARBY'S

BREAKFAST 400–1,930
BACON, EGG & CHEESE CROISSANT: w/o bacon & cheese [400] •
w/o cheese [600] • w/o bacon [640]
Outside-In Cinnamon Bites [480]

SANDWICHES/SUBS/ENTREES 350–2,270
Kid's Mac & Cheese [350] • Jr. Roast Beef [520] • Jr Deluxe Sandwich [560]
Jalapeno [600] • Loaded Potato Bites, 5 pc [650]
Kid's Prime-Cut Chicken Tenders [650] • Jr Chicken Sandwich [680]
CONDIMENTS. 65–180
Mayonnaise [65] • Ketchup [85] • Horsey Sauce [160]
DIPPING SAUCES 150–720
Honey Mustard [150] • Ranch Dipping Sauce [280]

SALADS *(w/o dressing)*. 15–1,000
CHOPPED SIDE SALAD: w/o cheese [15] • w/cheese [105]
Roast Chopped Farmhouse (w/o cheese & pepper bacon) [350]
DRESSINGS. 230–790
Dijon Honey Mustard [230] • Buttermilk Ranch [310]

SIDES 460–1,940
Potato Cakes (w/o ketchup), 2 pc [460]

DESSERTS/SHAKES 0–450
Apple Slices [0] • Yogurt Dip [30] • Apple Turnover [200] • Cherry Turnover [210]
SHAKES 210–450
Jr Orange Cream Shake [210] • Jr Vanilla Shake [230]

⬡ ARCTIC CIRCLE ⬡

BURGERS/FISH/CHICKEN. 290–1,283
Halibut, 2 pc [290] • Hamburger [497] • Double Burger [588]
Chicken Fingers, 2 pc [680]

SALADS *(w/o dressing)*. 826–1,806
Seafood Salad [826] • Taco Salad w/o Shell [864]
DRESSINGS. 380–480
Litehouse Ranch [380] • Litehouse Lite Ranch [400]

SIDES 124–656
French Fry, sm [124] • reg [180]

CONDIMENTS 99–400
White Sauce [99] • Tartar Sauce [170] • Sweet 'n Sour Sauce [190]

ICE CREAM/SHAKES 5–68
Vanilla Courtesy Cone [5] • Vanilla Ice Cream Cone [17] • Vanilla Sundae [23]
Vanilla Shake, sm/reg/lrg [38–68]

⬡ ATLANTA BREAD COMPANY ⬡

BREAKFAST. 390–2,040
Belgian Waffle w/maple syrup & whipped cream [390]
French Toast w/maple syrup [550] • Scrambled Eggs [620]

BAGELS. 420–1,660
Cinn Raisin [420] • Wheat [430] • Apple Spice [440] • Whole Grain [450]
CREAM CHEESE 150–570
Honey Raisin Walnut [150] • Chive Cream Cheese [180] • Plain [200]

MUFFINS 190–440
MUFFIN TOPS: Blueberry [190] • Banana Nut [200] • Choc Chip [220]
Blueberry Muffin [250]

PASTRIES/CROISSANTS 320–460
Bear Claw [320] • Sticky Bun [320] • Pecan Roll [320]
CROISSANTS: Apple [320] • French [320] • Cheese [320] • Almond [330] •
Choc [330] • Raspberry Cheese [340]
Apple Danish [340] • Raspberry Cheese Danish [340]

SANDWICHES **510–2,480**
Chicken Waldorf [510] • Chicken Salad on Sourdough [680]

ENTREES **480–2,630**
Kid's Penne & Cheese [480] • Fettuccine Salmone [560] • Penne Bolognese [670]

PIZZA **660–1,440**
Kid's Cheese Pizza, 1/2 [660] • Pepperoni Pizza, 1/2 [790]

SALADS **75–1,370**
House Salad [75] • Caesar Salad [390] • Balsamic Bleu Salad [410]
Chopstix Chicken Salad [530] • Salsa Fresca Salmon Salad [590]

SOUPS **1,010–1,750**

BAKED POTATO **1,260**

DESSERTS **130–440**
Creamy Caramel Brownie [130] • Double Choc Brownie [135]
COOKIES: Choc Toffee [160] • Choc Chunk [180] • White Choc Macadamia [190]
Key Lime Pie [190]

BREAD *(1 slice)* **170–790**
Rye [170] • Asiago loaf [180] • Sourdough [190]

AU BON PAIN

BREAKFAST **5–1,290**
Oatmeal or Apple Cinn Oatmeal, sm/med/lrg [5–15]
Museli, 8 oz [40] • Warm Apple Bake, 4 oz [220]
Sausage w/Peppers & Onions [320] • Scrambled Eggs, 4 oz [360]
Southwest Corn Casserole [400] • Roasted Potatoes, 4 oz [440]
Egg Whites & Cheddar Breakfast Sandwich [510] • Egg on a Bagel [580]

BAKED GOODS **160–820**
CROISSANT: Apple [160] • Choc [210] • Raspberry Cheese [280]
TORSADE: Golden Raisin/Creme [210] • Blueberry Lemon [220] • Choc/Creme [220]
BAGELS: Whole Wheat Skinny Bagel [230] • Cinn Crisp Bagel [410]
Cherry Strudel [270] • Apple Strudel [270] • Cherry Danish [340]
MUFFINS: Cranberry Walnut Muffin [500] • Blueberry Muffin [510]

SANDWICHES/WRAPS **480–1,960**
Kid's Hot Dog [480] • Classic Chicken Salad Sandwich, half [480]
Tuna Salad Sandwich, half [505] • Kid's Grilled Chicken on Multigrain [570]
Caprese w/Chicken [580] • Roast Beef & Herb Cheese Sandwich [620]
WRAPS (HALF): Chicken Caesar [650] • Mediterranean [655] • Moroccan Lemon [655]
　BREAD **490–720**
　Brioche Roll [490] • Country White Bread, 2 sl [580] • Tortilla Wrap [590]

SALADS *(w/o dressing)* **20–1,170**
Side Garden Salad [20] • Garden Salad [105]
Thai Peanut Chicken Salad [300] • Southwest Chicken Salad [360]
　DRESSINGS **190–740**
　FF Raspberry [190] • Balsamic Vinaigrette [360]

HARVEST RICE BOWLS **870–1,570**
Mayan Chicken w/Brown Rice [870]

SOUPS/STEWS **290–2,180**
SOUTHWEST VEGETABLE SOUP: sm [290] • med [430] • lrg [580]
TOMATO BASIL BISQUE: sm [360] • med [540]
Mediterranean Pepper Soup, sm [430] • Butternut Squash/Apple, sm [570]

HOT/COLD LUNCH BAR *(4 oz serving)* **60–600**
White Rice [60] • Tomato Cucumber Salad [160] • Broccoli & Carrots [160]
Pearl Barley w/Veg [180] • Roasted Chicken & Thyme [200]

Penne Marinara [200] • Green Beans [240] • Red Bliss Potato Salad [280]
Meatloaf w/Wine Sauce [300] • Vegetarian Lasagne [300]

TOPPINGS/CONDIMENTS/SPREADS **20–970**
Swiss Cheese [20] • Mozzarella Cheese [60] • Roasted Red Peppers [105]
Honey Pecan Cream Cheese [135] • Mayo [200] • Basil Pesto Sauce [210]

SWEETS/FRUIT/YOGURT **0–980**
Fresh Grapes [0] • Watermelon [0] • Choc Covered Almonds, 1/4 cup [10]
Fruit Cup [15] • Kind Bars, all varieties [25]
Mini Oatmeal Raisin Cookie [50] • Mini Choc Chip Cookie [115]
BLUEBERRY YOGURT (SM): w/Blueberries [135] • w/Blueberries & Granola [210]
Choc Mocha Whoopie Pie [150] • Chai Spice Whoopie Pie [190]

SPECIALTY DRINKS **25–180**
Iced Coffee, all (avg) [25] • Iced Chai Latte [90] • Ice Vanilla Latte [90]
BLASTS (MED): Mocha [95] • Vanilla [100] • Caramel [105] • Coffee [115]
SMOOTHIES (MED): Strawberry [110] • Peach [115]
Cappuccino [110] • Iced Mocha [110] • Caffe Latte [115]

AUNTIE ANNE'S

PRETZELS **210–1,180**
Cinn Sugar Party Pretzel [210] • Raisin Pretzel [390]
Almond Pretzel [400] • Cinn Sugar Pretzel [400] • Cinn Sugar Stix, 6 [400]
Original w/o Salt [400] • Garlic w/o Salt [400] • Sesame w/o Salt [400]
DIPPING SAUCES/CREAM CHEESE **0–580**
Sweet Dip [0] • Sweet Mustard [0] • Caramel Dip [95] • Cream Cheese [120]

DRINKS **10–510**
Icees, all sizes & flavors [10-20] • Lemonades, all sizes & flavors [10–30]
SMOOTHIES (14 OZ): Lemonade [120] • Kiwi-Banana [130] •
Pina Colada [130] • Strawberry [130] • Blue Raspberry [140]
LATTES (14 OZ): Mocha [160] • Caramel [170] • Coffee [180]
SHAKES: Vanilla [300] • Strawberry [300]

BACK YARD BURGERS

BURGERS/CHICKEN/SPECIALTY ITEMS **820–1,900**
BYB Mushroom Swiss Burger [820] • BYB Bak-Pak Dog [950]
CONDIMENTS **65–85**
Margarine Cup [65] • Mayonnaise, pkt [65] • Light Mayo, pkt [85]

SALADS *(w/o dressing)* **15–1,360**
Side Salad [15] • BYB Garden Fresh Salad [160] • BYB Grilled Chicken [950]
DRESSINGS **160–440**
Honey Mustard [160] • Balsamic Vinaigrette [330]

SIDES **690–1,740**
BYB Chili [690]

DESSERTS/SHAKES **55–390**
Ice Cream [55] • Blackberry Cobbler [170] • Blackberry Cobbler a la Mode [220]
Strawberry Shake [230] • Vanilla Shake [230]

BAHAMA BREEZE

APPETIZERS **140–2,980**
Tortilla Chips [140] • Flatbread Crisps [170] • Coconut Shrimp [220]
SAUCES/SALSAS **15–306**
Apple Mango [15] • Roasted Pineapple Salsa [50] • Sour Cream [65]
Black Bean & Tomato Salsa [126]

ENTREES **132–4,100**
Coconut Shrimp, 3 pc [132] • Salmon or Shrimp Saute, lunch [368]
JERK PAINTED (LUNCH): MahiMahi [285] • Halibut [293]
SIMPLY GRILLED (LUNCH): MahiMahi [293] • Salmon [300] • Halibut [308]
JERK PAINTED (DINNER): MahiMahi [375] • Halibut [385] • Salmon [395]
Center-Cut Filet Mignon w/Onion Ring & Grilled Tomato [400]

SOUPS **1,210–1,910**

SALADS *(w/o dressing)* **50–3,190**
House, side [50] • Caesar, side [210] • Grilled Chicken & Tropical Fruit [670]

DRESSINGS/ADDITIONS **125–600**
Citrus Mustard Dressing [125] • Croutons, 3 [180] • Blue Cheese Dressing [190]

SANDWICHES *(w/o sides)* **753–2,450**
Key West Fish Tacos, 3 [753] • Wood-Grilled Burger [830] • Hawaiian Burger [860]

SIDES **0–1,680**
Fruit Salad [0] • Plantains [0] • Seasonal Vegetables (Green Beans) [65]
Broccoli [125] • Black Bean and Corn Salsa [140]

DESSERTS **14–940**
Kid's Mango Sorbet [14] • Kid's Ice Cream [45] • Choc Island [440]

(BAJA FRESH MEXICAN GRILL)────────────────

TACOS **230–640**
ORIGINAL BAJA TACO: Chicken [230] • Steak [260] • Carnitas [280] • Shrimp [280]
Grilled Mahi Mahi Taco • Baja Fish Taco, Fried . . . . 300•420

BAJA FAVORITES **1,330–3,440**

SOUPS **2,600–2,760**

SALADS *(w/o dressing)* **430–2,520**
Side [430] • Baja, Charbroiled Shrimp [1,110] • Grilled Chicken Caesar [1,110]

DRESSINGS **290–470**
Olive Oil Vinaigrette [290] • FF Salsa Verde [370]

SIDE ITEMS **55–1,320**
Corn Tortilla Chips, sm [55] • Corn Tortilla Chips, lrg [170] • Guacamole [270]

(BASKIN ROBBINS)────────────────

CLASSIC FLAVORS *(small unless noted)* **10–210**
Daiquiri Ice, sm/lrg [10-35] • Sherbets, all flavors, sm/lrg [10–35]
Vanilla [45] • Very Berry Strawberry [45] • Cherries Jubilee [50]
Reduced Fat, No Sugar Added, all flavors [50]
Jamocha Almond Fudge [50] • Love Potion #3 [50] • Black Walnut [55]
Choc Chip [55] • Mint Choc Chip [55] • Egg Nog [55] • Peppermint [55]
Pistachio Almond [55] • Rum Raisin [55] • Winter White Choc [60]
Jamocha [60] • World Class Choc [60] • Creole Cream Cheese [60]
CONES: Waffle [5] • Cake [15] • Sugar [35]

SOFT SERVE/PARFAITS **75–630**
Vanilla, kids [75] • Strawberry 'n Almonds, mini [140] • w/M&Ms, mini [140]
Vanilla, reg [150] • Strawberry 'n Almonds, reg [240]

SUNDAES **200–950**
Banana Royale [200] • Two Scoop Sundae [200] • Classic Banana Split [240]

(BERTUCCI'S)────────────────

STARTERS **230–2,860**
Tuscan Chicken Wings [230] • Watermelon, Arugula & Feta [380]

PASTA *(lunch size)* 620–4,120
Rigatoni Broccoli Shrimp w/Wine Sauce [620]
Rigatoni Broccoli w/Wine Sauce [670] • Spaghetti Pomodoro [710]

MAIN ENTREE/POLLO/SEAFOOD 60–4,140
Kid's Rigatoni w/Butter [60] • Kid's Grilled Chicken w/Broccoli [180]
Kid's Grilled Chicken & Rigatoni w/Butter [230] • Pesto Grilled Salmon [260]
Kid's Crispy Chicken w/Broccoli [300] • Kid's Cheese Ravioli w/Butter [340]
Kid's Rigatoni w/Pasta Sauce [430] • Filet Mignon w/Chianti Sauce [440]

PIZZA *(1 slice)* 260–1,610
Margherita, individual or lrg [260] • Verde, individual or lrg [270]
Stella, individual [370] • Sofia, lrg [410] • Stella, lrg [420]
Plain Cheese, individual [430] • Plain Cheese, lrg [440]
Shrimp Belle Venezia, individual [470] • Sporkie, individual or lrg [470–480]

CALZONE/MENUCCI'S 860–1,180
Margherita Menucci [860] • Plain Cheese Menucci [910]

SANDWICHES 210–1,190
Italiano Rustic [210] • Americano Rustic [280] • Bello Rustic [300]

PANINI AL FORNO 1,000–1,960
Rosemary [1,000]

SALADS 170–1,280
Caesar, side [170] • Insalata (w/o dressing), side [180]
Caesar w/Chicken, side [290] • Insalata w/Chicken (w/o dressing), side [320]
Insalata w/Chicken [420] • Caesar Salad [500]

DRESSINGS 135–388
Lemon Dressing [135] • Lemon-Thyme Vinaigrette [135]

SOUPS 360–1,690
Tomato Florentine, cup [360] • Shrimp and Corn Chowder, cup [440]

SIDES 10–1,230
Rosemary Roasted Potatoes [10] • Roasted Green Beans [15]
Herb & Garlic Roasted Mushrooms [25] • Dinner Roll [40] • Asparagus [55]

SAUCES 10–610
Balsamic Nectar [10] • Marsala Sauce [65] • Piccata Sauce [70]
Roasted Tomato Sauce [80] • White Wine Sauce [85] • Pomodoro [95]

DESSERTS 0–420
Choc Budino [0] • Piccolo Budino [25] • Piccolo Tiramisu [30]
Hoodsie Ice Cream Cup [40] • Piccolo Limoncello Mascarpone Cake [40]
Tiramisu [55] • Full Limoncello Mascarpone Cake [80] • Tre Dolci [90]

BIG APPLE BAGELS/MY FAVORITE MUFFIN

BREAKFAST SANDWICHES 861–1,456
Morning Classic [861]

BAGELS 250–1,936
Quiche Lorraine Bagel [250] • Spinach Bagel [274]
Cinnamon Apple Pie Bagel [420] • Cinnamon Danish Bagel [428]
Cinnamon Bun Bagel [440] • Blueberry Cobbler Bagel [440]
Honey Oat Bagel [446] • White Choc Swirl Bagel [448]

CREAM CHEESE 65–200
Whipped Classic Plain [65] • Strawberry [65] • Whipped Brown Sugar Cinn [80]
Reduced Fat Spring Veggie [100] • Onion Chive [110] • Garden Veg [140]

MUFFINS 339–768
Deep Dish Apple Pie [339] • Banana Nut [363] • Cherry Cheesecake [372]
Pumpkin Spice [389] • Choc Cheesecake [399]

SANDWICHES/PIZZAAH **175–3,062**
Bruschetta Pizzaah [175] • Cheese Pizzaah [268] • Veggie Pizzaah [272]
Sausage Pizzaah [308] • Grilled Chicken Bruschetta Pizzaah [625]
Mediterranean Veg-Out Gourmet Sandwich [818]

SALADS **573–2,775**
Classic Caesar Cafe Salad [573] • Garden Mix Cafe Salad [684]

SOUPS **780–1,360**

SPECIALTY DRINKS **28–336**
Americano, 16 oz/20 oz [28–35] • Black Forest Coffee, 16 oz/20 oz [35–49]
Cafe Caramello, 16 oz/20 oz [40–49] • Strawberry Icepresso [120]
Italiano w/FF Milk, 16 oz [126] • Oregon Chai Tea Latte w/FF Milk, 16 oz [137]
Italiano w/2% Milk, 16 oz [138]

BLACK ANGUS STEAKHOUSE

STARTERS **1,000–4,090**

SANDWICHES *(w/o sides)* **535–2,810**
Kid's Hamburger [535] • Mushroom & Bleu Burger [1,442]
Filet Mignon Sandwich [1,563] • Chicken, Avocado & Bacon Sandwich [1,585]

ENTREES *(w/o sides)* **260–3,160**
FILET MIGNON, CENTER CUT: 6 oz [260] • 8 oz [286]
TOP SIRLOIN CENTER CUT: 8 oz [285] • 11 oz [320]
NY STRIP CENTER CUT: 12 oz [326] • 14 oz [349]
RIBEYE STEAK: 12 oz [329] • 16 oz [374]
Grilled King Salmon [387] • Bacon-Wrapped Filet, 6 oz [440]

SIDES **25–1,028**
Plain Baked Potato [25] • Classic Baked Potato [150]
Garden Salad (w/o dressing) [126] • Coleslaw [130]
  DRESSINGS **114–354**
    Honey Mustard [114] • Vinaigrette [154] • Cucumber [174]
  TOPPERS **121–140**
    Sauteed Sweet Onions [121] • Sauteed Mushroom & Onion [130]
    Sauteed Portabella Mushrooms [140]

BLIMPIE

BREAKFAST **240–2,570**
Bluffin, Plain [240] • Bagel [700] • Bagel w/Cream Cheese [780]
Cinn Roll [730] • Egg & Cheese on a Roll [740] • Bluffin, Egg & Cheese [770]

SANDWICHES/WRAPS **450–5,420**
Kid's Tuna Sub, 3" [450] • Tuna Sub, 6" [780]
BLT Sub, 6" [970] • Roast Beef & Provolone Sub, 6" wheat [970]

SANDWICH MAKINGS
BREADS: Pretzel Bread [75] • 6" Wheat [400] • 6" Honey Oat Bread [400] •
  6" White Bread [420] • Traditional Wrap, 12" [670] • Spinach Wrap, 12" [840]
  TOPPINGS/SAUCES **0–770**
    Lettuce [0] • Onion [0] • Tomato [0] • Blimpie Special Sauce [0]
    Swiss Cheese [45] • Honey Mustard [85] • Roasted Red Peppers [100]
    Sweet Pepper Strips, 6 [115] • Olives [125]
    Guacamole [135] • Pepper Jack [135]

SALADS *(w/o dressing)* **15–1,670**
Garden Salad [15] • Tuna Salad [370] • Chicken Caesar Salad [460]
  DRESSINGS **210–770**
    Peppercorn [210] • Dijon Honey Mustard [240] • Buttermilk Ranch [250]

FAST FOOD AND CASUAL DINING RESTAURANTS
Bob Evans

SOUPS **620–1,440**
Garden Veg [620] • Tomato Basil w/Raviolini [720] • Yankee Pot Roast [750]

SIDES/SNACKS **0–2,010**
POPCORN: reg [0] • lrg [5]
Multigrain SunChips [140] • Original SunChips [140] • Baked Potato [170]
Fritos [210] • Cole Slaw [240] • Baked BBQ Chips [240]

DESSERTS **0–210**
Cotton Candy [0] • Oatmeal Raisin Cookie [110] • Brownie [115]
White Choc Macadamia Nut Cookie [120] • Choc Chunk Cookie [125]

BOB EVANS

BREAKFAST **5–3,188**
Oatmeal, cup/bowl [5–9] • Fruit, dish/cup [7–8]
Hardcooked Egg, 1 [52] • Blueberry Banana Mini Fruit & Yogurt Parfait [61]
Fruit & Yogurt Plate [73] • Grits, cup [141] • Grits, bowl [252]
SCRAMBLED EGG WHITES: 1 Egg [90] • 2 Eggs [179] • 3 Eggs [269]
SCRAMBLED EGG LITES: 1 egg [119] • 2 eggs [238] • 3 eggs [362]
Multigrain Cranberry Sidecakes, 2 [234] • Scrambled Egg, 1 egg [238]
English Muffin [243] • French Toast, no topping, 1 slice [280]
Fruit & Yogurt Crepe, all varieties, 1 [275–292]
Multigrain or Cranberry Multigrain Hotcakes, 1 [468] • Be Fit Breakfast [537]
FFTF FRENCH TOAST: Strawberry-Blueberry [561] • Blueberry-Banana [613]
FFTF Veggie Omelet w/Fruit Dish & Wheat Toast w/Jelly [581]

ENTREES/MEALS **101–2,686**
Salmon, a la carte [101] • Garlic Butter Salmon, a la carte [174]
FFTF Grilled Salmon Fillet w/Baked Potato & Broccoli Florets [166]
Wildfire Salmon, a la carte [203] • FFTF Chicken-N-Noodles [365]
FFTF Chicken, Spinach & Tomato Pasta, Savor size [439]
FFTF Potato Crusted Flounder w/Baked Potato & Broccoli Florets [551]

SANDWICHES **491–3,122**
Kids Mini Cheeseburger [491] • Chicken Salad Sandwich, half [569]

SALADS **132–2,221**
Garden Salad (w/o dressing) [132] • Specialty Garden Salad [334]
FFTF Apple-Cranberry Spinach w/Reduced Fat Raspberry Dressing [463]
  DRESSINGS **105–741**
  Raspberry Reduced Fat [105] • Colonial [206] • Balsamic Vinaigrette [224]

SOUPS *(cup)* **365–1,593**
Roasted Chicken-N-Noodles [365] • Veg Beef Soup [526]

SIDES **0–1,564**
Baked Potato, plain [0] • Baked Potato w/margarine [32]
Lettuce & Tomato [4] • Tomato Slices [5] • Fruit, dish/cup [7–9] • Applesauce [11]
Broccoli Florets [33] • Glazed Carrots [99] • Corn [118] • French Fries [143]

DESSERTS/BAKERY **36–919**
Vanilla Ice Cream, 1 scoop [36] • Lemon Bundt Cake [90]
Double Choc Brownie [225] • Frosted Shortbread Cookie [229]

BOJANGLES

BREAKFAST **580–1,780**
Bo-Berry Biscuit [580] • Plain Biscuit [650]

CHICKEN/SANDWICHES **200–4,075**
Wing, 1 [200] • Breast, 1 [450] • Leg & Thigh [600]
Cajun Filet Sandwich [680]

SIDES **15–1,011**
Picnic Grits [15] • Botato Rounds, sm [312]

BOSTON MARKET

ENTREES *(w/o sides)* **310–1,640**
Kid's Turkey [310] • Kid's Beef Brisket [350] • Kid's Meatloaf [550]
Beef Brisket, reg [620] • Turkey Breast, reg [620]

SALADS. **650–1,640**
SW Santa Fe Salad, half [650] • Mediterranean Salad, half [690]

SOUPS. **1,300–3,060**

SANDWICHES **730–2,430**
Brisket Dip Carver, Au Jus [730] • All White Rotisserie Chicken Salad, half [780]

SIDES **55–1,050**
Sweet Corn [55] • Garlic Dill New Potatoes [80] • Green Beans [200]
Fresh Steamed Veggies [200] • Sweet Potato Casserole [250]

SAUCES. **85–240**
Poultry Gravy [85] • Honey Habanero [200]

DESSERTS. **330–460**

BREADSMITH

MUFFINS/SCONES. **140–710**
MUFFINS: Apple Cinn Walnut [140] • Choc [320] • Cranberry Orange [330]
Raisin Bran [350] • Zucchini [370]
SCONES: Pumpkin Choc Chip [370] • Pumpkin Cranberry [380] • Pumpkin Walnut [380]

BREAD. **10–260**
Reduced Carb, all varieties [10–15]
Stollen [45] • Vanilla Egg [50] • Egg [55] • Panettone [80]
French Baguette, 1" sl [90] • Greek Olive [95] • Pretzel Bread [95]
Apple Pie Bread [100] • Blueberry Pie [100] • Cherry Pie [100]
Honey Cake [110] • Icelandic Brown [110] • Austrian Pumpernickle [115]
Russian Rye [115] • Cherry Cordial [115] • Pain au Chocolat [125]
Bear Cheese [130] • Choc Cherry [130] • Farmer's Wheat [130]
Sweet Bellagio [130] • Poppyseed Babka [130] • Walnut Babka [130]
Rum Raisin Babka [135] • Potato Cheddar Chive [135] • Choc [130]
Cinn Spice [135] • English Muffin Bread [135] • Honey Raisin Pecan [140]
Maple Walnut [140] • Portuguese Sweet Bread [140] • Honey Challah [140]
Cherry Walnut [140] • Anise Sweet [140] • Granola Bread [140]
DESSERT BREAD **50–200**
Apple Cinn Walnut [50] • Choc Dessert Bread [95] • Cranberry Orange [100]
Zucchini Walnut [110] • Blueberry Corn Bread [135] • Lemon Poppyseed [140]

BUNS/ROLLS. **350–480**
Potato Flake Roll [350] • Soft Onion [410] • Soft Tomato Basil [410]
Soft Tomato Basil [410] • Soft Wheat Bun [410]

COOKIES/OTHER SWEETS **45–480**
Brownie w/Walnuts [45] • Brownie [55] • 1/2 Bostock [75]
BISCOTTI: Choc Hazelnut [70] • Almond [75] • Lemon Anise [90]
COOKIES: Choc Choc Chip [75] • Oatmeal Choc Chip [100] • Sugar [100] •
Oatmeal Raisin [100] • Lemon Sugar [100] • Orange Sugar [100]
1/2 Granola Bar [100] • 1/2 Choc Almond Stick [115]
COFFEE CAKE (1/2): Cherry [125] • Apple [130] • Blueberry [130]

OTHER ITEMS **70–270**
Almond Pecan Granola [70] • Cranberry Granola [70] • Vanilla Granola [80]

BRUEGGER'S

BREAKFAST. **170–1,670**
Whole Egg [170] • Egg White Patty [190] • Bacon [220]
Turkey Sausage [270] • Spinach & Cheddar Omelet [340]
BREAKFAST SANDWICH: Bagel w/Egg White & Sundried Tomato [870]

BAGELS. **152–1,540**
Bagel Bowl [152] • Trail Mix [340] • Cinn Sugar [420]
Choc Chip [480] • Cinn Raisin [480] • Cranberry Orange [480]
Honey Grain [490] • Blueberry [490] • Fortified Multi-Grain [500]
  CREAM CHEESE **100–150**
  Strawberry [100] • Onion & Chive [125] • Honey Walnut [125] • Plain [125]
  Light Herb Garlic [125] • Cucumber Dill [130] • Light Plain [130]
  Olive Pimiento [130] • Vermont Maple [135] • Pumpkin (seasonal) [135]

MUFFINS. **270–474**
Blueberry [270] • Cinn [280] • Corn [280] • Cranberry Nut [300]

SANDWICHES **540–2,430**
Garden Deli on Wheat [540] • Garden Deli on Bagel [550] • Tuna Salad on Bagel [870]
BREADS/WRAPS/SOFTWICHES: Bagel Bowl [152] • White Wrap [420]

SALADS *(w/o dressing)* **0–1,420**
Build Your Own Base [0] • Garden Salad, Cafe [90] • Caesar [220]
HARVEST CHICKEN SALAD: Cafe [350] • Entree [530]
SPICY THAI PEANUT CHICKEN SALAD: Cafe [400] • Entree [550]
Mandarin Medley, Cafe [530] • Mediterranean Mozzarella, Cafe [530]
  DRESSINGS **95–340**
  Asian Sesame Ginger [95] • Strawberry Vinaigrette [115]
  Romesco Red Pepper [140] • Spicy Peanut [140]

SOUPS. **570–1,240**
Spinach & Lentil [570] • New England Clam Chowder [600]
White Chicken Chili [630] • Butternut Squash [650]

CONDIMENTS/TOPPINGS **0–530**
Veggies (all except capers, jalapenos, pickles, roasted peppers) [0]
Cranberry Sauce [10] • Cranberry Horseradish Relish [20]
Sundried Tomato Spread [45] • Honey Mustard [45] • Swiss Cheese [60]
Pesto [70] • Chow Mein Noodles [70] • Mayo [100] • Hummus [120]
Chipotle Sauce [120] • Sundried Tomato Mayo [130] • Asiago Cheese [135]

DESSERTS. **25–340**
Choc Chunk Brownie [25] • Choc Chip Cookie [150]

BRUSTER'S REAL ICE CREAM

ICE CREAM/YOGURT/SORBET/SHERBET **15–105**
Strawberry Sorbet [15] • Orange Sherbet [20]
Vanilla Ice Cream [55] • Choc Ice Cream [60]
NO SUGAR ADDED: Vanilla [90] • Cinn [90] • Coffee [95] • Caramel Swirl [100] •
  Coffee Caramel Swirl [100] • Choc [100] • Choc Caramel Swirl [105] •
  Coffee Ripple [110] • Fudge Ripple [110]
Vanilla Yogurt [105] • Choc Yogurt [105]

BURGER KING

BREAKFAST. **100–2,920**
QUAKER OATMEAL: Original [100] • Maple & Brown Sugar Flavo [290]
French Toast Sticks, 3 pc [260] • French Toast Sticks, 5 pc [430]

Cini-minis, 4 [380] • Hash Brown Rounds, sm [410]
Croissan'wich, Egg & Cheese [620] • Breakfast Muffin, Egg & Cheese [650]

BURGERS/SANDWICHES/WRAPS/ENTREES 310–2,340
CHICKEN TENDERS: 4 pc [310] • 6 pc [460]
WHOPPER JR: w/o spread [450] • w/mayo [520]
Hamburger [460] • Double Hamburger [490]
Honey Mustard Crispy Chicken Wrap, half [495]
DIPPING SAUCE: Sweet & Sour Sauce [55] • Picante/Taco Sauce [115]

SALADS *(w/o dressing unless noted)* 100–1,750
Side Garden Salad [100] • Side Caesar Salad [250]
Chicken Apple/Cranberry Garden Salad w/Tendergrill (w/dressing) [950]

DRESSINGS/CROUTONS 115–440
Apple Cider Vinaigrette [115] • Croutons [160] • Lite Honey Balsamic [220]

SIDES 0–1,310
Apple Slices [0] • Applesauce [0] • French Fries, Value [330]

DESSERTS/SHAKES/SMOOTHIES........................... 20–550
SMOOTHIE (12–20 OZ): Strawberry Banana [20–50] • Tropical Mango [40–95]
Strawberry Sundae [125] • Soft Serve Cup [125] • Soft Serve Cone [130]
SHAKES (12 OZ): Vanilla [310] • Choc [310] • Strawberry [320]

(BURGERVILLE)

BREAKFAST..190–1,380
English Muffin [190] • English Muffin Sandwich w/Bacon [370]
Hash Brown Sticks [400] • Bagel [480]
Green Chili & Cheese Sandwich w/English Muffin [600]

BURGERS/CHICKEN/FISH................................410–1,400
ORIGINAL HAMBURGER: w/o spread [410] • w/spread [500]
Kid's Fish & Chips [470] • Kid's Chicken Tenders, 2 pc [520]
Classic Burger (w/o mayo) [660] • Turkey Club (w/o mayo, cheese & bacon) [660]
Original Cheeseburger [660] • Double Beef Cheeseburger (w/o spread) [660]
Spicy Anasazi Bean Burger (w/o mayo & cheese) [680]

SALADS *(w/o dressing)*................................100–1,750
Side Garden Salad [100] • Grilled Chicken Club Salad, half [390]
Wild Smoked Salmon Salad (w/o hazelnuts) [670]

DRESSINGS 105–430
FF Raspberry [105] • Balsamic Vinaigrette [135] • Honey Dijon [150]

SIDES 0–1,310
Apple Slices [0] • FRENCH FRIES: kids [55] • reg [100]

DESSERTS.. 100–160
Vanilla Ice Cream Cone [100] • Triple Berry YoCream Sundae [100]
Triple Berry Sundae [110] • YoCream Frozen Yogurt Cone [110]
Strawberry Splash Smoothie, 12 oz/16 oz [90–120]
MILKSHAKE (12 OZ): Fresh Strawberry [115] • Strawberry Splash [115]

(CAFE RIO MEXICAN GRILL)

BEANS/RICE 230–380
Black Beans [230] • Pinto Beans [230]

MEATS/ENTREES 40–370
Fire Grilled Steak [40] • Fire Grilled Chicken [45] • Fire Grilled Salmon [50]
Mahi Mahi [60] • Chile Roasted Beef [80] • Coconut Shrimp [140]
Pork Barbacoa [160] • Cancun Shrimp [170] • Chile Relleno [370]

SAUCES/TOPPINGS... 5–510
Lettuce [5] • Cabbage [5] • Salsa Fresca [5] • Sour Cream [10]
Pico de Gallo [40] • Cotija [110] • Cilantro Line Dressing [125]
Cheddar Jack Blend [170] • Guacamole [180] • Mango Sauce [190]

DESSERTS.. 110–195
Coconut Flan [110] • Choc Flan [130] • Tres Leche Cake [195] • Lime Pie [195]

CALIFORNIA PIZZA KITCHEN

APPETIZERS 501–2,079
White Corn Guacamole & Chips [501]

THIN CRUST PIZZA *(whole)* 1,840–4,163
Tricolore Salad [1,840] • Tricolore Salad w/Salmon [1.944] • Margherita [1,952]

PASTAS/SPECIALTIES/ENTREES.......................... 304–2,199
Kid's Buttered Fusilli [304] • Kid's Fusilli w/Meat Sauce [345]
Kid's Grilled Chicken Breast w/Broccoli [456]
Cedar Plank Salmon & Corn Succotash [558] • Kid's Fusille Alfred [559]
SMALL CRAVINGS: Crispy Mac 'N' Cheese [659] • Mediterranean Plate [690]

TACOS/SANDWICHES.................................... 369–2,862
Korean BBQ Steak Tacos (Small Cravings) [369]
Grilled Veg Sandwich w/Herb Onion [1,357] • Fish Tacos [1,410]
Fish Tacos w/Avocado [1,412]
Cranberry Walnut Chicken Salad Sandwich w/Herb Onion [1,420]
Steak Tacos [1,423] • Steak Tacos w/Avocado [1,426]

SALADS... 297–2,005
FIELD GREENS: half [297] • w/Sauteed Salmon, half [401] •
w/Grilled Shrimp, half [521]
CLASSIC CAESAR: half [343] • w/Sauteed Salmon [448] • w/Grilled Shrimp [568]
ROASTED VEG SALAD: half [396] • w/Sauteed Salmon, half [501]
The Wedge Salad [380] • Moroccan Chicken Salad, half [520]
THAI CRUNCH SALAD: half [538] • w/Avocado, half [543]
Caramelized Peach Salad, half [558]

SOUPS *(cup)* 617–1,373
Artichoke & Broccoli [617] • Smashed Pea & Barley [677] • Tortilla [695]

DESSERTS/SMOOTHIES/BLENDED BEVERAGES 2–643
Fresh Fruit [2] • Choc Souffle Cake [43] • Kid's Sundae [90]
APPLE CRISP: Plain [26] • w/Caramel [56] • w/Ice Cream [104]
Choc Souffle Cake w/Ice Cream [122] • Hot Fudge Sundae [170] • Tiramisu [213]
BLENDED DRINKS: Flavored Frozen Lemonade [9–28] • Flavored Coladas [27–39]
NF YOGURT SMOOTHIES: Strawberry Banana [98] • Mango Banana [98] •
Strawberry [130] • Mango [130] • Peach [130]

CALIFORNIA TORTILLA

BURRITOS/BOWLS 1,083–3,258
BURRITO IN A BOWL: Classic Steak [1,083] • Classic Veggie [1,267]
NOTE: Omitting rice reduces the amount of sodium by 480mg.

TACOS... 435–873
Steak Taco [435] • Chicken Taco [594] • Mesquite Chicken Taco [594]
Fish Taco [598] • Veggie & Bean Taco [631]

FAJITAS... 2,087–2,763

QUESADILLAS.. 863–1,896
Cheese Quesadilla [863] • Spinach Quesadilla [903]

SALADS...**546–1,961**
Southwestern Salad (w/o meat) [546]
DRESSINGS **97–350**
Honey Lime [97] • Fresh Salsa [106] • Lite Olive Oil Vinaigrette [159]
SIDES/EXTRAS **434–2,941**
Black Beans [434]

CAMILLE'S SIDEWALK CAFE

BREAKFAST...**12–2,059**
Seasonal Fruit Cup [12] • Breakfast on a Muffin w/Bacon [982]
WRAPS **1,330–2,864**
Poblano Chicken Natu [1,330] • Sonoma Veggie [1,441] • The Michelangelo [1,459]
SANDWICHES/PANINI *(w/o chips/salsa)*....................**836–1,910**
CAFE CHICKEN SALAD: on White [836] • on Rye [851] • on Wheatberry [881]
APPLE-WALNUT TUNA: on White [925] • on Rye [940] • on Wheatberry [970]
FLATBREAD PIZZA **937–1,676**
Rustic Italian [937] • Just a Cheese [1,028]
SOUPS *(small)* **920–1,860**
SALADS *(w/o dressing)*..................................**508–1,768**
The House Salad [508] • Bangkok Thai Salad [554] • Chef Salad [836]
DRESSINGS **390–911**
Honey Mustard [390]
DESSERTS.. **240–530**
White Choc Macadamia Nut Cookie [240] • White Choc Cherry Cookie [270]
SMOOTHIES **0–256**
Classic Blends, all [0–49]
YOGURT BLENDS: Blueberry Pie [101] • Strawberry Tweet [101] •
Island Time [105] • Get Going [131]

CAPTAIN D'S

FISH/SHRIMP/OTHER SELECTIONS **220–3,463**
Stuffed Crab Shell [220] • Premium Shrimp, 3 pc [323] • Chicken Tender, 1 pc [430]
Wild Alaskan Salmon, 1 pc [430] • Batter-Dipped Fish, 1 pc [454]
SANDWICHES **923–1,865**
Great Little Fish Sandwich w/o Cracklines [923]
SALADS *(w/o dressing)*................................... **9–497**
Side Salad [9] • Wild Alaskan Salmon [427]
Bite Size Shrimp Salad [437] • Fried Chicken Salad [497]
DRESSINGS **125–440**
Honey Mustard Dressing [125] • Ranch Dressing [210]
SIDES **10–1,200**
Corn on the Cob [10] • Plain Baked Potato [25] • Broccoli [30]
SAUCES..**360–1,300**
Scampi Sauce [360]
DESSERTS.. **220–270**
Cheesecake w/Strawberries [220] • Choc Cake [270]

CARL'S JR

BREAKFAST...**440–1,820**
Hash Brown Nuggets [440] • French Toast Dips, no syrup, 5 pcs [570]
Made From Scratch Biscuit [780] • Sunrise Croissant [810]

BURGERS/SANDWICHES/CHICKEN. 360–2,520
CHICKEN STARS: 4 pc [360] • 6 pc [540]
Kid's Hand-Breaded Chicken Tenders, 3 pc [520] • Kid's Hamburger [580]
Honey Mustard Hand-Breaded Chicken Tender Wrapper [640]
DIPPING SAUCES: Honey Mustard [190] • Buttermilk Ranch [300]

SALADS *(w/o dressing)*. 220–910
Side Salad [220] • Grilled Chicken Salad [850]

DRESSINGS 410–480

SIDES 490–1,710
Kid's Natural-Cut Fries [490] • Onion Rings [590]

DESSERTS/ICE CREAM DRINKS 230–420
Strawberry Swirl Cheesecake [230] • Oreo Ice Cream Sandwich [260]
Vanilla Shake [260] • Strawberry Shake [260]

CARROWS

BREAKFAST. 80–3,990
SR BREAKFAST: Oatmeal [80] • Cereal [105] • Potatoes & Toast [110] •
Fruit & Toast [130]
OMELETTE ONLY: Veg [460] • Spanish [600] • Bacon Avocado Jack [650]
Oatmeal w/Blueberries & Pecans [530] • Croissant French Toast [570]

MEALS *(w/o side dishes)*. . . . . .390 -4,170
Grilled Petite Sirloin Steak [390] • Grilled Cod [410] • Ribeye Steak [440]
Salmon Filet [450] • T-Bone Steak [470] • Sirloin Steak Dinner [680]

SANDWICHES/BURGERS. 660–2,790
Tuna Salad Croissant, half [660] • Turkey Bacon Avocado Stack, half [950]

SALADS. 160–1,750
Dinner Salad [160] • Southwest Chicken Salad, lunch [770]

DRESSINGS 230–520
Honey Mustard [230] • Chipotle Ranch [250]

SOUPS. 780–1,690
Chicken Tortilla [780]

SIDES 30–840
BAKED POTATO: Plain [30] • w/sour cream/butter/green onions [140]
Vegetable Blend [160]

DESSERTS/SHAKES 35–610
Ice Cream (all flavors): 1 scoop [35] • 2 scoops [70]
Root Beer Float [55] • Mini Hot Fudge Sundae [70]
Choc Cream Pie, slice [190] • Vanilla Malt [230] • Vanilla Shake [230]

CHARLEY'S GRILLED SUBS

BREAKFAST. 156–1,438
Two Eggs Scrambled [156] • Hash Browns [266] • Toast (2 pcs) [320]

SANDWICHES/CHICKEN *(w/o added salt)*. 755–1,890
Philly Veggie [755] • Mushroom Swiss Steak Sandwich [882]

SIDES 161–1,785
FRIES: Kids [161] • Regular [322]

SALADS *(w/o dressing)*. 383–1,333
Fresh Garden [383] • Grilled Chicken [533] • Grilled Steak Salad [693]

DRESSINGS 250

TOPPINGS. 0–470
Tomatoes/Lettuce [0] • Honey Mustard [30] • Spicy Brown Mustard [50] • Mayo [80]

CHECKERS/RALLY'S

BURGERS/HOT DOGS 570–1,610
Kid's Burger [570] • Chili Cheeseburger [620] • Checkerburger/Rallyburger [680]

CHICKEN/FISH/VEGGIE 710–3,420
Grilled Chicken Breast Sandwich [710] • Crispy Fish Sandwich [780] • BLT [830]
CLASSIC WINGS (5 PC): Honey BBQ [810] • Parmesan Garlic [830]

SIDES 700–1,880

SHAKES *(small)* 160–330
Banana [160] • Strawberry [170] • Choc [170] • Vanilla [180]

CHEVY'S

APPETIZERS 1,140–4,420

BURRITOS/TACOS/OTHER ENTREES (A LA CARTE). 200–4,590
Crispy Taco, Beef [200] • Beef Enchilada [300] • Crispy Taco, Chicken [350]
Crispy Carnitas Taco [370] • Salsa Chicken Enchilada [470]
Chicken Enchilada [470] • Carnitas Enchilada [490] • Soft Picadillo Beef Taco [500]
QUESADILLAS/SIZZLING FAJITAS 2,080–4,830

LUNCH BOWLS/BURGERS 1,000–3,270

SOUPS/SALADS *(w/o dressing)*. 100–2,636
Baby Greens, side [100] • Mixed Baby Greens [200] • Caesar Salad [310]
DRESSINGS 25–418
Apple Chipotle Vinaigrette [25] • Creamy Ranch [270] • Salsa Vinaigrette [280]
TORTILLA SOUP 1,180

SIDES 0–790
Tortilla Chips [0] • Sour Cream, 1 tbsp [10] • Sweet Corn Tamalito, 1 tbsp [15]
Pico de Gallo, 1 tbsp [40] • Guacamole, 1 tbsp [55]

DESSERTS. 125–1,070
Banana Brulee Split [125] • Flan [240]

CHICK-FIL-A

BREAKFAST. 45–1,910
Multigrain Oatmeal [45] • Multigrain Oatmeal w/toppings [290]
YOGURT PARFAIT: reg [60] • w/Choc Cookie Crumbs [85] • w/Granola [85]
Cinn Cluster [240] • Chick-n-Minis [370] • Hash Browns [380]
Sausage Breakfast Burrito [880]

SANDWICHES/CHICKEN 260–1,810
Chicken Nuggets, 8 pc [260] • Chicken Nuggets, 12 pc [400]
Chargrilled Chicken Sandwich [780]
DIPPING SAUCES 70–420
Honey Roasted BBQ [70] • Honey Mustard Sauce [150]

WRAPS 1,070–1,370
Chargrilled Chicken Cool Wrap [1,070] • Chicken Caesar Cool Wrap [1,290]

SALADS *(w/o dressing)*. 110–1,350
Side [110] • Chargrilled & Fruit Salad [450] • Chargrilled Chicken Garden [450]
DRESSINGS/TOPPINGS 25–510
Harvest Nut Granola [25] • Tortilla Strips [50] • Roasted Sunflower Kernels [55]
Spicy Dressing [130] • Reduced Fat Berry Balsamic Vinaigrette [150]

SIDES 0–1,130
Fruit, sm/med/lrg [0–5] • Waffle Potato Fries, sm [120]
Carrot & Raisin Salad, med [160]

DESSERTS/SHAKES **75–440**
Mini Sundae [75] • Icedream Cone [115] • Fudge Brownie [130]
SHAKES (SM): Vanilla [370] • Choc [380] • Strawberry [380]

CHICKEN EXPRESS

CHICKEN/FISH **40–1,120**
Catfish [40] • Hushpuppies, 3 pc [400] • Fried Chicken Liver [470]
Fried Chicken Wings [690]

SIDES **140–700**
Yeast Roll [140] • Cheese Sticks [280] • Cole Slaw [340]

DESSERTS.. **80–170**
Vanilla or Choc Soft Serve [80] • Fried Apple Pie [170]

CHILI'S

APPETIZERS **790–5,920**
Triple Dipper Hot Spinach/Artichoke Dip w/Chips [790]

SANDWICHES **440–6,510**
Kid's Pepper Pals Grilled Chicken Sandwich [440]
Pepper Pals Corn Dog [600] • Kid's Little Mouth Burger [630]
Southwestern BLT w/Fries [1,370] • Fajita Chicken Sandwich w/Fries [1,440]

ENTREES *(w/o sides)* **550–6,510**
Margarita Grilled Chicken [550] • Grilled Salmon w/Garlic & Herbs [570]

SALADS...**220–4,320**
House Salad (w/o dressing) [220] • Grilled Chicken Salad, lunch [610]
Caribbean Salad w/Grilled Chicken [810]

   DRESSINGS.. **220–510**
   Citrus Balsamic Vinaigrette [220] • Honey Lime [250]

SOUPS/CHILI **580–1,700**
Terlingua Chili w/toppings [580] • Loaded Baked Potato Soup, cup [590]

SIDES/ADDITIONS.....................................**0–1,300**
Avocado slices [0] • Sour Cream [55] • Swiss Cheese [105] • Cheddar [130]
Cinn Apples [130] • Guacamole [140]

SWEETS **210–930**
Frosty Choc Shake [210]

CHINESE GOURMET EXPRESS

ENTREES...**370–1,370**
Assorted Veg [370] • BBQ Pork [400] • Green Bean Chicken [410]
Curry Chicken [590] • Pineapple Chicken [650]

SIDES **0–1,230**
Steamed Rice [0] • Veg Egg Roll [95] • Pork [270]

CHIPOTLE MEXICAN GRILL

ENTREE *(before fillings/additions)* **0–670**
Burrito Bowl [0] • Salad [5]
TACOS: w/crispy corn tortillas [30] • w/soft corn tortillas [75]

   FILLINGS **0–540**
   Lettuce [0] • Sour Cream [30] • Brown Rice [150] • White Rice [200]
   Fajita Veg [170] • Cheese [180] • Guacamole [190]
   Tomatillo-Green Chili Salsa [230] • Black Beans [250] • Steak [320]
   Pinto Beans [330 • Chicken [370]

CHUCK E CHEESE

PIZZA *(1 slice)* **308–1,255**
  CHEESE: small [308] • medium [360] • large [404]
  VEGGIE COMBO: small [319] • medium [366] • large [402]
  SUPER COMB: small [393] • medium [453]
  BBQ CHICKEN: small [394] • large [447] • medium [460]
DESSERTS **6–1,308**
  Mandarin Oranges, side [6] • Cinnamon Sticks, 1 stick [87]
  Apple Dessert Pizza, 1 slice [164] • 1/4 Sheet Cake, Choc, 1 slice [200]

CHURCH'S CHICKEN

CHICKEN **160–1,980**
  Boneless Wing (w/o sauce) [160] • Original Leg [280] • Original Breast [440]
  Tender Strips [440] • Spicy Leg [470] • Spicy Tender Strips [480]
  Crispy Chicken Taco [600] • Original or Spicy Chicken Sandwich [660]
SIDES **15–800**
  Corn [15] • Cole Slaw [170] • Collard Greens [240]
SAUCES **35–570**
  Tartar Sauce [35] • BBQ Sauce [95] • Sweet & Sour Sauce [100]
  Honey Mustard [105] • Creamy Jalapeno Sauce [115] • Ketchup [150]
DESSERTS **360–790**
  Apple Pie [360]

CICI'S PIZZA

PIZZA *(1 slice)* **183–710**
  12" BUFFET PIZZA: Italiano Garlic [183] • Veg Italiano [210] • Pepperoni Flip [220] •
    Ole [240] • Mac & Cheese [250] • Italiano Pepperoni & Sausage [250] •
    The Meltdown [260] • Alfredo [270] • Spinach Alfredo [270] • Veggie [280] •
    Philly Cheesesteak [280] • Zesty Veggie [320] • Cheese [330] •
    Deep Dish Pepperoni [340] • Zesty Ham & Cheddar [340] •
    Zesty Pepperoni [340] • Ham & Pineapple [350] • Bacon Cheddar [350] •
    Classic Chicken [350] • Sausage [350]
  15" TO-GO PIZZAS: Macaroni & Cheese [310] • Veggie [340]
    Spinach Alfredo [380] • Zesty Veggie [390] • Lrg Pepperoni Deepdish [390]
PASTA W/MARINARA SAUCE **300**
SOUP/SALAD **180–520**
  Garden Salad [180] • Italian Salad [280] • Chicken Noodle Soup [520]
DESSERTS **100–290**
  Cinnamon Roll [100] • Brownie [125] • Bavarian Dessert [210]

CLAIM JUMPER

APPETIZERS **1,038–7,377**
BURGERS/SANDWICHES **777–4,030**
  Kid's Grilled Cheese [777] • Kid's Mini Corn Dogs [893]
ENTREES/MEALS **15–6,157**
  KID'S PASTA YOUR WAY: w/Butter [15] • w/Marinara [240] • w/Alfredo Sauce [375]
  Kid's Chicken Nuggets [468] • BBQ Chicken Breasts [583]
  Whiskey-Apple Glazed Chicken [591] • Kid's Mac 'n' Cheese [646]
PIZZA **1,096–3,346**
  Oven Roasted Tomato Flat Bread [1,096]

SOUPS **785–1,807**
Clam Chowder, cup [785] • French Onion, cup [952]

SALADS **200–2,090**
Vegetarian Chinese Salad [200] • Caesar, side [272] • Green Salad, sm [293]
House Salad [386] • Caesar, sm [481] • Chinese Chicken Salad [484]
BBQ Chicken Salad [518] • Spinach Salad [578] • California Citrus Salad [625]
  DRESSINGS **170–520**
    Citrus Vinaigrette [170] • Honey Mustard [231] • Ranch [233]

SIDES/BREADS **2–1,797**
Frozen Grapes [2] • Fruit, sm side [20] • Baked Potato [29] • Fruit, lrg side [48]
Apples & Caramel [77] • Green Beans [100] • Mashed Potatoes [160]
  BREADS **350–874**
    Sourdough Roll [350] • Blueberry Muffin [371]

DESSERTS **160–2,381**
Mini Hot Fudge Sundae [160] • Warm English Toffee Cake [326]

COLD STONE CREAMERY

ICE CREAM/SORBET **0–650**
Sorbet, all flavors & sizes [0–40]
SMALL ICE CREAM: Peach [45] • Strawberry Cheesecake [50] • Key Lime [50] •
  Blueberry [55] • Choc Dipped Strawberry [65] • Banana [70] •Mango [70] •
  Cotton Candy [75] • Macadamia Nut [75] • Orange Dreamsicle [75] •
  Mint [75] • Ghirardelli Choc [75] • Strawberry [75] • Raspberry [75] •
  Vanilla Bean [75] • White Choc [75] • Amaretto [80] • Irish Cream [80] •
  Choc Hazelnut [80] • Oreo Creme [80] • Coffee [80] • French Vanilla [80] •
  Coconut [80] • Cinnamon [80] • Sweet Cream [80] • Strawberry Basil [80] •
  Cheesecake [85] • Pistachio [85] • Pecan Praline [90] •
  Chocolate [95] • Dark Choc [95] • Mocha [95]
MEDIUM ICE CREAM: Peach [70] • Key Lime [80] • Strawberry Cheesecake [85] •
  Blueberry [90] • Choc Dipped Strawberry [100]

YOGURT *(like it)* **120–760**
Mango [120] • Pineapple [130] • Berry Tart [135] • Key Lime [140]
Blueberry Pomegranate [140] • Choc Hazelnut [140] • French Vanilla [140]
Blueberry Cheesecake [140] • Black Cherry [140] • Strawberry [140]
Amaretto [150] • Choc [150] • Cinnamon [150] • Coffee [150]
Cotton Candy [150] • Raspberry [150] • Mint [150] • Plain Tart [150]
Country Time Pink Lemonade [150] • Vanilla Bean [150] • White Choc [150]

CAKES **160–300**
BIRTHDAY CAKE: sm/med round [160] • rectangle [210]
Dark Peppermint Pleasure, sm round [200] • Choc Chipper, sm/med round [240]
Midnight Delight, sm/med round [240]

PIES/CUPCAKES/OTHER DESSERTS **135–1,610**
Sweet Cream Cupcake [135] • S'more Some More Pie [135]
Caramel Turtle Treat [140] • Mintastic Chip • Pumpkin Pie [140]
Caramel Apple Pie [160] • Double Choc Devotion [160]

SHAKES *(like it)* **240–1,120**
Creme de Menthe [240] • Savory Strawberry [260] • Cherry Cheeeshake [260]

SMOOTHIES **20–280**
Sinless, all varieties, all sizes [20–60] • Lifestyle, all varieties, sm [150–170]

COFFEE DRINKS **70–270**
Sweet Cream, all sizes [70–120] • Vanilla Creme Latte, all sizes [70–120]
Milk Caramel Latte, sm [110] • Rich Mocha Latte, sm [140]

CORNER BAKERY CAFE

BREAKFAST. **10–1,570**
Seasonal Fruit Medley [10] • Sweet Crisp [110] • Swiss Oatmeal [130]
Fresh Berry & Yogurt Parfait [170]
OATMEAL: w/o Toppings [230] • w/toppings [240]
Harvest Toast [270] • Breakfast Potatoes [290] • French Toast w/syrup [380]
Kid's Scrambler w/Toast/Fresh Fruit [540]
AVOCADO/SPINACH POWER PANINI THIN: w/egg whites [580] • w/whole eggs [590]
Kid's Cheesy Scrambler w/toast & fresh fruit [630]
FARMER'S SCRAMBLER: w/egg whites [660] • w/whole eggs [690]
   BAGELS/MUFFINS/PASTRIES **370–800**
      Croissant [370] • Blueberry Muffin [380]

SALADS. **240–2,800**
Caesar Salad, side [240]
AVOCADO WEDGE: cafe/combo [310] • entree [410]
MIXED GREENS: side [420] • cafe/combo [460]
Trio D.C. Chicken Salad [510] • Trio Egg Salad [520] • Trio Tuna Salad [530]
Trio Asian Edamame Salad [560] • Caesar, cafe/combo [660]
   DRESSINGS. **160–1,280**
      Balsamic Vinaigrette [160] • Light Ranch [220]

SOUP. **930–2,290**

PASTA **300–1,700**
Pasta w/Cream Sauce [290] • Kid's Pasta Marinara [360]
Penne w/Marinara, combo [450] • Kid's Half Moon Cheese Ravioli [640]
Half Moon Cheese Ravioli, combo [680] • Pesto Cavatappi, combo [690]

SANDWICHES *(on harveswt bread unless noted)*. **440–3,570**
Kid's Turkey [440] • Kid's Grilled Cheese [480]
Mom's Roasted Chicken, combo [580]
Mom's Tuna Salad, combo [620] • Calif Grille Panini, combo [630]
   BREADS **95–500**
      Traditional Sesame Baguette [95] • Raisin Pecan Miche [130]

SIDES . . . . **10 -330**
Seasonal Fruit Medley [10] • Baby Carrots [65] • Bakery Chips [120]

CAKES/SWEETS **120–650**
RUGALACH: Cinnamon Pecan [120] • Apricot Walnut [125]
COOKIES: Sugar [240] • Snickerdoodle [240] • Choc Chip [290] • Monster [300]
Lemon Bar [280] • Pumpkin Whoopee Pie [290]

HOT DRINKS **70–370**
Cappuccino, 12 oz/18 oz/20 oz [70–135] • Lattee, 12 oz/18 oz/20 oz [130–210]
Chai Latte: 12 oz [135] • 14 oz [180] • Truffle Mocha, 12 oz [150]
Truffle Hot Choc w/whipped cream, 12 oz [190]

COSI

BREAKFAST. **18–1,165**
Fruit Salad [18] • Cosi Break Bar [18] • Cosi Oatmeal [98]
FRESH FRUIT YOGURT PARFAIT: Strawberry [229]• Bananas Foster [238]
Veggie Quiche [466] • Spinach Florentine Breakfast Wrap [646]
   SQUAGELS **215–1,149**
      Whole Grain [215] • Plain [228] • Choc Chip [237]
      Cranberry Orange [239] • Cinn Raisin [239] • Sesame [241] • Poppyseed [242]
   MUFFINS/SCONES **280–470**
      Blueberry Scone [280]

MUFFINS: Carrot [420] • Raisin Bran [420] • Choc Choc Chip [420]

CREAM CHEESE **111–266**
Fruit Trio [111] • Plain [229]

SANDWICHES/MELTS **185–1,898**
Kid's Peanut Butter & Jelly [185] • TBM Sandwich [252] • Kid's Turkey [262]
Fire-Roasted Veggie [291] • Kid's Gooey Grilled Cheese [314] • TBM Light [326]
Chicken TBM [364] • Chicken TBM Light [437] • Steak TBM [449]
Tuscan Pesto Chicken [454] • Kid's Tuna [462] • TBM Melt [472]
Pesto Chicken Melt [508] • Turkey Light [526] • Hummus & Veggie [532]
Grilled Chicken TBM Melt [570] • Steak TBM Melt [665]

FLATBREAD PIZZA **198–1,455**
Kid's Traditional Cheese [198] • Traditional Cheese [397]
Margherita [410] • Kid's Pepperoni [467] • Margherita w/Chicken [521]

FLATBREADS **72–82**

SALADS *(w/o dressing)* **504–1,543**
Signature Salad Light [504] • Signature Salad [682]

DRESSINGS **151–749**
Sherry Shallot [151] • Balsamic Vinaigrette [169] • LF Sherry Shallot [170]

SOUP *(side)* **460–2,082**
Pollo e Pasta Soup [460] • Southwestern Corn & Turkey Chili [477]
Chicken Queso Tortilla [509] • New England Clam Chowder [571]

DESSERTS **233–1,065**
Cosi Bread Pudding [233] • S'mores [234]

COUSINS SUBS

SUBS **330–4,000**
5" Mini Garden Provolone (Better Bunch) [330] • 5" Mini Tuna [531]
5" Mini Ham & Provolone (Better Bunch) [740]

SOUPS **753–1,695**
Cream of Potato, reg [753] • Cream of Broccoli w/Cheese, reg [823]

SALADS *(w/o dressing)* **30–1,330**
BETTER BUNCH: Gourmet Garden [30] • Almond Berry Chicken [240] •
Gourmet Garden w/Chicken [610]
Almond Berry Chicken Salad [560]

DRESSINGS **370–400**

SIDE ITEMS **150–288**
French Fries, small [150]

COOKIES **60–260**
Snickerdoodle [60] • Oatmeal Cranberry Walnut [100] • Oatmeal Raisin [110]
Choc Chip [120] • Choc Chip w/M&Ms [125] • White Chunk Macadamia [125]
Double Choc Chip [130] • Peanut Butter w/Reese's Pieces [140]

CULVER'S

BURGERS **440–1,831**
BUTTERBURGER "THE ORIGINAL": single [440] • double [470]
Kid's Chicken Tenders, 2 pc [576] • Cheddar ButterBurger, single [580]
Mushroom & Swiss ButterBurger, single [581]
Sourdough Melt, single [600] • Wisconsin Melt, single [605]

SANDWICHES/FAVORITES **816–2,010**
Grilled Chicken [816] • Beef Pot Roast [948] • No Atlantic Cod Filet [979]

DINNERS **1,276–3,616**
Chopped Steak [1,276] • Beef Pot Roast [1,710]

SALADS. **102–1,445**
Side Salad [102] • Side Caesar [169] • Garden Fresco [375]
DRESSINGS **170–500**
Raspberry Vinaigrette [170] • French Dressing [320]

SOUPS. **650–2,010**
Tomato Basil Ravioletti [650]

SIDE ITEMS. **10–1,740**
Applesauce [10] • CRINKLE CUT FRIES: sm [40] • reg [56] • lrg [72]
Green Beans [115] • Dinner Roll [200] • Mashed Potatoes [204]

DESSERTS. **4–608**
Lemon Ice, 1, 2, or 3 scoops [4–6] • Vanilla Cake Cone, mini scoop [63}
Choc Cake Cone, 1 scoop [77] • Vanilla Dish, 1 scoop [84]
Vanilla Cake Cone, 2 scoops [99] • Choc Dish, 1 scoop [118]
Vanilla Waffle Cone, 1 scoop [119] • Choc Cake Cone, 1 scoop [123]

SPECIALTY DRINKS. **7–566**
Lemon Ice Cooler (no topping), med [7] • Lemon Ice Smoothie (no topping), med [76]
ROOT BEER FLOAT: short [108] • med [120]

D'ANGELO

SUBS/POKKET SANDWICHES. **340–5,980**
Kidz Turkey Sub [340] • Turkey Pokket, sm [360] • Turkey Pokket, med [380]
Hamburger Pokket, sm [420] • Turkey Sub, sm [510] • Hamburger Sub, sm [540]
Kidz Tuna Sub [550] • Mushroom Swiss Burger Pokket [550]
Cranberry Pecan Chicken Salad Pokket [590]

WRAPS/QUESADILLAS. **640–2,590**
Turkey Wrap [640] • Cranberry Wrap [790] • Mushroom Swiss Wrap [800]
Veggie Quesadilla [810] • Turkey Club Wrap [880]

SOUPS. **270–1,380**
HEARTY VEGETABLE: sm [270] • lrg [400]
Tuscan Pasta & Bean, sm [430] • Butternut Squash & Apple, sm [540]

SALADS *(w/o dressing)*. **25–2,040**
Tossed Salad [25] • Pokket Salad [310] • Cobb Salad [610]
DRESSINGS **510–1,260**
Honey Mustard [510]

BREADS/TOPPINGS. **310–930**
White Pokket Bread [310] • White Sub, sm [470] • Multigrain Sub, sm [470]
TOPPINGS **0–2,860**
Cucumber, lettuce, mushrooms, onions, sweet peppers, or tomato [0]
Swiss Cheese [60] • Mayonnaise [65]

DESSERTS. **180–500**
Choc Brownie [180]

DAPHNE'S GREEK CAFE

STARTERS. **520–1,302**
Orig Hummus & Pita [520] • Orig hummus & Multigrain Pita Chips [540]

MEALS/ENTREES/SANDWICHES. **230–2,332**
Grilled Steak Kabob [230] • Falafel [320] • Kid's Fresh-Carved Gyros [340]
Kid's Fresh-Carved Gyros Street Pita [340] • Kid's Grilled Chicken Street Pita [350]
Crispy Shrimp [410] • Grilled Salmon Plate [490] • Kid's Grilled Cheese [500]
Fresh-Carved Gyros Plate [520] • Grilled Chicken Kabob Plate [560]
STREET PITAS (1): Falafel [590] • Fresh-Carved Gyros [640] • Grilled Chicken [650]
Falafel & Spanakopita dinner [640]

SALADS *(w/o dressing)*.. 230–1,190
   Side Greek Salad [230] • Side Greek Salad w/Lite Dressing [350]
   Classic Greek Salad [590] • Chicken Pine Nut Salad [950]

   DRESSINGS 150–410
     Pomegranate Dressing [150] • Greek Lite Dressing [180]

SIDES/TOPPINGS 40–600
   Gaucamole [40] • Orig Hummus [130] • Tzatziki Sauce [140] • Fire Feta [180]
   Tabouli [230] • Multigrain Pita Chips [270] • Fire-Roasted Veg [270]

DESSERTS... 35–320
   Caramel Pecan [35] • Shortbread Cookie [65] • Baklava [170]

(DEL TACO)

BREAKFAST.. 180–1,440
   HASH BROWN STICKS: 5 pc [180] • 8 pc [290]
   Sausage Biscuit [370] • Sausage, Egg & Cheese Muffin [480]
   Sausage, Egg & Cheese Biscuit [480] • Breakfast Burrito [570]

TACOS... 180–790
   Taco [180] • Deluxe Taco [260] • Chicken al Carbon Taco [300]
   Classic Taco [320] • Crispy Fish Taco [320] • Soft Taco [330]
   Chicken Asado Taco [380] • Steak Taco al Carbon [400]
   Classic Soft Taco [470] • Steak Asada Taco [480] • Grilled Chicken Taco [490]

BURRITOS/QUESADILLAS.................................... 540–3,460
   Kid's Quesadilla (2 pack) [540] • Spicy Jack Quesadilla [820]
   Cheddar Quesadilla [840] • Classic Grilled Chicken Burrito [870]

BURGERS/SALADS/NACHOS.................................. 530-2,470
   Nachos [530] • Hamburger [560] • Tostada [850]

SIDES 5–3,490
   Sour Cream [5] • Guacamole [65] • Kid's Fries [190] • Chips & Salsa [200]

DESSERTS/SHAKES 0–600
   Churro w/Cinnamon & Sugar [0] • Choc Chip Cookie [85]

   SHAKES 300–350

(DENNY'S)

BREAKFAST.. 7–3,410
   Seasonal Fruit [7] • Grits w/Margarine [15] • Yogurt, LF, 6 oz [100]
   Toast w/Margarine, 2 slices [110] • 2 egg whites [180] • 2 eggs [235]
   Oatmeal w/Milk [220] • English Muffin w/o margarine [250]
   Bagel & Cream Cheese [560] • Harvest Oatmeal Breakfast [600]
   Red-Skinned Potatoes [630] • Hash Browns [650]
   Veggie-Cheese Omelette [680] • Senior Fit Fair Omelette [690]

APPETIZERS 225–930
   Smothered Cheese Fries, 1/4 [225]

BURGERS/SANDWICHES...................................... 620–3,760
   Bacon, Lettuce & Tomato (no condiments) [620]

ENTREES/DINNERS.. 290–2,920
   Senior Starter [290] • Kid's Spaghetti [430] • Kid's Mac & Cheese [570]
  Senior Grilled Chicken w/Bread [710]

SALADS *(w/o dressing unless noted)* 150–1,180
   Garden Salad [150] • Grilled Chicken Deluxe Salad [530]
   CRANBERRY APPLE CHICKEN W/BALSAMIC VINAIGRETTE: half [590] • full [610]

SOUPS.. 1,150–1,710

SIDES **3–750**
    Tomato Slices [3] • Broccoli [20] • Corn [45] • Fit Fare Veggies [85]
    Kid's French Fries [95] • Salted French Fries [95] • Sauteed Spinach [125]

DESSERTS/SPECIALTY DRINKS **25–740**
    Desert Blush [25] • Strawberry Banana Bliss [30] • Ice Cream, all flavors [87]
    Kid's Vanilla Yogurt w/Strawberry [100] • Floats, all flavors [120]
    Milk Shakes, all flavors [170] • Banana Split [190]

DICKEY'S BARBECUE PIT

BREAKFAST. **240–1,200**
    Scrambled Eggs [240] • French Toast [270] • Breakfast Burrito [500]

MEAT. **105–2,390**
    Turkey Breast [105] • Brisket [120] • Turkey [130] • Half Chicken [260]
    Chicken Breast [290]

SALADS. **20–850**
    Fresh Fruit Salad [20] • Original Potato Salad [55] • Broccoli Salad [200]
    CAESAR SALAD: w/o croutons [280] • w/croutons [310]
    Taco Salad [400]
    OLIVE VINAIGRETTE DRESSING **100**

SIDES/BREADS **15–2,960**
    Baked Potato [15] • Corn on the Cob [15] • Fries [50]
    Texas Toast w/Pan & Grill [85] • Jalapeno Beans [125] • Mashed Potatoes [140]
    Black Eyed Peas [160] • Stir Fried Broccoli [200]

SAUCES. **90–350**
    Basting Sauce [90] • Barbecue [110] • Low Carb Barbecue Sauce [120]

DESSERTS. **150–580**
    Soft Serve Ice Cream [150] • Banana Pudding [230] • Peach Cobbler [230]

DOMINO'S PIZZA

PIZZA **250–11,130**
    ARTISAN (1/8 SL): Spinach & Feta [250] • Tuscan Salami & Roasted Veggie [280] •
      Italian Sausage & Pepper Trio [330] • Chicken & Bacon Carbonara [360]
    Cheese w/Garlic Parmesan Sauce, Thin Crust, sm, 1/4 [302]
    MADE TO ORDER
      CRUSTS **75–258**
        Gluten Free, 10", 1/6 [75] • Thin Crust, sm, 1/4 [85] • Thin, med 1/4 [120]
        Thin Crust, lrg, 1/4 [180] • Thin crust, extra lrg, 1/4 [230]
      SAUCES **77–176**
        BBQ Sauce: sm [77] • med [128]
        Garlic Parmesan, sm [85] • New Pizza Sauce, sm [113]
        Hearty Marinara, sm [133]
      TOPPINGS (FOR ENTIRE SMALL PIZZA) **0–414**
        Onions, Green Peppers, Pineapple, Green Chile Pepper, or Garlic [0–5]
        Mushrooms [15] • Spinach [35] • Roasted Red Pepper [70]
        Cheddar Cheese [180] • Banana Peppers [200] • Tomato [220]
        Provolone Cheese [240] • Feta Cheese [250] • Black Olives [310]

SALADS *(w/o dressing)*. **160–590**
    Garden Fresh [160] • Grilled Chicken Caesar [590]
    DRESSINGS **360–770**

DESSERTS. **86–340**
    CinnaStix, 1 [86] • Choc Lava Crunch Cake, 1 [170]

DONATOS PIZZERIA

PIZZA **959–2,932**
HAND TOSSED (2 SL): Margherita [959] • Chicken Vegy Medley [1,038]
NO DOUGH (WHOLE PIZZA): Margherita [1,044] •
   Chicken Spinach Mozzarella [1,147] • Hawaiian [1,199]
HAND TOSSED (2 SL): Chicken Spinach Mozzarella [1,061]
THIN CRUST (INDIVIDUAL OR 1/4 LRG): Margherita [1,164]

STROMBOLI. **784–1,877**
Deluxe, half [784] • Cheese, half [887] • Pepperoni, half [888]

SUBS *(1/2 on wheat)* **764–3,108**
Fresh Vegy [764] • Chicken Bacon Cheddar [903]

SALADS. **25–1,190**
Harvest Salad, side [25] • Italian Salad, side [290] • Chef [1,040]
DRESSINGS **40–790**
   Apple Cider Vinaigrette [40] • Dijon Honey Mustard [250]

SIDE ITEMS **195–1,032**
3 Cheese Garlic Bread, 1 pc [195]

DESSERTS. **90–478**
Cinnamon Twists, 2 [90] • Choc Chunk Cookie [330]

DON PABLO'S

APPETIZERS *(1/4)* **64–2,473**
Chips & Salsa [64] • Guacamole Appetizer [204]

MEALS/ENTREES **307–6,232**
Chicken Tamale [307] • Pecos Valley Veggie Fajita [315] • Beef Crispy Taco [406]
Chipotle Portabella Mushroom Fajita [545] • Chicken Enchilada [560]
Mama's Skinny Enchilada [570] • Cheese & Onion Enchilada [583]
Chicken Crispy Taco [583] • Steak Fajita, lunch sized [622]
Steak & Chicken Fajita, lunch size [641] • Chicken Fajita, lunch size [642]

SANDWICHES **805–2,506**
The Don's Chicken Sandwich [805] • The Don's Burger [839]

SALADS. **58–4,877**
Tortilla Salad: w/o shell [58] • w/shell [407] • Side Salad [104]
DRESSINGS **119–718**
   Ranch [119] • Cilantro Ranch [121] • Honey Lime Dressing [152]

SOUPS. **674–3,691**
White Chicken Chili, cup [674]

SIDES **21–1,138**
Mexican Rice [21] • Seasoned Vegetables aka Pecos Valley Veggies [83]

DESSERTS. **31–1,324**
Vanilla Ice Cream, 1 scoop [31]

DQ/DAIRY QUEEN

BREAKFAST. **210–2,200**
Hash Browns [210] • Pancake Platter [740] • Sausage Biscuit Sandwich [930]

BURGERS/SANDWICHES/ENTREES. **450–3,650**
Corn Dog [450] • Deluxe Hamburger [680] • BBQ Beef Sandwich [700]
Deluxe Double Hamburger [750] • Kids' Chicken Strip, 2 [750]
Grilled Chicken Wrap [800] • Crispy Chicken Wrap [820]
1/4 lb Mushroom Swiss Grillburger [820]

SALADS **20–1,230**
  Side Salad [20] • Grilled Chicken Salad [890]
  DRESSINGS **320–430**
    FF Red French [320]

SIDE ITEMS **400–2,360**
  French Fries, Kids' [400]

DESSERTS **0–580**
  Banana [0] • Starkiss Bar, all flavors [10] • Applesauce [30]
  Vanilla Orange Bar [40] • No Sugar Added Dilly Bar [60] • Choc Dilly Bar [70]
  Choc Mint Dilly Bar [70] • Fudge Bar [70]
  VANILLA CONE: Kids [70] • sm [100] • med [140]
  CHOC DIPPED CONE: Kids [75] • sm [105]
  CHOC CONE: Kids [80] • sm [115]
  Cherry Dilly Bar [80] • Heath Dilly Bar [95] • Butterscotch Dilly Bar [105]
  DQ Sandwich [135] • Plain Waffle Cone w/Soft Serve [135]
  SUNDAES *(sm unless noted)* **90–540**
    Banana [90] • Cherry [100] • Pineapple [100] • Marshmallow [105]
    Strawberry [105] • Choc [115] • Banana, med [130] • Hot Fudge [135]
    Caramel [140] • Cherry, med [140] • Pineapple, med [140] • Strawberry, med [140]
  BLIZZARDS *(mini)* **115–1,000**
    Banana Split [115] • Hawaiian [125] • Choco Cherry Love [125]
    M&Ms Choc Candy [125] • Midnight Truffle [150]
    Butterfinger, mini [160] • Strawberry CheeseQuake, mini [160]

SPECIALTY DRINKS **0–900**
  Arctic Rush Frozen, all flavors, all sizes [0] •
  Arctic Rush Float, all flavors, sm/med [95–115]
  Arctic Rush Freeze, all flavors, sm [140]
  SHAKES (SM): Banana [190 • Cherry [200] • Vanilla [200] • Strawberry [200]
  Banana Malt, sm [230]

(**DUNKIN' DONUTS**)───────────────────────────

BREAKFAST **340–1,380**
  Egg White Veggie Wake-Up Wrap [340] • Egg White Western Wake-Up Wrap [340]
  Egg White Turkey Sausage Wake-Up Wrap [400] • Egg Wake-Up Wrap [470]
  Egg w/Bacon Wake-Up Wrap [580] • Egg w/Sausage Wake-Up Wrap [730]

DONUTS **105–540**
  French Cruller [105] • Sugared Cocoa [240] • Vanilla Frosted Cocoa [250]
  Triple Cocoa [260] • Vanilla Cocoa Kreme [260] • Dad's Heart [270]
  Cocoa Glazed [280] • Powdered Cocoa [280] • Glazed Cocoa Jelly [280]

MUNCHKINS **35–85**
  Cocoa Glazed Cocoa Kreme Puff [35] • Double Cocoa Kreme Puff [45]

DANISHES/FRITTERS/OTHER BAKERY **250–620**
  Brownie [250] • Strawberry Cheese Danish [260] • Cheese Danish [270]
  Apple Cheese Danish [270] • Fritters, all varieties [360–380]
  MUFFINS: Honey Bran Raisin [410] • Blueberry Muffin [450]

BAGELS **500–3,350**
  Cinn Raisin [500] • Wheat [500] • Multigrain [500] • Cinn Bagel Twist [510]

SANDWICHES **750–1,560**
  Tuna Salad on English Muffin [750]

COOKIES **220–380**
  Oatmeal Raisin Cookie [220]

FAST FOOD AND CASUAL DINING RESTAURANTS
East of Chicago

BEVERAGES **5–650**
Tea [5] • Coffee [5] • Espresso, no added milk [20]
SPECIALTY COFFEE *(small)* **70–220**
Cappuccino [70] • Mocha Spice Latte (or Iced) [95]
CARAMEL MOCHA LATTE (OR ICED): w/skim [105] • reg milk [115]
LATTE (OR ICED): w/skim [105] • reg milk [110]
Latte Lite (or Iced) [110] • Vanilla Latte Lite (or Iced) [110]
Mocha Raspberry [110] • Mocha Swirl Latte (or Iced) [115]
COOLATTAS **15–350**
Orange or Strawberry Coolatta, sm/med/lrg [15–70]
FROZEN BEVERAGES *(small)* **70–440**
Frozen Coffee [70] • Frozen Coffee, med [130] • Frozen Mocha [130]
HOT CHOCOLATE/CHAI **180–650**

EAST OF CHICAGO

PIZZA **160–1,210**
9" THIN CRUST (1/6): PBJ [160] • Cheese [260] • Taco [290] •
Dutch Crunch [310] • Garden Veg [350] • BBQ Chicken [370]
14" PAN PIZZA (1/12): PBJ [160] • Dutch Crunch [380] • Chees [410]
6" PAN PIZZA (1/4): PBJ [210] • Cheese [270] • Taco [270] •
Dutch Crunch [310] • Garden Veg [330] • BBQ Chicken [350]
14" CRISPY (1/12): Cheese [220] • Taco [290] •
Garden Veg [330] • BBQ Chicken [360]
9" PAN PIZZA (1/6): PBJ [230] • Cheese [320] • Taco [330] •
Dutch Crunch [370] • Garden Veg [390]
12" THIN CRUST (1/8): PBJ [230] • Dutch Crunch [340] • Cheese [400]
14" THIN CRUST (1/12): PBJ [230] • Dutch Crunch [350] • Cheese [380]
12" CRISPY (1/8): Cheese [240] • Taco [280] • Garden Veg [370]
12" PAN PIZZA (1/8): PBJ [300] • Dutch Crunch [410]

EINSTEIN BROS

BREAKFAST EGG SANDWICHES/WRAPS **420–1,660**
Asparagus, Mushroom & Swiss Bagel Thin Egg White Sandwich [420]
Cheese Only Egg Sandwich [710] • Spicy Elmo Breakfast Wrap [820]
Spinach/Mushroom/Swiss Sandwich [820] • Bacon/Cheddar Sandwich [840]
BAGELS **120–770**
BAGEL THIN SINGLES: Honey Whole Wheat [120] • Plain [240] • Everything [400]
Power Bagel [280] • Apple & Cinn Oatmeal [410] • Cranberry [420]
Choc Chip [430] • Good Grains [440] • Cinnamon Raisin [450]
CREAM CHEESE **80–210**
WHIPPED REDUCED FAT: Honey Almond [80] • Blueberry [90] • Strawberry [90] •
Onion & Chive [105] • Plain [115]
SANDWICHES/WRAPS **410–3,000**
Asparagus, Mushroom & Swiss Bagel Thin Sandwich [410]
California Chicken Wrap, half [565] • Veg Out on Sesame Seed Bagel [610]
Chicken Salad Sandwich [630] • Tuscan Chicken Pesto Bagel Thin [750]
SALADS **220–1,940**
STRAWBERRY CHICKEN: half [220] • full [340]
CHIPOTLE CHICKEN: half [460] • full [620]
DRESSINGS **210–1,180**
Raspberry Vinaigrette [210]
SOUPS **1,120–1,910**

SIDES **25–360**
Fruit Cup [25] • Fruit & Yogurt Parfait [115] • Potato Salad [360]

DESSERTS **0–490**
Cinn Twist [0] • Choc Mudslide Cookie [75] • Marshmallow Crispy Treat [125]

SPECIALTY BEVERAGES **95–320**
CAPPUCCINO: reg [95] • med [125]
LATTE (REG): Caffe Latte [115] • Vanilla [115] • Chai Tea Latte [115] •
Vanilla Hazelnut [120] • Sugar Free Vanilla or Vanilla Hazelnut [125]
Caramel Macciato, reg [115] • Fruit Smoothies, all flavors [115]
Frozen Blended Drinks [125] • Iced Caramel Macchiato, med [130]
Iced Latte, med [140] • Iced Vanilla Latte, med [140]

(ELEPHANT BAR)

OPENERS **860–4,540**

ENTREES/MEALS **1,070–5,460**
Moroccan Chicken Breast [1,070]

SANDWICHES/BURGERS *(no sides)* **1,420–2,780**
Veg Gardenburger [1,420] • NY Steak Sandwich [1,430]

SALADS *(w/o dressing)* **85–4,220**
Garden Salad, side [85] • Citrus Salad, side [320]
Iceberg Wedge Salad, side [340] • Organic Field Greens, side [370]
   DRESSINGS **110–1,250**
   Balsamic Mustard [110] • Walnut Cider Vinaigrette [150]
   Tropical Honey Citrus [160] • Bleu Cheese [180]

SOUPS **710–1,710**
Thai Style Chicken & Veg w/2 pita chips [710] • Baked Onion [820]

SIDES **0–770**
Steamed White Rice [0] • Steamed Brown Rice [10] • Coleslaw [200]

DESSERTS **270–1,380**
Citrus Cheesecake Brulee [270] • Creamy Creme Brulee [290]

(EL POLLO LOCO)

TACOS/BURRITOS **290–2,490**
Taco Al Carbon [290] • Crunchy Chicken Taco [440]
Chicken Taquito w/Avocado Salsa [550] • BRC Burrito [1,020]

CHICKEN **170–690**
FLAME GRILLED CHICKEN: Leg [170] • Wing [290] • Thigh [320]
Chopped Breast Meat [330] • Chicken Breast, skinless [560]

SALADS *(w/o dressing)* **260–1,430**
Loco Side Salad [260] • Grilled Chicken Salad [520]
   DRESSINGS **260–770**
   Creamy Cilantro Dressing [260] • Thousand Island [350]

SIDES **35–730**
FRESH VEGETABLES: (w/o margarine) [35] • (w/margarine) [65]
Corn Cobbette, 2 pc [45] • Cole Slaw [220]

(ERBERT & GERBERT'S)

SANDWICHES **440–2,680**
Kid's Mini Pudder: on Honey Wheat [440] • on French bread [460]
HALF PINT HAM & CHEESE: on Honey Wheat [660] • on French bread [690]
LI'L TYKES TURKEY & CHEESE: on Honey Wheat [680] • on French bread [710]

CALLY: on Honey Wheat [1,090] • on French Bread [1,150]
HALLEYS COMET: on Honey Wheat [1,140] • on French Bread [1,140]

SOUP...870–2,400
Beef Chili [870] • Minnesota Wild Rice/Chicken [870] • Cheesy Asparagus [870]

SIDES...61–1,481
Avocado [61] • Deli Pickle [350]

DESSERTS...185–887
Oatmeal Raisin Cookie [185] • Frosted Brownie [190] • Choc Chip Cookie [198]

FATBURGER

BURGERS/SANDWICHES..................................780–2,160
Hot Dog [780] • Fish Sandwich [850] • Grilled Chicken Sandwich [860]

SALADS *(w/o dressing)*...............................140–610
Fat Salad Wedge [140] • Fat Salad Wedge w/Chicken [610]

SIDES...40–1,280
Fat Fries [40] • Chili Fat Fries [410]

CONDIMENTS/TOPPINGS.................................0–710
Lettuce, Onions, or Tomato [0] • Mayo [80] • Mustard [80] • Relish [115]

SWEETS/SHAKES.......................................140–810
Big Fat Float [140] • Vanilla Shake [350] • Maui-Banana Shake [350]

FATZ CAFE

APPETIZERS...119–4,542
8 Chicken Wings (w/o sauce), half [119] • Lite Shrimp Skewer [396]

MEALS/ENTREES.......................................190–7,449
Grilled Shrimp Skewer [190] • Fried Shrimp, 3 pc [359]
Kid's Grilled Salmon w/Broccoli [360] • Kid's Pasta w/Alfredo [417]
Lite Chopped Steak w/Steamed Broccoli [473]
ANGUS BEEF SIRLOIN: 6 oz [528] • 10 oz [588]
Lite Grilled Top Sirloin w/Broccoli, lunch [612]
Chopped Steak w/Broccoli, lunch [612]
Lite Grilled Shrimp Skewer, lunch [627] • Calabash Popcorn Shrimp [648]

BURGERS/SANDWICHES/WRAPS.........................327–5,103
Kid's Hamburger [327] • Grilled Cheese Sandwich, lunch [399]
Kid's Grilled Chicken Sandwich [399] • Chicken Salad Sandwich, half [416]
Popcorn Shrimp Wrap, half [714] • Old Fashioned Hamburger [762]

SOUPS..532–1,024
Loaded Potato Soup, cup [532]

SALADS...23–2,020
Side Veggie Salad [23] • Veggie Salad [29] • Side Caesar Salad [128]
Traditional Caesar Salad [187] • Lite Grilled Chicken Salad, lunch [386]
Side House Salad [402] • Seabreeze Spinach [437] • Asian Chicken [493]
Seabreeze Spinach w/Grilled Aloha Chicken [647]

DRESSINGS...90–490
Raspberry Walnut Vinaigrette [90] • Sweet Vidalia Onion [115]

SIDES..38–3,076
Steamed Broccoli [38] • Poppyseed Roll [111] • Grilled Asparagus [126]
Steamed Veggies [135] • Plain Baked Potato [140]
Plain Baked Sweet Potato [143]

DESSERTS...397–1,894
Poppyseed Bread Pudding [397]

FAZOLI'S

PASTA/ENTREES 330–2,740
Roasted Chicken [330] • Kid's Spaghetti w/Marinara [370]
Kid's Fettuccine Alfredo [470] • Kid's Spaghetti w/Meat Sauce [560]
Kid's Spaghetti w/Meatballs [570] • Spaghetti or Penne Marinara [970]
TOPPINGS 20–700
Broccoli [20] • Broccoli & Fire Roasted Tomatoes [85]
Mushroom, Pepper & Onion Blend [115]
PIZZA 710–880
Margherita [710] • Triple Cheese [730]
SUBS 2,550–2,970
SALADS 130–2,880
Side Chopped Salad [130] • Cherry Almond Chicken Salad [1,190]
DRESSINGS/TOPPINGS 100–760
Croutons [100] • Cherry Vinaigrette [180] • Honey French [310]
BREADSTICKS 160–290
Breadstick, dry, 1 [160]
DESSERTS 330–630
Turtle Cheesecake [330] • Choc Chunk Cookie [350]

FIREHOUSE SUBS

SUBS 7000–4,230
Kid's Ham [700] • Kid's Roast Beef [800] • Kid's Turkey [820]
Veggie, med white (w/o mayo/cheese) [1,140]
Tuna, med white (w/o mayo/cheese) [1,230]
Ham, med white (w/o mayo/cheese) [1,240]
SOUPS/CHILI 960–1,113
Chili [960]
SALADS *(w/o dressing)* 740–1,230
Chief's Salad Chicken Salad [740]
DRESSINGS 110–550
FF Raspberry Vinaigrette • Ranch . . . . 110•240
DESSERTS 160–240
Choc Chip Cookie [160] • Macadamia Cookie [170]

FIVE GUYS

BURGERS/DOGS/SANDWICHES 380–240
Little Hamburger [380] • Hamburger [430] • Little Bacon Burger [640]
Bacon Burger [690] • Little Cheeseburger [690]
FRIES/TOPPINGS 0–400
Hot sauce, Lettuce, Tomatoes, Onions , or Green Peppers [0–3]
Mustard [55] • Mayonnaise [75] • Relish [85] • Mushrooms [100]
FRIES: reg [90] • lrg [213]

FLAMERS

BURGERS 514–1,444
Charbroiled Chicken [514] • Cajun Chicken [514]
Lemon Pepper Chicken [514] • BBQ Chicken [641] • Hamburger [684]
NOTE: Removing pickles reduces sodium by 212mg.

FREDDY'S FROZEN CUSTARD & STEAKBURGERS

BURGERS/SANDWICHES **305–1,623**
CALIF STYLE STEAKBURGER: w/o cheese or sauce [305] • w/o cheese [517] •
w/o sauce [665]
DOUBLE CALIF STYLE STEAKBURGER: w/o cheese or sauce [341] • w/o cheese [552]
TRIPLE CALIF STYLE STEAKBURGER: w/o cheese or sauce [376] • w/o cheese [588]
Patty Melt Single (w/o cheese) [378] • Patty Melt (w/o cheese) [414]
GRILLED CHICKEN BREAST SANDWICH: w/o mayo [354] • w/mayo [467]
Single Steakburger (w/o cheese) [466] • Reg Steakburger (w/o cheese) [502]
Veggieburger (w/o cheese or sauce) [620]

SIDES **530–1,515**
Fries, reg [530]

SWEETS **79–841**
SUNDAES (MINI): Hawaiian [79] • Choc [133] • PBC&B [180]
SINGLE CUP: Choc [114] • Vanilla [122]
SINGLE CAKE CONE: Choc [121] • Vanilla [127]
SINGLE SUGAR CONE: Choc [159] • Vanilla [167]
CONCRETES (MINI): PBC&B [185] • Hawaiian Delight [189] • Dirt & Worms [264]
SHAKES/MALTS (MINI): Choc Shake [154] • Vanilla Shake [164] • Choc Malt [200]

FRESH CHOICE

SALADS *(1/2 cup unless noted)* **4–500**
Marinated Cucumber [4] • Fresh Italian Bruschetta [22]
Fresh Peach & Berry Toss [25] • Ocean Mist Asparagus Toss [40]
Autumn Greens w/Roasted Beets [43] • Cool Napa Crunch [53]
Classic Picnic Slaw [61] • Tabbouleh [78] • Confetti Orzo [83]
HUMMUS (2 TBSP): Sundried Tomato [80] • Roasted Red Pepper [80] •
Squash Hummus [80] • Roasted Garlic [90] • Regular [104]
Sundried Tomato & Basil Couscous [88] • Apple Walnut Blues [94]
Summer Endives & Apple Medley [94] • Almond Craisin Delight [94]
Roasted Squash Medley [101] • Roasted Potato & Veg Bistro [101]
Strawberry Fields Spinach Salad [104] • Classic Carrot Raisin [105]
Cravin' Broccoli Bacon Raisin [113] • Ginger Soy Long Noodles [118]
Roasted Butternut Squash w/Cranberries [120]
Mandarin Spinach w/Toasted Almonds [133] • Insalata Caprese [134]
Saida's Mediterranean Lentils [135] • Bartlett Blue w/Champagne Vinaigrette [137]
Broccoli Obsession [140] • Cilantro, Black [140]
Southern Creamy Dill Potato [152] • Cayley's Classic Caesar [164]
Classic Shrimp Louie [178] • Crunchy Quinoa [195]

DRESSINGS **0–410**
VINAIGRETTES: Raspberry [0] • Poppy-Sesame Seed [20] • Champagne [35] •
Cal-Bistro Balsamic [61] • Orange Maple [61] •
Roasted Garlic [111] • Roasted Garlic Balsamic [111]
Azteca Dressing [124] • Thousand Island [140] • Blue Cheese [142]

SOUPS **98–1,261**
Old World Veg Minestrone [98] • Summer Veg Dumplings [102]
Fresh Harvest Veg Soup [102] • Garden Patch Lentil & Barley [118]
Hearty Garden Veg Barley [122] • Sweet Potato Corn Chowder [124]
Butternut Squash Bisque [136] • Cream of Broccoli • Cream of Spinach [139]
Roasted Veg & Butternut Squash Medley [148] • Rustic Country Veg [174]
Creamy Irish Potato Leek [201] • Broccoli Cheese Soup [215]

PASTAS/FARM FAV'S

PASTA/RICE. **1–847**
Plain Pasta [1] • White Rice [1] • Springtime Veg [32]
Roasted Fingerling Potatoes [43] • Squash Ratatouille [51]
Roasted Winter Veg [101] • Chicken Marinara [197
Chicken & Bowtie Primavera [250]

SAUCES **52–450**
Garden Marinara [52] • Pomodoro [52] • Italian Meat Sauce [149]
Creamy Garlic Alfredo [177]

PIZZA. **180–322**
Grilled Onion Focaccia [180] • Cheese Pizza [212] • Fresh Tomato/Basil [218]
Pepperoni Pizza [219] • Peppery Onions & Sausage [245]

BAKERY **99–696**
Cherry Vanilla Chip [99] • Pumpkin Choc Chip Bread [99]
Kiwi Strawberry Bran Loaf [110] • Citrus Carrot Raisin Bread [120]
Caribbean Banana Nut [121] • Zucchini & Carrot Nut Spice Bread [121]
Peach Cardamon Loaf [125] • Lemon Poppy Seed Loaf [130]
Lemon Raspberry Loaf [130] • Italian Dinner Roll [166] • Wheat Dinner Roll [166]

SPREADS **25–32**

DESSERTS. **0–344**
Sugar Free Gelatin [0] • Georgia Peach Cobbler [21] • Choc Raspberry Silk [83]
Triple Decdence Choc Brownie [84] • Soft Serve Choc or Vanilla [100]
Bread Pudding w/Citrus Rum Sauce [107] • Old Fashion Bread Pudding [107]
Mom's Caramel Apple Cobbler [125] • Spiced Apple Cranberry Cobbler [125]

GODFATHER'S PIZZA

PIZZA **230–1,310**
THIN CRUST, MED, 1/8: Cheese [230] • Hawaiian [330] • Veggie [280] •
Super Hawaiian [330] • Pepperoni [350]
ORIGINAL CRUST, MINI, 1/4: Cheese [250] • Hawaiian [270] • Super Hawaiian [270] •
Veggie [300] • Pepperoni [310]
THIN CRUST, LRG, 1/10: Cheese [270] • Hawaiian [380] • Veggie [340] •
Super Hawaiian [380] • Pepperoni [400]
GOLDEN CRUST, SM, 1/6: Cheese [360]
GOLDEN CRUST, MED, 1/8: Cheese [380]
GLUTEN-FREE CRUST, SM, 1/6: Cheese [380] • Hawaiian • Super Hawaiian [380]

CALZONES **2,540–2,920**

SIDES **160–1,440**
Breadsticks, 1 [160] • Cheesestick, 1/6 [210] • Breadstick w/Cheese, 1 [220]

DESSERTS. **160–970**
Apple Cinnamon Streusel, 1/6 [160] • Cherry Cinn Streusel, 1/6 [160]

GOLDEN CHICK

ENTREES. **472–1,489**
Golden Roast Chicken Wing [472] • Fried Chicken Tenders, 4 [490]
Fried Chicken Wing [541] • Fried Chicken Leg [550]

SANDWICHES **573–905**
Chunky Chicken Salad Sandwich [573]

SIDES **11–923**
Tropical Fruit Salad [11] • Coleslaw [20] • Corn on the Cob [52]
Fresh Baked Yeast Roll [182] • Chunky Chicken Salad [212]

DESSERTS. **110–125**

GREAT STEAK

BREAKFAST. **890–1,540**
Egg & Cheese Sandwich [890]

SANDWICHES/BURGERS **470–4,780**
Hamburger [470] • Philly Burger [500] • Cheeseburger [730]
Chili Burger [800] • Steak Philly Slider [850] • Chicken Philly Slider [880]
Veggie Delight, 7" [950]

BAKED POTATOES. **15–923**
Plain [15] • Sour Cream & Chive [45]

SALADS *(w/o dressing)* **20–1,520**
Side Salad [20] • Garden Salad [40]
GREAT SALAD: w/Grilled Chicken [460] • w/Grilled Steak [590]
WEDGE SALAD: w/Grilled Steak [550] • w/Grilled Chicken [610]

> **DRESSINGS** **160–280**
> Ranch Dressing [160]

SIDES **680–6,810**
Great Fry, Kid's [680]

HAPPY JOES

PIZZA *(1 slice)* **310–468**
Cheese Original [310] • Cheese Pan [326] • Pepperoni Original [409]
Taco Pan [412] • Pepperoni Pan [425] • Taco Original [428]
Sausage Original [451] • Sausage Pan [468]

HARDEE'S

BREAKFAST. **360–2,130**
Hash Rounds, sm [360] • Grits [490] • Hash Rounds, med [490]
Cinn 'N' Raisin Biscuit [680] • Scratch Biscuit [750] • Pancakes, 3 [830]

BURGERS/CHICKEN **480–2,840**
Hamburger, sm [480] • Fried Chicken Leg [570] • Cheeseburger, sm [710]
Fried Chicken Wing [740] • Hand Breaded Chicken Tenders, 3 pc [770]
Double Cheeseburger [820] • Regular Roast Beef Sandwich [850]

> **DIPPING SAUCES** **190–330**
> Honey Mustard Dipping Sauce [190]

SIDES **140–410**
Cole Slaw [140]

DESSERTS/SHAKES **85–330**
Single Scoop Ice Cream Cone [85] • Single Scoop Ice Cream Bowl [140]
Choc Chip Cookie [170] • Peach Cobbler, sm [230] • Ice Cream Shake [260]

HAWAIIAN BARBECUE

ENTREES. **130–2,339**
Garlic Ahi, 1 pc [130] • Healthy Garlic Ahi [167] • Katsu Musubi [305]
Healthy Garlic Shrimp [367] • Healthy Salmon Patty [367]
Mahi, 1 pc [410] • Chicken Katsu, 1 pc [430] • Short Rib, 1 pc [430]
Spam Musubi [483] • Chicken Musubi [486] • BBQ Chicken, 1 pc [486]
Healthy BBQ Chicken [517] • Mini Garlic Ahi [520]

SANDWICHES **633–853**
Hamburger [633] • BBQ Hamburger [712] • Mahi Mahi Sandwich [741]

SIDES **0–390**
Brown or White Rice, 1 scoop [0] • French Fries [240]

270

HONEY DEW DONUTS

BAGELS.. 650–760
Wheat Bagel [650] • Cinnamon Raisin Bagel [670]
CREAM CHEESE.................................... 95–250
Veggie [95] • Strawberry [200]
SANDWICHES/WRAPS................................ 670–1,630
ENGLISH MUFFIN SANDWICH: Egg White & Cheese [670] • Egg & Cheese [680]
CROISSANT SANDWICH: Egg White & Cheese [720] • Egg & Cheese [730]
Egg White & Cheese Wrap [810] • Egg & Cheese Wrap [820]
DONUTS 85–640
French Cruller [85] • Dew Drops, all varieties [85–90]
Honey Dip [330] • Sugar Raised [330] • Vanilla Frosted [340] • Jelly [340]
Apple Filled [340] • Choc Frosted [340] • Choc Frosted w/Jimmies [340]
MUFFINS... 410–630
Raisin Bran Muffin [410] • Cranorange Nut Muffin [410]
PASTRIES/COOKIES/YOGURT 60–580
Mini Cranberry Orange Scone w/Orange Glaze [60]
Mini Lemon Scone w/Lemon [70] • Glaze Cinnamon Burst [86]
Strawberry Yogurt Parfait [200] • Vanilla Yogurt Parfait [200]
Choc Chip Cookie [210] • Oatmeal Raisin Cookie [210]
SPECIALTY DRINKS................................ 70–300
Iced Mocha Madness [70] • Cappuccino [80] • Mocha Madness [90]
Latte w/whole or skim milk [95] • Mocha Latte w/whole [105] or skim milk [110]
Iced Latte w/whole milk [115] or skim milk [120]
Iced Mocha Latte w/whole [130] or skim milk [135]
Caramel Latte w/skim milk [140] • Iced Caramel Latte w/skim milk [140]

HOT DOG ON A STICK

HOTDOGS/ENTREES................................ 410–1,220
Fish Platter [410] • Veggie Dog on a Stick [570]
Pepperjack Cheese on a Stick [590] • American Cheese on a Stick [640]
SIDES 75–200
French Fries Funnel [75] • Cake Sticks [200]

HOULIHAN'S

APPETIZERS 777–4,911
Seared Rare Tuna Wontons [777] • Bruschetta [822]
MEALS/ENTREES 307–3,827
Vietnamese Spring Spring Eggrolls [307] • Kid's Pasta w/Marinara Sauce [351]
Grilled Shrimp Azteca [442] • Grilled Atlantic Salmon, 4 oz [486]
5 oz Atlantic Salmon, Simply Prepared, w/Salad & Asparagus [572]
Petite Sirloin, 5 oz [602] • Spicy Chicken & Avocado Eggrolls [610]
Seared Sea Scallops [610] • Fancy Spaghetti Small Plate [641]
SANDWICHES/BURGERS............................. 391–2,744
Kid's Grilled Chicken Sandwich [391] • Kid's Cheeseburger [469]
Kid's Corn Dog [570] • Honey Dijon Chicken Salad Sandwich [696]
SOUPS.. 1,284–2,108
Original Baked Potato Soup [1,284]
SALADS... 110–3,703
SPINACH SALAD: side [110] • w/Berries {220} • w/Berries & Chicken [406] •
w/Berries, Chicken & Feta [536]

271

Grilled Asparagus Salad [287] • House Salad w/Cheddar Cheese, side [295]
House Salad w/Bleu Cheese, side [343] • Signature Tuscan Salad [497]
Caesar Salad [545] • House Salad w/Cheddar Cheese, lrg [591]

DRESSINGS **121–464**
 Poppyseed [121] • Napa Dressing [220] • LF Ranch [370]

SIDES **209–705**
Peanut Ginger Slaw [209] • French Green Beans [292]
Tortilla Chips w/Salsa [365] • French Fries [373]

DESSERTS **27–992**
Creme Brulee [27] • White Choc Banana Cream Pie [192]

HUNGRY HOWIES PIZZA

PIZZA **256–1,472**
CHEESE, THIN CRUST: med, 1/8 [256] • lrg, 1/10 [323]
Cheese, small, 1/6 [370] • Cheese, med, 1/8 [437]

ADD TOPPINGS (FOR MEDIUM PIZZA) **0–736**
Mushrooms, Onions, Green Peppers, Pineapple, or Bacon [0–1]
Olives [47] • Pepperoni [75] • Ham [81] • Beef [96]

SUBS . . . .**895 -1,722**
Vegetarian Sub [895] • Steak & Cheese Sub [914]

CHICKEN **520-760**
Boneless Wings [520]

SALADS *(w/o dressing)* **10–581**
Garden [10] • Chef [396] • Antipasto Salad [554] • Greek Salad [581]

DRESSINGS **70–560**
Greek [70] • French Style [170]

IHOP RESTAURANT

BREAKFAST **0–4,310**
Seasonal Fruit [0] • Simple & Fit Oatmeal [25]
Create Your Own Omelette w/Egg Substitute [320]

ADD FILLINGS **0–480**
Green Peppers & Onions, Mushrooms, or Tomatoes [0]
Fresh Spinach [45] • Swiss Cheese [90] • Oven-Roasted Tomatoes [125]
Stuffed French Toast, side [370]
Simple & Fit Veggie Omelette w/Fresh Fruit [420]
Simple & Fit Seasonal Fresh Fruit Crepes [440]
BELGIAN WAFFLE: w/Strawberry & Whipped Topping [540] • w/Butter [580]
Kid's Cheese Omelette [580]
Simple & Fit Spinach, Mushroom & Tomato Omelette w/Fresh Fruit [690]

SANDWICHES/BURGERS **760–2,930**
Cheeseburger [760] • Simple & Fit Chicken Sandwich w/Fresh Fruit [840]

ENTREES/DINNERS **340–3,580**
Kid's Crispy Chicken Strips [340] • Kid's Jr Fish [520]
Kid's Mac & Cheese [580] • Simple & Fit Grilled Balsamic-Glazed Chicken [940]

SALADS **50–2,430**
Simple & Fit Fresh Fruit & Yogurt Bowl [50] • Simple & Fit House Salad [140]
House Salad (w/o dressing) [170] • Caesar Salad Side [860]

DRESSING **105–550**
Reduced-Fat Italian [105] • Honey Mustard [200]

SOUPS **1,040–1,640**
New England Clam Chowder [1,040]

DESSERTS. **25–660**
ICE CREAM, 1 SCOOP: Vanilla [25] • Strawberry [30] • Choc [30]
ICE CREAM SUNDAE: Reg [70] • w/Strawberry Topping [75] • w/Hot Fudge [165]

IN-N-OUT BURGER

BURGERS **370–1,520**
Hamburger, Protein Style *(bun replaced w/lettuce)* [370] • Hamburger [650]

FRENCH FRIES **245**

SHAKES **270–320**
Strawberry [270] • Vanilla [300] • Chocolate [320]

JACK IN THE BOX

BREAKFAST. **350–1,650**
Mini Pancakes [350] • Hash Brown Sticks, 5 pc [400]
Sausage Croissant [776] • Breakfast Jack [780] • Bacon Breakfast Jack [790]

BURGERS/CHICKEN & MORE **320–2,440**
1 Beef Taco [320] • 1 Egg Roll [320] • Kid's Grilled Chicken Strips, 2 pc [540]
Hamburger [660] • Deluxe Hamburger [680] • Jack's Spicy Chicken [820]
Chicken Fajita Pita w/Whole Grain (no salsa) [870] • Chicken Sandwich [880]

DIPPING SAUCES **160–840**
Sweet & Sour [160] • Zesty Marinara [200] • Honey Mustard [210]

SALADS (W/O DRESSING) **10–1,260**
Side Salad [10] • Grilled Chicken Salad [660]

DRESSINGS. **360–740**
LF Balsamic Vinaigrette [360]

SIDES **410–1,690**
Kid's French Fries [410]

CONDIMENTS **5–1,950**
Syrup [5] • Sour Cream [25] • Mayonnaise [40] • Margarine Spread [45]
Mayo-Onion Sauce [50] • Mustard [50] • Taco Sauce [80]

DESSERTS/SMOOTHIES/SHAKES **69–555**
SMOOTHIES, 16 OZ/24 OZ: Strawberry [69–98] • Strawberry Banana [72-103] •
Mango [73–104]
Vanilla Shake, 16 oz [250] • Strawberry Shake, 16 oz [260]
NY Style Cheesecake [260] • Mini Churros, 5 pc [280]

JAMBA JUICE

OATMEAL **20–50**
Steel-Cut Oatmeal, as served, all varieties [20–50]

WRAPS/FLATBREADS **530–910**
Spinach n' Cheese Wrap [530] • Turkey Sausage n' Cheese Wrap [610]
SW Chicken Chorizo Wrap [620] • Smokehouse Chicken [690]

BAKED GOODS **90–640**
Berry Agave Bar [90] • Cinn Swirl [230] • Apple Cinnamon Pretzel [250]
Sweet Belgian Waffle [290]

FROZEN YOGURT *(small)*. **100–220**
Blueberry Pomegranate Peaks [100] • Magnificent Mango Pineapple [100]
Swirly Strawberry Vanilla [100] • Wildly Watermelon [100]

SMOOTHIES **5–490**
CLASSIC, ALL SIZES: Strawberry Surf Rider [5–15] • Mango [35–65] •
Peach [35–65] • Caribbean Passion [35–70] • Pomegranate [35–70] •
Razzmatazz [40–75] • Aloha Pineapple [50–70]

273

ALL FRUIT SMOOTHIES: all flavors & sizes [10–45]
PRE-BOOSTED, ALL SIZES: Coldbuster [15–40] • Acai Super-Antioxidant [45–95]
CLASSIC, 16 & ORIG: Banana Berry [65–90] • Orange [85–125] •
  Strawberries Wild [95–140]
FRUIT & VEGGIE: Orange Carrot, 16/Orig [90–120] • Apple 'n Greens, 16 [115]
MAKE IT LIGHT (16/ORIG): Strawberry Surf Rider [90–125] • Peach [95–125] •
  Caribbean Passion [95–125] • Pomegranate [100–135] • Razzmatazz [100–130]
PROBIOTIC FRUIT & YOGURT BLEND: Thrivin' Mango, 16/Orig [120–135]

OTHER DRINKS **0–460**
Orange Berry Antioxidant, 12/16 [0] • Tropical Kick-Start, 12/16 [5]
HOT BLENDS: The Chillbuster, 12/16 [20–30] • Orig Spiced Chai, 12 w/2% milk [140]
Triple Revitalizer, 12/16 [35–65]
FRUIT & YOGURT PARFAIT, 12/16: Berry Topper [80–110] • Mango Peach Topper [85–115]
CREAMY TREATS: Apple Cinn Cheer, 16/Orig [95–120]
FRUIT REFRESHERS: Watermelon Splash, 16/Orig [95–135]
  Strawberry Lemonade, 16/Orig [105–140] • Tropical Mango, 16 [120]

JASON'S DELI

BREAKFAST **370–1,380**
BAGELS: Cinn Raisin [370] • French Toast [370] • Plain [380] • Multi Grain [380]
MUFFINS: Banana Nut [390] • Morning Glory [400] • Blueberry [440]
COFFEE CAKES: Red/White/Blue [440] • Choc Chip [450] • Lemon Poppy [450]
Cheese Danish [450] • Apple Danish [480]
Mini Croissant Breakfast Sandwich w/Cheddar (or Jalapeno) & Ham [520]

PASTA/POTATOES **590–3,110**
Kid's Pasta Alfredo (w/o chicken) [590] • Kid's Baked Potato [600]
"Lighter" Zucchini Garden Pasta (w/o bread) [640]

SANDWICHES/WRAPS **450–10,390**
KID'S PEANUT BUTTER & JELLY SANDWICH: on Wheat [450] • on White [540]
Spinach Veggie Wrap [570] • Chicken Club Wrapini, half [580]
"Lighter" NY Yankee, half [625] • Chicken Panini, half [660]

BUILD YOUR OWN
MEATS **190–1,247**
  Homemade Chicken Salad, slim or 1/2 sandwich portion [190]
  Grilled Chicken Breast, slim or 1/2 sandwich portion [260]
  Homemade Tuna Salad, 1/2 or lighter sandwich portion [320]
  Roast Beef, slim or 1/2 sandwich portion [350] • Chicken Salad [370]
BREADS/WRAPS **130–657**
  Organic Wheat Wrap, half [130] • Multigrain Ciabatta Bun, half [140]
  All Butter Croissant, half [150] • Gourmet Onion Bun, half [180]
  Herb Focaccia Bun, half [210]
SPREADS/TOPPINGS **0–220**
  Lettuce, Tomato, Onions, Avocado, or Homemade Pico de Gallo [0] • Spinach [10]
  Swiss Cheese [50] • Guacamole [60] • Mayo [75] • Chipotle Aioli [75] •
  Basil Pesto [120]

SALADS *(w/o dressing)* **170–2,060**
"LIGHTER" NUTTY MIXED UP SALAD: w/o chicken [170] • w/chicken [430]
Nutty Mixed Up Salad (w/o chicken) [380]
SALAD BAR **0–870**
  Sunflower Seeds [0] • All fresh lettuces, fruits & veggies [0–35]
  Hard Boiled Egg [60] • Homemade Chicken Salad [190]
DRESSINGS **160–720**
  1,000 Island (Russian) [160] • LF Raspberry Vinaigrette [170] • Ranch [260]

SOUPS (CUP) **410–2,040**
Chicken Noodle Soup [410] • SW Chicken Chili [570]
Red Bean/Rice w/Sausage [580] • Tomato Basil [600] • Seasonal Beef Stew [660]

SIDES **25–870**
Fresh Fruit Cup w/Creamy Fruit Dip [25] • Gingerbread Muffin [35]
Garlic Toast [45] • Steamed Veggies [55] • Cornbread Muffin [75]
Organic Blue Corn Tortilla Chips [90] • Baked Lays [115]

DESSERTS **5–550**
Ice Cream Cone, plain or w/choc topping [5–20] • Cranberry Walnut Mix [25]
Fudge Nut Brownie [25] • Mixed Fruit & Yogurt [35] • Mixed Berry Granola [85]
Soft Serve Vanilla [75] • Soft Serve Choc [80] • Choc Mousse [85]
Banana Pudding [125] • Choc Chip Cookie [135] • Cream Cheese Pecan Bar [140]

JERRY'S SUBS & PIZZA

PIZZA *(1/4 of 8" small)* **255–553**
Classic White [255] • Veggie Supreme [284] • Phillips Crab [325] • Wildfire [329]

SUBS *(small)* **678–5,265**
Veggie Melt [678] • Tuna [812] • Phillips Crabcake [859]
Grilled Chicken [863] • Philly Cheesesteak [872]

TOPPINGS/CONDIMENTS **0–641**
Green Peppers [0] • Swiss Cheese [23] • Mushrooms [28]
Jerry's Mayo [45] • Sweet Peppers [63] • Mustard [100]

SALADS **233–1,589**
Side Salad [233] • House Salad [469]

DRESSINGS **234–700**
Bleu Cheese [234] • Honey Mustard [345]

SIDES **120–2,070**
Choc Chip Cookie [120] • Chicken Nuggets, 2 pcs [200]
CHIPS: Baked Lays [202] • Plain Lays [270]

JERSEY MIKE'S SUBS

SUBS/WRAPS **690–8,510**
ROAST BEEF & PROVOLONE: Wheat Mini [690] • Flour Wrap [860] • Wheat Wrap [930]
VEGGIE: Wheat Mini [720] • White Mini [750] • Flour Wrap [960]

TOPPINGS **0–330**
Lettuce, Onions, or Tomatoes [0–20]

SALADS *(w/o dressing)* **20–1,480**
Tossed Salad [20] • Tuna Salad [740]

DRESSINGS **150–410**
Chipotle Mayo [150] • Russian [200] • Ranch [240]

SOUPS **680–2,320**
Timberline Chili w/Beans, cup [680]

DESSERT **100–250**
COOKIES: White Chip Macadamia Nut [100] • Choc Choc Chip [110]
Oatmeal Raisin [115] • Choc Chunk [140]
Choc Chip [150] • Choc Chip Walnut [150]

JIMMY JOHN'S

SANDWICHES **873–2,166**
8" Vegetarian [873] • Slim Double Provolone [991] • Slim Roast Beef [996]

SIDES **80–2,314**
Reg Potato Chips [80] • BBQ Potato Chips [90] • Thinny Chips [105]

KFC

CHICKEN. **140–1,480**
WINGS (1): Hot [140] • HBBQ Hot [240] • Fiery Buffalo Hot [270]
GRILLED CHICKEN: Whole Wing [250] • Drumstick [290] • Thigh [530]
ORIG RECIPE: Drumstick [310] • Whole Wing [380] • Breast w/o skin/breading [580]
EXTRA CRISPY: Drumstick [360] • Whole Wing [410]
SPICY CRISPY: Drumstick [440] • Whole Wing [470]

SANDWICHES/POTPIE/BOWLS **470–1,880**
KFC SNACKER: Honey BBQ [470] • w/Crispy Strip (w/o sauce) [550]
Snack-Size Bowl [760] • Honey BBQ Sandwich [770]

SALADS *(w/o dressing and croutons)* **10–1,220**
House Side Salad [10] • Caesar Side [90] • Grilled Chicken Caesar [740]

DRESSINGS/TOPPINGS. **160–540**
Parmesan Garlic Croutons [160] • Buttermilk Ranch Dressing [220]

SIDES **0–870**
Sweet Kernel Corn [0] • Corn on the Cob [5] • Cole Slaw [135]

SAUCES/OTHER **0–1,130**
Honey Sauce Packet [0] • Colonel's Buttery Spread [30]
DIPPING SAUCE CUP: Sweet/Sour [95] • Honey Mustard [110] • KFC Signature [135]

DESSERTS. **85–260**
Choc Chip Cookie [85] • Oatmeal Raisin Cookie [90]
Lil' Bucket Strawberry Shortcake Parfait Cup [140] • Apple Turnover [160]

KRISPY KREME DOUGHNUTS

DOUGHNUTS. **40–320**
Mini Original Glazed [40] • Mini Choc Iced Glazed w/ or w/o Sprinkles [45]
Sugar Doughnut [85] • 4 Original Glazed Doughnut Holes [90]
Choc Iced Banana Filled Eclair [90] • Original Glazed [90] • Glazed Cinn [90]
Choc Iced Glazed [95] • Choc Iced w/Sprinkles [95]
White Iced Strawberries & Kreme Filling Eclair [110] • Apple Fritter [110]
White Iced Heart w/Valentine Sprinkles [115] • Choc Iced Choc Filled Eclair [120]
Pumpkin, Football, Iced & Stamped [120] • White Iced Glazed Hearts [120]
Snowman [120] • White Iced Egg [120] • Shamrock [120]
Star w/Sprinkles [120] • Cinn Bun [125] • Baseball [125]
Tennis Ball Doughnut [125] • Choc Iced Glazed Football [125]
Choc Iced Raspberry Filled [125] • Glazed Raspberry Filled [125] • Cinn Twist [130]
Powdered Strawberry [135] • Glazed Lemon Filled [135] • Blueberry Filled [135]
Choc Iced Kreme Filled [140] • Glazed Kreme Filled [140]

BAGELS/MUFFINS/SWEET ROLLS. **65–400**
Classic Cinnamon Roll [65]
MUFFINS: Blueberry [280] • Cinn Coffee Cake [290] • Choc Chip [300]
 Lemon Poppy Seed [310] • Corn Muffin [340]
 Whole Wheat Blueberry [380] • Banana w/Oat Crisp Crunch Topping [390]
BAGELS: Cinnamon Raisin [440] • Sesame [460] • Blueberry [470]

CREAM CHEESE **100–150**
Reduced Fat Strawberry [100] • Plain [115] • Reduced Fat Plain [130]

CHILLERS (12 OZ) **10–580**
Very Berry [10] • Orange You Glad [10]
Orange & Cream [220] • Berries & Cream [220] • Lemon Sherbert [220]

KOOL KREME **170–690**
Choc Cone [170] • Swirl Cone • Vanilla Cone [180]
SUNDAES: Strawberry [200] • Orig Glazed Doughnut [230] • Hot Fudge [250]

BEVERAGES **10–290**
Iced Coffees, all sizes [10–40] • Iced Latte, 12 oz/16 oz [80–125]
Iced Hazelnut or Vanilla Latte, 12 oz/16 oz [80–125]
Iced Kaffe Kreme, 12 oz/16 oz [80–125] • Iced Mocha, 12 oz/16 oz [110–160]
Cappuccino, 12 oz/16 oz [105–150] • Latte, 12 oz/16 oz [105–150]
Mocha, 12 oz [150] • Hot Chocolate, 12 oz [150]

KRYSTAL

BREAKFAST. **220–1,650**
Toast [220] • Kryspers [270]
Sausage on Toast [420] • Bacon on Toast [450]
4 Pancakes [500] • Pancake Scrambler [530]
One Egg Custom Breakfast (Sr Meal) [550] • Grits w/Margarine [570]
Egg on Toast [580] • Krystal Sunriser [620]

LUNCH/DINNER. **330–1,580**
Krystal [330] • Bacon Cheese Krystal [430] • Cheese Krystal [470]
Plain Pup [450] • Corn Pup [520] • Chili Pup [560]
Double Krystal [580] • Bacon Cheese Krystal [580]

SALADS **95–890**
Side Salad [95] • Crispy Chicken Salad [890]

SIDE ITEMS **40–720**
FRIES: reg [40] • med [65] • lrg [80] • Chili Fries, lrg [200]

DESSERTS/SHAKES **105–700**
Oreo Choc Sandwich Cookie [105] • Lemon Ice Box Pie [230] • Sweet Bites, 3 [230]
MILKQUAKES: Choc [250] • Strawberry [250] • Vanilla [280]

LAMAR'S DONUTS

DONUTS **250–1,190**
Apple Spiced Cake [250] • Ray's Orignal Glazed [260] • Choc Glazed Donut [260]
Blueberry Cake [280] • Choc Iced Cake [320] • White Iced Cake Donut [320]

LITTLE CAESAR'S

PIZZA **440–730**
14" ROUND HOT-N-READY, 1/8: Cheese [440] • Veggie [560] • Pepperoni [560]
Deep Dish, Cheese, 1/8 [510] • Baby Pan!Pan!, Cheese [520]

CHICKEN. **150–350**
CAESAR WINGS (1): Oven Roasted [150] • BBQ [220] • Mild [250] • Hot [350]

SIDES **140–540**
Buttery Garlic Caesar Dip [140] • Crazy Breadstick, 1 [150]

LONG JOHN SILVER'S

ENTREES. **250–1,190**
Grilled Tilapia, 1 filet [250] • Langostino Lobster Stuffed Crab Cake, 1 [390]
Grilled Pacific Salmon, 2 filets [440] • 3 Battered Shrimp [480]
Chicken Strip, 1 [480] • Baja Fish Taco [810] • Freshside Grille Tilapia Entree [820]

SANDWICHES **880–1,500**
Zesty Chicken Strip Sandwich [880] • Alaskan Pollock Sandwich [1,100]

SIDES **0–730**
CORN COBBETTE: w/o Butter Oil [0] • w/Butter Oil [30]
Hushpuppy [200]

DESSERTS. **230–250**

MANCHU WOK

ENTREES/APPETIZERS **170–730**
Sweet & Sour Chicken Tenders [170] • Seafood Rangoon [240]
Pineapple Chicken [260] • Chicken Egg Rol [350]l • Vegetable Egg Roll [380]
Sweet & Sour Pork [470] • Pepper Steak [510] • Mixed Vegetables [510]
Kung Pao Chicken [540] • Spicy Beef [560] • Green Bean Chicken [580]

RICE/NOODLES **3–1,620**
Steamed Rice [3] • Lo Mein Noodles [850]

MARIE CALLENDER'S

BREAKFAST **15–4,400**
Fresh Fruit [15] • English Muffin [220] • English Muffin w/Butter [280]
French Toast [440] • Buttermilk Pancakes [490] • Buttermilk Pancake Stack [700]
MUFFINS: Coconut Pineapple [500] • Banana [530] • Blueberry Streusel [560]
2 Eggs, Any Style (w/o hashbrowns) [700] • Veg Quiche, slice [780]

SANDWICHES/BURGERS **1,670–3,620**
Kid's Moo Burger [1,670] • Meatloaf on Grilled Parmesan Sourdough [1,910]

ENTREES/MEALS **120–4,110**
Skewer of Shrimp [120] • Cajun Atlantic Salmon w/Broccoli [210]
Angus Sirloin w/Potato & Asparagus [410] • Grilled Mahi Mahi Cabo Tacos [420]
Avocado Shrimp Stack [450] • Grilled Shrimp Street Tacos [660]
GRILLED ATLANTIC SALMON: Cajun Seasoned [560] • Lemon Pepper [600]

SOUPS **80–2,910**
Vegetarian Veg, cup [80] • Vegetarian Veg, bowl [120]
Chicken Noodle, cup [520] • Chili, cup [630]

SALADS **160–5,000**
Spring Mix Salad, side [160] • House Salad, side [200]
Caesar Salad, side [560] • Gorgonzola, Pecan & Field Greens Salad [910]

SIDES **180–550**
Rice Pilaf [180] • Cole Slaw [200] • Happy Hour Chips & Salsa [260]

DESSERTS **125–600**
COOKIES: Sugar [125] • Oatmeal Raisin [150] • Choc Chunk [170]
PIE (SLICE): Fresh Berry [150] • Fresh Peach [160] • Fresh Strawberry [160] •
Fresh Wildberry [160]
Cheesecake, all varieties, slice [180]

MCALISTER'S DELI

SANDWICHES *(half)* **440–10,000**
CHOOSE 2 PORTION: Harvest Chicken Salad [440] • Veggie Club [540] • Tuna [570] •
Grilled Chicken [590] • Deli Roast Beef [610]

BREAD **230–940**
Wheat Hoagie, 1/2 [230] • Wheat Hoagie, whole [360] • Baguette, 1/2 [360]

CHEESE/MEATS **30–300**
Swiss [30] • Sharp Cheddar [90] • Provolone [125] • Smoked Bacon [170]
Harvest Chicken Salad [410] • Grilled Chicken Breast [430]

SPREADS/TOPPINGS **0–1,280**
Cucumbers [0] • Avocado [5] • Lite Sour Cream [35] • Roasted Red Peppers [45]
Spicy Guacamole [90] • Light Mayo [125] • Spicy Brown Mustard [150]

SOUPS/CHILI *(cup)* **600–2,010**
White Chicken Chili [600] • Fire Roasted Veg [700] • Country Potato [820]

SALADS *(w/o dressing, choose 2 portion unless noted)* **240–2,290**
GARDEN SALAD: Choose 2 portion [240] • whole [470]
Savannah Chopped Salad [410] • Grilled Chicken Salad [540] • SW Cobb [640]
DRESSINGS **300–1,050**
Sherry Shallot Dressing [300] • Lo Cal Italian Dressing [410]

SPUDS **0–1,620**
WHOLE: Justaspud [0] • Cheese Spud [350] • Veggie Spud [620]
CHOOSE 2 PORTION: Cheese Spud [180] • Veggie Spud [310] •
Bacon Spud [420] • Grilled Chicken Spud [420] • Spud Ole [480]

NACHOS *(1/4 serving)* **740–970**

SIDES **10–750**
Applesauce [10] • Fruit [15] • Plain Potato Chips [300]

DESSERTS **70–660**
COOKIES: Sugar [70] • Oatmeal Raisin Walnut [85] •
White Choc Macadamia Nut [85] • Heath [105] • Choc Chip [125]
Double Fudge Brownie [100] • Magic Bar [210]

MCDONALD'S

BREAKFAST **15–2,260**
Seasonal Fruit [15] • Snack Size Fruit & Walnuts [60] • Fruit 'n Yogurt Parfait [70]
OATMEAL: Fruit & Maple (w/o brown sugar) [115] • Fruit & Maple [160]
Hash Browns [310] • Cinn Melts [370] • Hotcakes [590] • Egg McMuffin [820]

BURGERS/SANDWICHES/CHICKEN **360–2,020**
Chicken McNuggets, 4 pc [360] • Chicken McBites Snack Size [490]
Hamburger [490] • Filet-O-Fish [610] • Honey Mustard Snack Wrap (Grilled) [650]
Chipotle BBQ Snack Wrap (Grilled) [670] • Mac Snack Wrap [690
DIPPING SAUCES **0–800**
Honey [0] • Honey Mustard Sauce [115] • Sweet 'N Sour Sauce [150]

SALADS *(w/o dressing)* **10–1,010**
Side Salad [10] • Bacon Ranch w/o chicken [300]
SW SALAD: w/o Chicken [150] • w/Chicken [650]
CAESAR SALAD: w/o Chicken [180] • w/Grilled Chicken [650]
DRESSINGS/TOPPINGS **140–730**
Garlic Croutons [140] • Creamy SW Dressing [340] • LF Italian [390]

SIDES **70–350**
FRENCH FRIES: Kids [70] • sm [160]

DESSERTS/SMOOTHIES/SHAKES **20–510**
Kiddie Cone [20] • Vanilla Reduced Fat Cone [70] • Dipped Cone [80]
Smoothies, all flavors, all sizes [30–65] • Fruit 'n Yogurt Parfait [70]
Strawberry Sundae [85] • Choc Chip Cookie [90] • Sugar Cookie [120]
M&Ms Candies McFlurry, snack size [120] • Oatmeal Raisin Cookie [135]
MCCAFE SHAKES (12 OZ): Vanilla [160] • Strawberry [170]

COFFEE DRINKS/FRAPPES **40–260**
ICED COFFEES (REG, HAZELNUT, OR VANILLA): sm [40] • med [60] • lrg [85]
ICED COFFEE: Sugar Free Vanilla, sm [70] or med [100] • Caramel, sm [80]
CAPPUCCINO (SM): Hazelnut or Vanilla [70] • Reg [85] • Sugar Free Vanilla [105]
Latte, Hazelnut or Vanilla, sm [90] • Latte, sm [105]
Iced Mocha, sm [120] • Frappe Mocha, sm [130] •

MILIOS SANDWICHES

SUBS/SANDWICHES **1,019–2,273**
Texas Longhorn [1,019] • Cheddar Beef Classic [1,105] • Veggie Delite [1,109]

CHIPS **170–350**
Baked Lays [170]

COOKIES **230–260**

MOE'S SOUTHWEST GRILL

BUILD YOUR OWN MEAL **0–3,150**
TORTILLAS/SHELLS/CHIPS **0–550**
Corn Tortilla [0] • Chips [84] • 6" Flour Tortilla [200] • 10" Flour Tortilla [220]
Crispy Bowl [250] • 12" Flour Tortilla [350]
MEAT **135–510**
Fish [135] • Chicken [240] • Tofu [290] • Steak [380]
ADDITIONS **0–590**
Grilled Mushrooms, Cucumbers, or Shredded Lettuce [0–1] • Sour Cream [23]
SW Slaw [45] • Grilled Peppers [50] • Grilled Onions [55] • Pinto Beans [129]
Rice [135] • Cheese [180] • Corn Pico [200] • Guacamole [220]
*Note: Tacos have less meat and additions, reduce above sodium amounts by
half for each taco; rice bowls have more rice, double rice to 270mg sodium.*

COOKIES **125–140**

MRS FIELDS COOKIES

COOKIES **65–210**
Enrobed Cookies, Semi Sweet [65]
BITE-SIZE NIBBLERS (3): White Chunk Macadamia [140] • Semi-Sweet Choc [140] •
Debra's Special Nibbler [150] • Triple Choc [160]
Semi-Sweet Choc Cookie w/Walnuts [160] • Semi-Sweet Choc Cookie [170]
Triple Choc [170] • White Chunk Macadamia [170]

BROWNIES **15–110**
BITES (3): Butterscotch Blondie [15] • Double Fudge [75] • Toffee Fudge [85]
Butterscotch Blondie [20] • Special Walnut Fudge & Blondie [55] • Pecan [95]
Pecan Fudge [95] • Walnut Fudge [95] • Double Fudge [95]

MUFFINS/CAKES **270–330**
Choc Chip Muffin [270] • Blueberry Muffin [280] • Choc Chip Cake [330]

MY FAVORITE MUFFIN

(See Big Apple Bagels, pg 249 for menu items)

NATHAN'S FAMOUS/ARTHUR TREACHERS

BREAKFAST **660–1,020**
Egg & Cheese on an English Muffin [660]

HOT DOGS/SANDWICHES **400–2,600**
Hot Dog Nuggets, 6 pc [400] • Hot Dog Nuggets, 9 pc [600]
Hamburger [700] • Natural Casing Hot Dog [710] • Corn Dog on a Stick [730]

CHICKEN/SEAFOOD **380–8,680**
Shrimp, 4 pc [380] • Fish Sandwich [440] • Shrimp, 5 pc [470]
Filet of Flounder Sandwich [580] • Honey BBQ Chicken Wings, 4 pc [810]

SOUPS **680–2,300**
Manhattan Clam Chowder, 12 oz [680]

SIDES **20–1,760**
Corn on the Cob [20] • FRENCH FRIES: reg [65] • lrg [100] • family [135]

DESSERTS **230–360**
Hot Cherry Pie [230] • Hot Apple Pie [250]

NOODLES & CO

ENTREES *(small)* 430–2,400
Bangkok Curry [430] • Chinese Chop Salad [440] • The Med Salad [500]
Wisconsin Mac & Cheese [520] • Penne Rosa [530] • Buttered Noodles [530]
Caesar Salad [530] • Pesto Cavatappi [550] • Mushroom Stroganoff [550]
• Spaghetti • Pasta Fresca .... 550•570•610

PROTEINS 310–860
Organic Tofu [310] • Meatballs [360] • Chicken Breast [370]

SANDWICHES 770–2,170
Spicy Chicken Caesar (w/o dressing) [770]

SIDES 140–1,080
TOSSED GREEN SALAD: w/Balsamic [140] • w/FF Asian [420]

DESSERTS.. 140–680
Choc Chunk Cookie [140] • Snoodledoodle Cookie [220]

OLD CHICAGO PASTA & PIZZA

STARTERS...129–2,430
Chips & Salsa, 1/4 [129] • Nachos Grande (Half), 1/2 [351]

BURGERS/ SANDWICHES *(w/o sides)*..................437–3,820
Kid's Mighty Cheeseburger [437] • Calif Chicken Sandwich [595]
Kid's Cheesy Chicken Sandwich [736] • Burger, Old Chicago Plain [805]

PIZZA *(1 slice)* 206–1,175
DEEP DISH: Cheese Only, express [206] • Cheese Only, individual [349] •
Malibu Veggie, individual [365] • Vegetarian 7, individual [376]
NY THIN CRUST: Cheese Only, express [219]
ARTISAN: Cheese Only [215] • Roasted Chicken & Mushroom [326] •
3 Cheese, Tomato & Pepperoni [332]

PASTAS/CALZONES/ENTREES 624–3,640
Cheese Calzone, lunch [624] • Spaghetti Marinara, lunch [890]

SALADS *(w/o dressing)*............................. 92–3,314
House, side [92] • Mediterranean [324] • Roasted Chicken w/Bacon/Apple, half [512]
HARVEST W/BALSAMIC CHICKEN: half [298] • full [594]
DRESSING: Honey Mustard [270] • Ranch [320]

SOUPS *(cup)* 753–2,330
Beef Chili Soup [753] • Potato Chowder [795]

SIDES 33–1,745
Side Veggies [33] • Steamed Veggies [93] • Cole Slaw [257]

DESSERTS... 82–354
Little Big Cookie, 1/2 [82]• Turtle Choc Brownie [194]

OLD SPAGHETTI FACTORY

APPETIZERS 1,120–2,540

ENTREES..390–3,530
SENIOR: Spaghetti Marinara [390] • Fettucine Alfredo [400] • Marinara/Clam [420]
Marinara/Mushroom [420] • Spaghetti Clam [440] • Mushroom/Clam [450]
Spaghetti Mushroom [450] • Marinara/Meat [460] • Clam/Meat [490]
Spaghetti Meat Sauce [530]
Mushroom/Meat [530] • Fettucine Alfredo [560]

PASTA 0–5

SANDWICHES 980–2,620
Grilled Cheese [980]

SOUPS/SALADS **280–2,470**
HOUSE SALAD: w/FF Honey Mustard [280] • w/Balsamic [300] •
w/Creamy Pesto [360] • w/Caesar [390] • w/Blue Cheese [430] •
w/1,000 Island [560]
SOUP: Minestrone [660]

DESSERTS **70–220**
Choc Truffle Mousse Cake [70] • Vanilla Ice Cream [80]
Spumoni Ice Cream [90]

OLIVE GARDEN

APPETIZERS **630–2,860**
Fried Zucchini [630] • Stuffed Mushrooms [720]

MEALS/ENTREES **470–3,380**
Kid's Cheese Ravioli [470] • Linguine alla Marinara, lunch [670]
Herb-Grilled Salmon, dinner [760] • Fettuccine Alfredo, lunch [810]

FLATBREADS/PIZZA **1,500–3,200**
Grilled Chicken Flatbread [1,500] • Caprese Flatbread [1,520]

PANINI **635–1,440**
Grilled Chicken Florentine, half [635] • Grilled Steak & Portobello, half [675]

SOUPS/SALADS **530–1,530**
Garden Fresh Salad (w/o dressing) [530] • Pasta e Fagioli Soup [680]

DESSERTS **50–590**
DOLCINI: Amaretto Tiramisu [50] • Limoncello or Strawberry Mousse [70] •
Choc Mousse [120] • Dark Choc Cake, Choc Mousse & Caramel Cream [140]
Tiramisu [75] • Warm Apple Crostata [240]

ORANGE JULIUS

JULIUS FRUIT DRINKS **30–1,290**
ALL SIZES: Lemon, Mango, Orange, Peach, Pineapple, or Pomegranate [30–75]
Raspberry or Strawberry [30–75] • Tropical Tango [50–105] •
Orange Swirl, Strawberry Banana, Tripleberry, or Tropical [70–150]
Bananarilla, Blackberry, or Pina Colada [80–160]
Eggnog, sm [100] or med [125]

SMOOTHIES **0–790**
Raspberry Crush or Berry Banana Squeeze, all sizes [0–20]
Light Premium Fruit Smoothies, all flavors & sizes [45–115]
Berry Lemon Lively or Blackberry Toner, sm/med [95–140]
Banana Chill or Strawberry Sensation, sm/med [100–150]
3-Berry Blast or Pomegranate & Berries, sm/med [100–150]
Mango Passion, Peaches & Cream, or Strawberry Xtreme [105–160]
Raspberry Creme, Blackberry Storm, or Tropi-Colada, sm [135–140]

SANDWICHES/HOT DOGS **810–2,120**
Grilled Chicken Sandwich [810] • Garden Veggie Pita [810] • Classic Dog [900]

OUTBACK STEAKHOUSE

APPETIZERS **403–683**
Coconut Shrimp [403] • Grilled Shrimp on the Barbie [433]

ENTREES *(w/o sides)* **159–3,864**
Joey Sirloin [159] • VICTORIA'S FILET: 6 oz [206] • 8 oz [283]
OUTBACK SPECIAL: 6 oz [226] • 9 oz [339] • 12 oz [452]
Norwegian Salmon [295] • NY Strip, 10 oz [394] • Ribeye, 10 oz [405]

SANDWICHES/BURGERS *(w/o sides)* 787–3,977
Joey Boomerang Cheese Burger [787]
Grilled Chicken Sandwich w/Broccoli [793]

SOUPS *(cup)* 1,021–2,733

SALADS 336–2,168
HOUSE SALAD (SIDE): w/Mustard Vinaigrette [336] • w/Tangy Tomato [410]
Caesar Salad, side [699] • Grilled Chicken Cobb Salad w/Oil & Vinegar [902]

SIDES 153–894
Seasonal Veggies [153] • Sweet Potato [172]
Steamed French Green Beans [193]

DESSERTS 115–226
Classic Cheesecake [115] • Sydney's Sinful Sundae [136]
Choc Thunder from Down Under [140]

PANDA EXPRESS

APPETIZERS 180–540
Cream Cheese Rangoon, 3 pc [180] • Chicken Potsticker, 3 pc [280]

ENTREES 260–1,310
Mixed Vegetables [260] • Sweet & Sour Chicken Breast [320]
SweetFire Chicken Breast [370] • Sweet & Sour Pork [460]
Honey Walnut Shrimp [470] • Golden Treasure Shrimp [500]

RICE/NOODLES 0–980
Steamed Rice [0] • Fried Rice [820]

SAUCES/COOKIES 8–340
Fortune Cookie [8] • Sweet & Sour Sauce [115]

PANERA BREAD

BREAKFAST 10–1,350
Summer Fruit Cup [10] • Strawberry Granola Parfait [100]
STEEL CUT OATMEAL: w/Pecans [160] • w/Blueberries & Granola [160]
Four Cheese Egg Souffle [690] • Egg & Cheese on Ciabatta [710]

BAGELS 400–640
Whole Grain [400] • Cinnamon Crunch [440] • Plain Bagel [460]
Sesame [460] • Cinnamon Raisin Swirl [470] • Choc Chip [480]
CREAM CHEESE 200–370
Reduced Fat Raspberry [200] • Reduced Fat Honey Walnut [200]
Veggie [210] • Reduced Fat Hazelnut [210]
Plain [210] • Reduced Fat Plain [230]

PASTRIES/SWEETS 100–900
Strawberry Granola Parfait [100] • Pastry Ring [160]
COOKIES: Flower [150] • Shortbread [160] • Peanut Butter Dream [200]
MUFFINS: Choc Chip Muffie [200] • Pumpkin Muffie [240] • Wild Blueberry [320]
French Croissant [220] • Choc Pastry [250] • Pecan Braid [270]
SCONES (MINI): Strawberries & Cream [260] • Orange [270] • Blueberry [300]
Apple Pastry [290] • Fruit Pastry [290] • Cherry Pastry [310] • Pecan Roll [310]

SANDWICHES 450–2,800
Roasted Turkey & Avocado BLT on Sourdough (w/o salt), half [450]
Tuna Salad Sandwich on Honey Wheat (w/o salt), half [550]
Napa Almond Chicken Salad on White [610]

SOUPS 580–2,320
CREAMY TOMATO: w/o Croutons [580] • w/Croutons [720]
Vegetarian Summer Corn Chowder [730]

SALADS **280–1,690**
Classic Salad [280] • Strawberry Poppyseed & Chicken Salad [330]
BBQ Chopped Chicken [770] • Asian Sesame Chicken [810]

SIDES **0–410**
Apple [0] • Panera Potato Chips [130] • Baked Lays Potato Chips [200]

PAPA GINO'S PIZZA

APPETIZERS/SIDES **180–1,800**
French Fries [180] • Toasted Ravioli [430]

PIZZAS *(1 slice)* **470–1,640**
THIN CRUST (SMALL): Cheese [470] • Hawaiian [520] • Super Veggie [530]
Works [560] • Pepperoni [570] • Chicken & Roasted Garlic [570]
RUSTIC: Cheese [520] • Super Veggie [560] • Hawaiian [570 •
Garlic Chicken [600]

PASTA **560–2,040**
Penne Alfredo [560] • Spaghetti Alfredo [560]

SUBS/SANDWICHES **480–3,870**
Hamburger [480] • Double Hamburger [560] • Cheeseburger [720]
Steak Sub, sm [750] • Double Cheeseburger [790]

SALADS *(w/o dressing)* **105–1,170**
GARDEN SALAD: side [105] • full [300]
CAESAR SALAD: side [135] • full [380]
  DRESSINGS **250–400**
  Honey Mustard [250] • Balsamic [330]

DESSERTS **15–500**
Cinnamon Stick [15] • Choc Brownie [180] • Blondie Brownie [270]

PAPA JOHN'S PIZZA

PIZZA *(1 slice)* **350–1,100**
THIN CRUST (LRG): Spinach Alfredo [350] • Garden Fresh [360] •
Cheese [380] • Tuscan Six Cheese [460]
ORIGINAL CRUST (SM): Garden Fresh [350] • Cheese [440] • Spinach Alfredo [460]
PIZZA FOR ONE: Garden Fresh [440] • Cheese [450] • Spinach Alfredo [460]

SIDES **430–1,070**
Chickenstrips, 2 [430] • Breadsticks, 2 [540]
  DIPPING SAUCES **120–310**
  Honey Mustard [120] • Cheese Sauce [160]

DESSERTS **540**

PAPA MURPHY'S

PIZZAS **202–980**
LARGE SIZE DELITE (1/10 SLICE): Cheese [202] • Veggie [219] •
Veggie Combo [267] • Hawaiian [280] • Pepperoni [300] •
Gourmet Vegetarian [306] • Gourmet Chicken Garlic [311] •
Herb Chicken Mediterranean [344] • Specialty of the House [351] •
Rancher [371] • BBQ Chicken [374] • Cajun Combo [376] • Thai Chicken [385] •
Chicken Pesto [386] • Chicken Bacon Ranch [386] • Chicken Bacon Artichoke[389]
FAMILY SIZE DELITE (1/12 SLICE): Cheese [227] • Veggie [247] •
Vegetarian Combo [297] • Hawaiian [324] • Gourmet Vegetarian [349] •
Specialty of the House [399] • Herb Chicken Mediterranean [401] •
Gourmet Chicken Garlic [408] • Pepperoni [08] • Chicken Pesto [420]

CALZONES 899–1,153
Vegetarian, lrg, 1/6 [899] • Vegetarian, family, 1/8 [944]

SALADS *(w/o dressing)* 117–495
Caesar [117] • Garden [231] • Italian [368] • Club [482] • Chicken Caesar [495]
DRESSING (1/2 PKT) 170–330
Caesar [170] • Buttermilk Ranch [210]

DESSERTS *(1/8)* 222–415
Cookie dough w/Hershey's Choc Chips [222] • S'Mores Dessert Pizza [291]

PERKINS

BREAKFAST. 10–6050
Seasonal Fresh Fruit [10] • Oatmeal [90]
MINI MUFFIN: Choc Choc Chip [105] • Blueberry [110] • Apple Cinn [110] •
Banana Nut [120]
CEREAL: Frosted Flakes [240] • Special K [240] • Raisin Bran [330]
English Muffin [410] • TOAST (2 SL): White [450] • Whole Wheat [530]
Mushroom 'n Swiss Omelette (w/o potatoes) [460] • Breakfast Potatoes [460]
BUILD YOUR OWN OMELETTE 0–490
2 eggs [130] • 3 eggs [200]
ADDITIONS: Diced Tomatoes [0] • Asparagus [0] • Garden Mix [15] •
Broccoli [25] • Swiss Cheese [35] • Mushrooms [110] • Bacon Pieces [140]

SALADS. 530–2,510
Side Salad (w/o croutons & cheese) [530]
DRESSING. 480–1,230
Balsamic Vinaigrette [480]

SOUPS. 220–1,480
HOMESTYLE CHICKEN NOODLE: Cup [220] • Bowl [340]
Loaded Baked Potato Soup, cup [540]

SANDWICHES/WRAPS *(includes french fries)*. 950–5,270
Hamburger (w/o pickles & whipped butter) [950]

LUNCH/DINNERS 470–4,940
Top Sirloin Steak [470] • 55 Plus Top Sirloin Steak [980]
Island Tilapia Dinner [1,060] • Salmon Dijon [1,080]

DESSERTS. 25–600
MINI COOKIE: Oatmeal Raisin Walnut [25] • Choc Chip [25] •
White Choc Macadamia Nut [25] • Sugar [30] •
Peanut Butter Choc Chip [30] • Double Choc Chip [45]
Ice Cream, 1 [70] or 2 scoops [140] • Ice Cream Sundae, 1 scoop [85]
COOKIES: Oatmeal Raisin Walnut [100] • White Choc Macadamia Nut [105] •
Choc Chip [110] • Sugar [115] • Peanut Butter Choc Chip [125]

PETER PIPER PIZZA

APPETIZERS 190–2,341
Wings [190]

PIZZA *(1 slice)* 270–970
THIN CRUST (XL): Calif Veggie [270] • Cheese [290] • Ham & Pineapple [320} •
Pepperoni [340] • Chicago Classic [350] • Sausage [370] • The Werx [440]
THIN CRUST (LRG): Calif Veggie [290] • Cheese [290] • Ham & Pineapple [320] •
Chicago Classic [340] • Pepperoni [340] • Sausage [360] •
Pepperoni & Sausage [370] • The Werx [420] • NY 3 Cheese w/Pepperoni [440]
ORIG CRUST (XL): Calif Veggie [400] • Cheese [420] • Ham & Pineapple [470]
ORIG CRUST (LRG): Calif Veggie [430] • Pepperoni [460] • Cheese [470]

SALADS. 30–1,910
Side Salad [30] • Garden Salad [45]

CINNAMON CRUNCH DESSERT 220

(PIZZA HUT)

PIZZA *(1 slice)* 400–2,110
FIT N' DELICIOUS PIZZA: Green Pepper, Red Onion & Diced Red Tomato [400] •
Chicken, Red Onion & Green Pepper [510]
PAN PIZZA (MEDIUM): Veggie Lover's [500] • Ham & Pineapple [520] •
Pepperoni & Mushroom [520] • Cheese Only [530]
THIN 'N CRISPY (MED): Veggie Lover's [530] • Ham & Pineapple [540] •
Pepperoni & Mushroom [540] • Cheese Only [550]
HAND TOSSED (MED): Veggie Lover's [530] • Pepperoni & Mushroom [540] •
Ham & Pineapple [550] • Cheese Only [550]

CHICKEN WINGS (2 PC). 290–1,020
TRADITIONAL: All American [290] • Lemon Pepper [430] • Spicy Asian [500]
Baked, Hot or Mild [430] • Bone Out, All American [490]
Crispy Bone In, All American [500]

SIDES 260–450
Breadsticks, 1 [260]

DESSERTS. 190–220
Apple Pie [190] • Cinn Sticks, 2 [210] • Hershey's Choc Dunkers, 2 [220]

(POLLO CAMPERO)

CHICKEN. 304–5,538
Traditional Drumstick [304] • Traditional Whole Wing [337]
Chicken Strips, 1 [553] • Chicken Crispers [668]
CHICKEN BOWLS 3,033–3,146

SANDWICHES/WRAPS. 613–1,749
Grilled Chicken Wrap [613] • Grilled Cilantro Mayo Chicken Sandwich [1,301]

BURRITOS. 1,048–3,213
Kid's Grilled Chicken Burrito [1,048]

SALADS. 1,071–2,581
Campero Salad [1,071]

SIDES 0–2,295
Tomatoes [0] • Tortilla Chips [22] • SWEET PLANTAINS: 4 [22] • 12 [66]
Yuca Fries [144] • Sweet Campero Cole Slaw [297] • French Fries [325]

SAUCES. 108–960
Beef Gravy [108] • Mayonnaise [111] • Cilantro Garlic Mayo [137]
Fire Roasted Chipotle Salsa [125] • Chipotle Honey Mustard [129]

DESSERTS. 90–290
SOFT SERVE NF YOGURT (CUP): Choc Swirl, Mocha Swirl, or Strawberry Swirl [90] •
Blue Goo Swirl, Orange Swirl, Mango Swirl, or Caramel Swirl [90]
SOFT SERVE NF YOGURT (CONE): Choc Swirl, Orange Swirl, or Mocha Swirl [105] •
Blue Goo Swirl, Strawberry Swirl, Mango Swirl, or Caramel Swirl [105]

(POPEYES)

BREAKFAST. 30–1,520
Grits [30] • Hashbrowns [450] • Bacon Biscuit [780]

CHICKEN/BIG EASYS/SEAFOOD 230–2,165
CHICKEN NUGGETS: 4 pc [230] • 6 pc [350]

SPICY CHICKEN: Leg [360] • Wing [410] • Thigh [460]
Mild Chicken Leg [460]
BIG EASYS: Chicken & Sausage Jambalaya [760] • Loaded Chicken Wrap [890]
Butterfly Shrimp, 8 [820]

SIDES 0–2,208
Corn on the Cob [0] • Cole Slaw [300]

SAUCES. 90–320
Confetti Sauce [90] • Spicy Honey Mustard Sauce [170]

DESSERTS. 210–340
Mississippi Mud Pie [210] • Sliced Pecan Pie [220]

POTBELLY SANDWICH SHOP

BREAKFAST. 1–1,464
Irish Oatmeal, cup or bowl [1–2] • Banana Nut Muffin Top [295]
Blueberry Muffin Top [303] • Egg & Cheddar on Square Bread [618]

SANDWICHES 603–2,668
Vegetarian on Thin-Cut w/Mayo/Swiss [603] • Chicken Salad Square Meal [614]
Skinnys, Mushroom Melt w/Swiss [507] • Skinnys, Mushroom Melt [673]

SALADS *(w/o dressing)*. 167–1,685
Waldorf Salad [167] • Tomato Cucumber Salad [144] • Chicken Salad Salad [270]
  DRESSING. 300–1,120
  Potbelly Vinaigrette [300] • Buttermilk Ranch [380]

SOUPS. 686–2,700
Loaded Baked Potato, cup [686]

SIDES 3–615
Seasonal Fruit [3] • Pickle [237] • Potato Salad [310]

SWEETS 60–615
COOKIES: Mini Oatmeal Choc Chip [60] • Cherry Choc Granola [105]
Yogurt Parfait [120]

SHAKES/MALTS/SMOOTHIES 189–550
SHAKES: Vanilla [189] • Mixed Berry [213] • Strawberry Banana [219]
SMOOTHIES: Mixed Berry [262] • Banana [274] • Coffee [284] • Strawberry [286]
  MALTS 1,084–1,343

QDOBA

BREAKFAST. 350–2,460
BREAKFAST BURRITO, W/POTATOES & EGG (W/O TORTILLA): sm [350] • lrg [540]

TACOS/BURRITOS/OTHER ENTREES *(w/o tortilla)* 630–2,900
Fajita Ranchera Burrito w/Grilled Chicken or Steak [630]
Queso Burrito w/Grilled Chicken or Steak[640] • Grilled Veggie Burrito [690]
  BUILD YOUR MEAL
  Soft Corn Tortilla [0] • Crispy Taco Tortilla [25] • Soft Flour Tortilla [200]
  MAIN INGREDIENT 35–190
  Grilled or Fajita Veg [35] • Grilled Steak [80] • Grilled Chicken [115]
  Pulled Pork [130] • Ground Beef [180] • Shredded Beef [190]
  ADDITIONS 0–180
  Lettuce [0] • Sour Cream [15] • Crispy Tortilla Strips [30]
  Black Beans [75] • Pinto Beans [85] • Cheese [85] • Guacamole [100]

SALSAS. 45–200
Roasted Chile Corn [45] • Mango Salsa [50] • Pico de Gallo [70]
Fiery Habanero [80]

SOUPS/SALADS **590–2,280**
Grilled Veg w/Black Beans & Cheese (w/o shell) [590] • Tortilla Soup [740]

CHIPS *(small/large)* **115–230**

QUIZNOS

SUBS/WRAPS **400–3,770**
KIDZ FLATBREAD FOLDABLES: Triple Play Cheese Melt [400] • Marinara Melt [500]
SUB SLIDERS BASE (1): BLT Classic [420] • Turkey Club [535] • Chipotle Turkey [540]
Kidz Monster Meatball Sub Slider [660] • Pestos Sub, sm [735]
Lobster & Seafood Salad Sub, sm [750] • Harvest Chicken Wrap, half [760]

BREADS (SMALL) **370–900**
Rosemary Parmesan [370] • Italian White [380]

MEATS (SMALL) **190–570**
Bacon [190] • Tuna Salad [400] • Turkey Breast [440]

ADDITIONS (SMALL) **0–280**
Lettuce, Tomato, Onion, Cucumber, Mushroom, or Green Pepper [0]
Swiss [10] • Mozzarella [60] • Black Olives [75] • Cheddar [90] • Guacamole [105]

CONDIMENTS **125–340**
Honey Dijon [125] • Buttermilk Ranch [150] • FF Balsamic [190]
Mayo [200] • Chipotle Mayo [210] • Yellow Mustard [220]

GRILLED FLATBREADS *(small)*. **780–2,400**
BASIL PESTO CHICKEN: Base [780] • w/Cheese & Dressing [1,020]
SONOMA TURKEY: Base [880] • w/Cheese & Dressing [1,170]

SALADS *(w/o dressing)*. **140–1,011**
Harvest Chicken, sm [140] • Harvest Chicken, lrg [300]
Lobster & Seafood, sm [310] • Chicken Caesar, sm [330] • Cobb, sm [390]

DRESSINGS **250–970**
Acai Vinaigrette, sm [250] • Honey Mustard, sm [290]

SOUPS. **985–2,520**

DESSERTS. **80–370**
Qkidz Cookie [80] • Choc Brownie [220] • Ultimate Choc Chunk Cookie [220]

RED BURRITO

BURRITOS. **480–2,,820**
Make It Wet [480] • Bean & Cheese [1,200]

TACOS. **410–700**
HARD TACO: Beef [410] • Chicken [410]
DELUXE HARD TACO: Beef [430] • Chicken [470]
SOFT TACO: SW Chicken [630] • Beef [650] • Chicken [650]

OTHER ITEMS **1,140–2,410**
Quesadilla [1,140]

SIDES/CONDIMENTS. **60–1,000**
Sour Cream [60] • Guacamole [100] • Hot Sauc [200] • Chips & Salsa [230]

RED LOBSTER

STARTERS. **125–3,380**
Oysters on the Half Shell, 6 [125] • Grilled Jumbo Shrimp Cocktail [580]

DINNER ENTREES *(w/o condiments)*. **240–4,300**
Wood-Grilled Salmon [240] • Blackened Walleye [410] • Rock Lobster Tail [490]
OVEN-BROILED/GRILLED/BLACKENED FRESH FISH: Cobia [310] • Barramundi [350]
MahiMahi [360] • Grouper [370] • Opah [380] • Monchong [390]

288

SALADS *(w/o dressing)* **105–1,620**
Garden Salad, side [105] • Garden w/Shrimp, side [230] • Caesar, side [560]
DRESSINGS **180–560**
Thousand Island [180] • Balsamic Vinaigrette [190]

SOUPS *(cup)* **680–2,370**
CLAM CHOWDER: New England [680] • Manhattan [690]

SIDES **250–1,100**
Coleslaw [250] • Fresh Asparagus [270]

DESSERTS **270–980**
NY-Style Cheesecake w/Strawberries [270]

RED ROBIN

APPETIZERS **173–3,430**
JUMP STARTER: Mushrooms [173] • Zucchini [354] • Sweet Potato Fries [423]

BURGERS/SANDWICHES **250–2,390**
Kid's Chick on a Stick [250] • Kid's Red Robin Burger [381]
Lettuce-Wrapped Burger [441] • Kid's Rad Chicken Burger [510]
Kid's Rad Turkey Burger [605] • Grilled Turkey Burger [898]
Keep It Simple Burger [991] • Simply Grilled Chicken Sandwich [993]

WRAPS **914–2,349**
Caesar's Chicken Wrap, half [914]

ENTREES/COMBOS **243–4,970**
Kid's Parmesan Noodles [243] • Kid's Chick on a Stick [250]
Kid's Red Robinetti Spaghetti [521] • Kid's Carnival Corn Dog [75]

SALADS **195–2,520**
House Salad, side [195] • Caesar Salad, side [299]
Simply Grilled Chicken Salad (w/o croutons & garlic bread) [478]
DRESSINGS **0–983**
Italian (Oil & Vinegar) [0] • Baja Ranch [285] Honey Mustard Poppyseed [376]

SIDES **1–846**
Freckled Fruit Salad [1] • Steamed Broccoli [30] • Steak Fries [444]

SOUPS **562–3,074**
Roasted Veg, cup [562]

DESSERTS/SHAKES **55–580**
BOOZY SHAKES: Kahlua [55] • Baileys [64] • Jungle [77]
CLASSIC MILKSHAKES: Banana, Vanilla, Peach, or Strawberry [110] •
Raspberry [130] • Choc [146]
Birthday Sundae [119 • Kid's Sundae [119]
CLASSIC MALTS: Strawberry, Peach, Vanilla, or Banana [195]

ROCK BOTTOM RESTAURANT BREWERY

BRUNCH **396–3,508**
Kid's Pancakes [396] • Eggs Benedict, Vegetarian w/Side of Fruit [744]

APPETIZERS *(1/4 serving)* **243–1,432**
Jumbo Lump Crab Cake [243] • Crab & Shrimp Tower [339]

ENTREES **521–3,818**
TEXAS FIRE STEAK: Top Sirloin [521] • NY Strip [536] • Filet [663]
OFF THE HOOK: w/Trout [662] • w/Grouper [664] • w/Cod or Halibut [666]

PIZZA *(1 slice)* **203–360**
Roasted Veg [203] • Margherita [204] • Fab Five [294]
Pepperoni [309] • BBQ Chicken [360]

BURGERS/SANDWICHES **1,034–4,457**
Kid's Rocky Burger [1,034] • Patty Melt [1,195] • Roasted Turkey Sandwich [1,420]

SOUPS/SALADS *(w/o dressing)*. **211–2,927**
Greenhouse Salad [211] • Seafood Chef Salad [369] • Caesar, side [491]
SOUP (CUP): Beer Cheese [375] • Brewery Chili [474] •
  Cream of Chicken/Artichoke [485] • Lobster Bisque [530] •
  Minestrone [546] • SW Chicken & Corn Chowder [601]

DRESSINGS **62–260**
Tangy Vinaigrette [62] • Balsamic Vinaigrette [117] • Honey Mustard [124]

SIDES **10–1,632**
Fresh Fruit [10] • Brewery Slaw [63] • Veggies [218]

DESSERTS (1/4) **80–282**
Pint Glass Sundae [80] • Triple Choc Brownie [86] • White Choc Bread Pudding [177]

ROMANO'S MACARONI GRILL

TAPAS/ANTIPASTI. **580–2,150**
Lobster-Stuffed Clams [580] • Zucchini Fritti [630]

PIZZA **1,310–1,960**

PASTA **570–3,640**
Kid's Spaghetti & Meat Sauce [570] • Kid's Spaghetti & Pomodoro [680]
Mushroom Ravioli [1,020] • Lobster Ravioli [1,030]

ENTREES. **480–3,600**
Kid's Chicken Strips w/Broccolini [480] • Shrimp Portofino [760]

SALADS. **120–1,200**
Fresh Greens [120] • Caesar [330]

SOUPS. **790–1,380**
Lentil [790] • Pomodorna [790]

SANDWICHES **650–1,890**
Caprese Panini, half [650] • Roasted Turkey, half [840]

DESSERTS. **0–660**
White Peach Sorbet [0] • Gelato, all flavors [40] • Quattro Cannoli [110]

ROUND TABLE PIZZA

APPETIZERS **115–460**
Garlic Bread [115] • Garlic Bread w/Cheese [180] • Honey BBQ Wings, 1 [180]

PIZZAS *(1 slice)* **250–980**
SKINNY (PERSONAL): Fire Roasted Veggie [250] • Guinevere's Garden [270] •
  Cheese [290] • Fire Roasted Chicken & Bacon [310] •
  Fire Roasted Pepperoni [320] • Hawaiian [330] • Gourmet Veggie [330] •
  Gourmet Veggie [350] • Chicken & Garlic [350]
ORIGINAL (PERSONAL): Fire Roasted Veggie [300] • Guinevere's Garden [320] •
  Cheese [340] • Fire-Roasted Chicken & Bacon [360]
SKINNY CRUST (SM): Fire-Roasted Veggie [350] • Cheese [350]

FLATBREADS *(6" x 12" slice)* **400–560**
Tomato Pesto [400] • Roasted Veggies & Mozzarella [430]

PASTA **1,760–3,090**

SANDWICHES **1,600–2,440**
Turkey Pesto [1,600]

SALADS. **95–350**
GARDEN SALAD: sm [95] • lrg [190] • CAESAR SALAD: sm [170] • lrg [350]
NOTE: Adding chicken to salad increases the sodium by 590mg.

RUBIOS FRESH MEXICAN GRILL

TACOS *(made w/corn tortilla)* 160–1,840
STREET TACOS Carnitas [160] • Grilled Chicken [180] • Grilled Steak [190]
Chile-Lime Salmon [190] • Grilled Mahi Mahi [240]
HealthMex Grilled Mahi Mahi [290] • Grilled Portobello & Poblano Gourmet [330]
Grilled Steak [340] • HealthMex Grilled Chicken [340]
Blackened Mahi Mahi [360] • Grilled Chicken [380] • World Famous Fish [430]
Fish Taco Especial [520] • Blackened Salmon [540] • Garlic Herb Shrimp [570]
NOTE: If made with flour tortillas instead of corn, add 340mg sodium.

KID'S MEALS 350–1,710
2 Chicken Taquitos [350] • Fish Taco [510] • 2 Chicken Taquitos w/Rice [550]

BURRITOS/OTHER FAVORITES 1,180–3,260
Chile-Lime Salmon Burrito [1,180] • HealthMex Grilled Veggie Burrito [1,260]

SALADS 180–1,490
Side Salad [180] • Chicken Balsamic & Roasted Veggie Salad [950]

SIDES 10–940
Applesauce [10] • Rice, reg [220] • Chips, reg [290]

CHURRO 140

RUBY TUESDAY

SHARABLES *(1 serving)* 231–2,285
Jumbo Lump Crab Cake [231] • Chicken Tenders [250] • Guacamole Dip [269]

BRUNCH 127–3,478
Berry Good Yogurt Parfait [127] • Garlic Cheese Biscuit [310] • French Toast [943]

ENTREES 71–4,746
Plain Grilled Chicken [71] • Plain Grilled Salmon [163] • Creole Catch [200]
Blackened Tilapia w/Mango Salsa [235] • Plain Grilled Petite Sirloin [240]
Petite Creole Catch [397] • Asian Sesame Glazed Half-Rack Ribs [460]
New Orleans Seafood [472] • Petite Sirloin [492] • Classic BBQ Half-Rack [500]
Barbecued Grilled Chicken [500] • Grilled Salmon [553]

BURGERS/SANDWICHES/WRAPS 309–2,186
Asian Lettuce Wraps [309] • Avocado Grilled Sandwich, half [593]
Turkey Burger Wrap, half [748] • Triple Prime Burger [757]

SALADS *(w/o dressing)* 346–2,318
Petite Grilled Chicken [346] • Petite Carolina Chicken Salad [346]
Petite Creole Catch [397] • Petite Sliced Sirloin [664]

DRESSINGS 150–540
Honey Mustard [150] • Blue Cheese [220] • Lite Ranch [230]

SOUPS 1,117–2,240

SIDES 69–1,769
Roasted Spaghetti Squash [69] • Fresh Steamed Broccoli [82]
Baked Potato, plain [103] • Grilled Green Beans [145] • Sugar Snap Peas [164]

DESSERTS 60–950
Tiramisu [60] • Berry Good Yogurt Parfait [127] • Carrol Cake Cupcake [170]

RUNZA

SANDWICHES/BURGERS/ENTREES 230–2,300
Kid's Jr Hamburger, plain [230] • 5 Mini Corn Dogs [530]
Kid's Junior Cheeseburger, plain [530] • Kid's Jr Hamburger The Runza Way [530]
2 Piece Chicken Strip [600] • Mini Original Runza Sandwich [700]
1/4 lb Hamburger The Runza Way [770] • Ranch Mini Chicken Wra [750]

SALADS *(w/o dressing)* **10–2,110**
Side Salad [10] • Sweet Berry Chicken, half [590]

DRESSING **220–1,040**
FF Raspberry Vinaigrette [220] • Poppyseed [310]

SOUPS **980–2,140**
Potato Bacon [980]

SIDES **260–690**
Onion Rings, med [260] • French Fry, sm [310] • Frings!, med [350]

DESSERTS/SHAKES **10–520**
Applesauce [10] • Kids Cake Cone w/Vanilla Ice Cream [60]
Dish of Ice Cream, all [105] • Choc Sundae [115] • Ice Cream Cone, all [130]

SHAKES (REG) **250–510**
Vanilla [250] • Strawberry [250] • Cappuccino [260] • Choc [280]

SCHLOTZSKY'S DELI

SANDWICHES/WRAPS **607–4,084**
Homestyle Tuna Wrap, half [607] • Fresh Veggie Sandwich, sm [690]

PIZZA *(1 slice)* **419–2,455**
GOURMET (14"): Double Cheese [419] • Fresh Veggie [478] •
Chipotle Chicken [521] • Grilled Chicken & Pesto [527] • Combo Special [537]

SALADS *(w/o dressing)* **292–2,132**
Garden Salad [292] • Pasta Salad [293] • Potato Salad [514]
Cranberry, Apple, Pecan & Chicken Salad [872]

DRESSINGS **227–1,015**
FF Raspberry Vinaigrette [227] • Freshly Prepared Ranch [595]

SOUPS **568–2,535**
Hearty Vegetable Beef, cup [568] • Red Beans & Rice, cup [813]

CHIPS **190–310**
Regular (Plain) [190] • Sour Cream & Onion [220] • Jalapeno [220]

DESSERTS **50–767**
COOKIES: Choc Chip [50] • Oatmeal Raisin [50] • Macadamia Nut [50] • Sugar [65]

SHAKEYS PIZZA

SHAREABLES **547–4,984**
Mojo Potatoes, approx 5 [547]

PIZZA (1 SLICE) **258–898**
THIN CRUST (LRG): Margherita [258] • Garden Veggie [299] • Cheese [301] •
Rustic Garlic Chicken [335]
PAN PIZZA (LRG): Margherita [338] • Garden Veggie [380] • Cheese [381]

ADDITIONAL TOPPINGS **0–305**
Mushrooms, Onions, Green Peppers, Pineapple, or Tomato [0]
Beef [35] • Chorizo [57] • Black Olives [62]
Chicken [80] • Pepperoni [88] • Jalapenos [90] • Ham [91]

CHICKEN **317–1,383**
Fried Chicken Wing, 1 [317] • Fried Chicken Leg, 1 [542]

SHEETZ

BREAKFAST **115–2,212**
Oatmeal [115] • Hashbrownz [280]

SANDWICHEZ
BREADS: Pretzel Roll [239] • English Muffin [267] • Croissant [282]

EGGS/MEATS: Fried Egg Patty [120] • Scrambled Egg Patty [1]
Pepperoni [107] • Steak [113] • Ham [248] • Bacon [271]
CHEESE: Swiss [21] • Cheddar [72] • Mozzarella [86] • Pepper Jack [91]
TOPPINGS: Onions, Green Peppers, Lettu, or Tomatoes [0–1]
CONDIMENTS: Sour Cream [0] • Pico de Gallo [9] • Tabasco Sauce [38] •
Basil Pesto [103] • Chipotle Ranch Dressing [104]
Bacon, Egg, Cheese & Salsa Burrito [568] • Western Burrito [618]

SANDWICHES/SUBS
Roast Beef [283] • Steak [349] • Tuna Salad [399]

BREAD **239–630**
Pretzel Roll, sm [239] or lrg [341] • Croissant [282] • Wheat Bread [320]
Corn Dusted Deli Bun [352] • White Bread [359] • Wheat Burger Bun [390]
Wheat Sub Roll [418] • White Sub Roll [454]

CHEESE **41–366**
Swiss [41] • Parmesan [139] • Cheddar [144] • Mozzarella [172]

TOPPINGS/EXTRAS **0–330**
Cooked Peppers, Onions, Green Peppers, Lettuce, or Tomatoes [0–2]
Black Olives [58] • Coleslaw [77] • Dill Pickle Chips [225]

CONDIMENTS **38–816**
Tabasco Sauce [38] • Marinara Sauce [74] • Honey Mustard Sauce [128]
Buttermilk Ranch [142] • Mayo [182] • Ketchup [321] • Mustard [330]

BURGERZ/DOGZ/WRAPZ **484–1,147**
JR BURGERZ: w/Mustard & w/o Cheese [484] • w/Mustard & w/Swiss [510]
GOURMET BURGERZ: w/Honey Mustard & w/o Cheese [552] •
w/Honey Mustard & Swiss Cheese [578]
WRAPZ: Burger (Schnack) [573] • Veggie [630] • Crispy Chicken (Schnack) [702]

SALADS **27–2,930**
Garden Salad Base [27] • Steak Salad Base [376] • Grilled Chicken Base [636]
DRESSINGS (1 OZ): Honey Mustard [128] • Buttermilk Ranch [142]

PRETZELS **716–2,238**
Plain [716] • Cinnamon Sugar [716]

NACHOS/QUESADILLAS **657–3,148**
Nachoz Side, cheese (no extra cheese sauce) [657] • Cheese Quesadillaz [868]

PIZZA *(1 slice)* **1,091–1,749**

FRYZ/SIDES **0–2,734**
Apple Slices [0] • Hard Boiled Egg [94] • Coleslaw [191]
Rice & Beans [445] • Onion Rings, bag [448] • Fryz, bag [577]

BURRITOS **1,295–2,340**

◖ SIZZLER ◗

ENTREES **683–4,567**
Malibu Chicken, single [683] • Petite Steak [819] • Classic Steak [847]

SALAD BAR ITEMS **0–638**
Grapes, Strawberries, Pineapple, Watermelon, or Bell Peppers [0–1]
Cucumbers, Green Beans, Jicama, Mushrooms, Onions, or Tomatoes [1–2]
Zucchini, Broccoli, Raisins, Cabbage, or Spinach [3–6]
Cauliflower, Lettuce, Honeydew Melon, Cantaloupe, or Radishes [8–11]
Bean Sprouts or Carrots [19] • Roasted Corn/Peppers [27] • Chopped Eggs [42]
Pickled Beets [53] • Croutons [90] • Cottage Cheese [95] • Sunflower Seeds [115]

PREPARED SALADS **15–638**
Asian Chopped Salad [15] • Ambrosia [30] • Caesar Salad [35]
Carrot Raisin Salad [70] • Creamy Cole Slaw [104] • Greek Salad [190]

DRESSINGS **156–355**
Blue Cheese [156] • Ranch [197] • Caesar [240]

SOUPS *(6 oz bowl)* **400–1,080**
Navy Bean [400] • Menudo [426] • Chicken Noodle [490]
Veg Steak [550] • Chicken Tortilla [560] • Garden Veg [590]

BURGERS/SANDWICHES **680–2,475**
Malibu Chicken Sandwich, half [680] • Sizzler Burger (1/3 lb) [1,344]

SIDES/SAUCES **15–783**
Baked Potato, plain [15] • Broccoli [38] • Roll [67]
Vegetable Medley [70] • Sweet Potato, whole [83]
BUTTER: Savory Butter [67] • Maple Butter [67] • Honey Butter [67]
SAUCES: Burger Sauce [195] • Malibu Sauce [241]

SKYLINE CHILI

BURRITOS/WRAPS **450–2,070**
Chilito [450] • Classic Chicken Wrap w/Chili Ranch Dressing, half [835]
Vegetarian Black Bean Burrito Deluxe [920]

POTATOES. **25–1,100**
Plain Potato [25] • Sour Cream Potato [310] • Cheddar Potato [650]

BOWLS **710–2,120**
Vegetarian Black Beans & Rice [710]

SANDWICHES/CONEYS **510–934**
Kid's Double Weiner Hog Doggy (w/o cheese) [510]
Reg Coney (w/o cheese) [660] • Regular Chili Sandwich (w/o cheese) [700]

WAYS/PASTA. **260–2,830**
Kids P'sghetti [260] • Chili Spaghetti, sm [510]
Vegetarian Black Bean & Rice 3-Way, sm [640]

SALADS *(w/o dressing)*. **250–1,190**
Garden, side [250] • Garden, reg [270]

DRESSINGS. **260–770**
Dijon Honey Mustard [260] • Chunky Blue Cheese [280]

SONIC DRIVE-IN

BREAKFAST. **460–2,580**
French Toast Sticks, 4 [460] • Jr Breakfast Burrito [820]

BURGERS/SANDWICHES. **380–2,020**
Crab Sandwich [380] • Jr Deluxe Burger [470] • Corn Dog [530]
Jr Burger [640] • Chicken Strip Sandwich [740] • Sonic Burger w/mayo [760]

CHICKEN/WRAPS **470–1,890**
Chicken Strips, 2 [470] • Crispy Chicken Wrap, half [640]

SAUCE **190–380**
Honey Mustard Sauce [190]

SIDES **0–1,820**
Apple Slices [0] • Apple Slices w/Caramel Sauce [60] • French Fries, sm [270]

DESSERTS/SHAKES/MALTS **140–890**
Vanilla Dish [140] • Vanilla Cone [150] • Banana Split {210]
Strawberry Sundae [230] • Pineapple Sundae [230]
SHAKES (MINI): Strawberry, Banana, or Pineapple [230] • Vanilla [250] •
Hot Fudge [270] • Chocolate [280]
MALTS (MINI): Strawberry, Banana, or Pineapple [240] • Vanilla [260] •
Chocolate [270] • Hot Fudge [280]
SONIC BLASTS (MINI): M&Ms [210] • Snickers or Reese's Peanut Butter Cup [270]

294

SPECIALTY BEVERAGES **25–690**
REAL FRUIT SLUSHES (ALL): [25–100] • FAMOUS SLUSHES (ALL): 43–168
FLOATS (MINI): [150–180] • CREAM SLUSHES (MINI): [150–160]
Iced Lattes 90–250

SONNY'S REAL PIT BAR-B-Q

BIG DEALS/BURGERS **496–1,400**
Sliced Pork Sandwich on Bun [496] • Hamburger on Bun [560]
Sliced Pork Sandwich on Garlic Bread [696] • Pulled Pork Sandwich on Bun [702]

SALADS *(w/o dressing)*..............................**10–2,916**
Backyard Garden Salad [10]
BIG SALAD: w/Sliced Beef [343] • w/Sliced Pork [358] • w/Pulled Pork [564] •
w/Pulled Chicken [603]

DRESSINGS.. **180–420**
Ranch [180] • French [240] • Lo-Cal Red French [240]

SIDES **14–2,913**
Baked Potato [14] • Corn on the Cob [20] • Cinnamon Apples [23]
Broccoli [55] • Baked Sweet Potato [117] • French Fries [148]

SAUCES.. **80–480**
Brisket Finishing Sauce [80]

DESSERT.. **228–446**
Banana Pudding [228]

SOUPLANTATION/SWEET TOMATOES

BREAKFAST....................................... **160–590**
Zucchini Fritatta [160] • Potatoes O'Brien [190] • Homemade Oatmeal, plain [240]
Belgian Waffles [270] • French Toast w/Blueberry Sauce [280]
Egg Scramble Focaccia w/Bacon [330] • Mediterranean Sunrise Pasta [330]
Scrambled Eggs [360] • Sweet Pepper & Sausage Egg Breakfast Burrito [360]
Country Ham & Egg Breakfast Burrito [450]

PASTA/ENTREES *(1 cup)* **250–990**
Steamed Veg w/Lemon Herb Butter [250] • Sauteed Balsamic Veg [250]
Carbonara Pasta w/Bacon [250] • Creamy Herb Chicken [360]
Italian Sausage w/Red Pepper Puree [380] • Lemon Cream w/Capers [390]
Smoked Salmon & Dill [290] • Nutty Mushroom [410] • Bruschetta [450]

SALADS

TOSSED SALADS (1 CUP) **75–730**
Strawberry Fields w/Caramelized Walnuts [75] • Greens w/Sweet Maple [80]
Honey Minted Fruit Toss [80] • Cambay Curry w/Almonds & Coconut [90]
Greens w/Citrus Vinaigrette [110] • Mandarin Spinach w/Walnuts [110]
Outrageous Orange w/Cashews [110] • Crunchy Island Pineapple [130]
Cherry Chipotle Spinach [170] • Bartlett Pear & Caramelized Walnut [220]
San Marino Spinach w/Pumpkin Seeds [220] • Azteca Taco w/Turkey [230]

PREPARED SALADS (1/2 CUP) **40–780**
Dijon Potato w/Vinaigrette [40] • Carrot Raisin [80] • Ambrosia w/Coconut [80]
Oriental Slaw [80] • Herb Thai Slaw [120] • Poppyseed Coleslaw [130]
Tabouli [120] • Sweet/Sour Broccoli Slaw [140] • Confetti Avocado Slaw [140]

SOUPS *(1 cup)*.................................**230–1,470**
Classic Shrimp Bisque [230] • Basmati Lentil [380] • X-treme Spice Veg Chili [420]
Big Chunk Chicken Noodle [440] • Tomato Parmesan & Veg [460]
Split Pea & Potato Barley [470] • Island Coconut Chicken Soup [480]
Potato Tomato & Spinach [490] • Continental Lentil & Spinach [490]
Turkey Veg [490] • Spicy Navajo Veg [490]

BAKERY **120–580**
MUFFINS: French Quarter Praline [120] • Cappuccino Chip [160] •
Spiced Pumpkin w/Cranberries [170] • Wildly Blue Blueberry [180} •
Pauline's Apple Walnut Cake [180] • Apple Raisin [190] • Banana Nut [190] •
Date N' Honey Bran [190] • Zucchini Nut [190] • Tangy Lemon [190] •
Country Blackberry [190] • Choc Chip [190] • Choc Brownie [190] •
Taffy Apple [190] • Black Forest [190] • Cherry Nut [190]

DESSERTS.. **5–580**
Apple Medley [5] • Banana Royale [5] • GELATIN: Sugar-Free or Regular [5]
SUGAR-FREE MOUSSE: Cherry Choc [20] • Lemon [20] • Raspberry [20] •
Strawberry [20] • Choc [65]
Cran-Raspberry Gelatin [45] • Rice Pudding [50] • Vanilla Frozen Yogurt [55]
COOKIES: Sugar [60] • Oatmeal Raisin [90] • Holiday w/sprinkles [90] •
Choc Chip [100]
Choc Frozen Yogurt [65] • Nutty Waldorf Salad [80]

SPICY PICKLE

BREAKFAST.. **432–1,063**
Rio [432] • Garden of Eden [451] • Alamo [531]

PANINIS/SANDWICHES/WRAPS *(w/o salt)* **806–3,307**
Coliseum Wrap [806] • Deli Tuna Sandwich [968] • Deluca Panini [1,047]

PIZZA **1,629–2,166**

SALADS *(w/o dressing)*.................................. **840–1,472**
Spinach (w/o salt) [840] • Chicken Caesar (w/o salt) [952]

DRESSINGS.. **0–660**
Apple Cider Vinaigrette [0] • Greek Dressing [160]

STEAK ESCAPE

SANDWICHES/BURGERS..................................... **310–5,200**
Jr Veggie Sandwich [310] • Philly Char-Burger [600]
Double Philly Char-Burger [660] • Philly Burger [680] • Double Philly Burger [700]
Jr Steak Sandwich [710] • 6" Grand Escape Sandwich [910]

WRAPS **1,160–2,930**
Grand Escape [1,160] • Wild West BBQ [1,270]

SALADS.. **100–1,980**
Side Salad [100] • One Killer (w/o meat) [1,070] • Grilled Salad (w/o meat) [1,090]
DRESSING: Ranch Dressing [250] • French Dressing [290]

POTATOES.. **210–1,670**
Plain Potato [210] • Veggie Killer Potato [210] • Chicken Killer Potato [980]

SIDES/EXTRAS **55–2,090**
CHEESE: Swiss [55] • Cheddar [135] • Parmesan [135]
FRIES: Kid's [120] • sm [390]

CONDIMENTS **0–490**
Lettuce, Tomato, or Cucumbers [0] • Sour Cream [25]
Ketchup [105] • Mayonnaise [150]

STEAK 'N SHAKE

BREAKFAST... **15–1,130**
Mandarin Oranges, cup [15] • Yogurt Parfait [95]
1 or 2 Eggs, Scrambled or Over Easy [70–140]
Perfect Start Oatmeal [260] • Cinn Roll [270] • Shredded Hashbrowns [300]
BUTTERED TOAST: Wheat [270] • White [360] • Sourdough [370]

Sausage, Egg & Cheese Taco [360] • Potato & Egg Taco [370]
Shooter w/Sausage [400] • Shooter w/Bacon [420]
KID'S SCRAMBLED EGG & TOAST: w/Sausage [460] • w/Bacon [510]

BURGERS **210–1,130**
STEAKBURGER SHOOTERS: Plain [210] • BBQ [250] • Chipotle [260] •
Frisco [280] • Ketchup & Mustard [290] • Ketchup & Onion [290]
STEAKBURGERS: Single [310] • Double [330] • Triple [350] •
Kid's w/Fries [360] • Single w/cheese [570] • Double w/cheese [590]

SANDWICHES/CHICKEN/MELTS **520–1,610**
Kid's Mini Corn Dogs & Fries [520] • Kid's 2 Chicken Fingers & Fries [660]
3 Chicken Fingers [920] • Bacon, Lettuce, 'n Tomato [950]
Grilled Chicken Sandwich [980] • Patty Melt [1,000]

STEAK FRANKS **1,120–1,590**

CHILI **1,010–2,560**

SALADS *(w/o dressing)* **105–1,050**
Small Garden [105] • Apple Pecan Grilled Chicken Salad [640]
DRESSINGS **115–480**
Honey Mustard [115] • Berry Balsamic Vinaigrette [160]

SIDES **0–2,150**
Applesauce [0] • Mandarin Oranges [15] • Apples & Caramel [75]
FRENCH FRIES: sm [80] • med [140]

DESSERTS/SHAKES **140–1,360**
Coke Float [140] • Strawberry Sundae [140] • Root Beer Float [170]
SHAKES (KID): Strawberry Banana [170] • Orange Freeze [180] •
Ultimate Banana [180] • Strawberry, Vanilla, or Very Berry Strawberry [190] •
Banana, Choc Banana, or Mocha [200]
SHAKES (SM): Orange Freeze [240] • Strawberry Banana [240]

(SUBWAY) ───────────────────────────────────

BREAKFAST **460–1,680**
MUFFIN MELTS: Egg & Cheese [460] • Egg White & Cheese [480]
Bacon, Egg & Cheese [550] • Bacon, Egg White & Cheese [580]
FLATBREAD (3"): Egg & Cheese [520] • Egg White & Cheese [540]

SANDWICHES **310–1,810**
6" Veggie Delite [310] • 6" Ultimate Veggie w/Avocado [440] • 6" Tuna [620]
6" Oven Roasted Chicken [640] • 6" Oven Roasted Chicken w/Spinach [650]

SOUPS **410–990**
Fire-Roasted Tomato Orzo [410] • Chicken Tortilla [440]

SALADS **65–660**
Veggie Delite [65] • Oven Roasted Chicken [270]
Grilled Chicken & Baby Spinach [330] • Roast Beef [450]
DRESSINGS **560–720**

BREADS **190–1,260**
Mini Italian (White) [190] • Mini Wheat [200] • 6" Sourdough [210]

TOPPINGS/CONDIMENTS **0–200**
VEGGIES: Avocado, Lettuce, Tomato, Onions, Green Peppers, or Spinach [0] •
Cucumbers [0] • Banana Peppers [20] • Olives, 3 rings [25] •
Jalapenos, 3 rings [70]
CHEESE: Swiss • Shredded Monterey • Cheddar • Provolone . . . . . 30•90•95•125
CONDIMENTS: Mayo • FF Sweet Onion Sauce • Light Mayo . . . . 80•85•100
Mustard • FF Honey Mustard Sauce . . . . 115•125

COOKIES/DESSERTS.. 0–130
Apple Slices [0] • Yogurt Parfait [75] • Choc Chunk Cookie [100]
M&M® Cookie [100] • Raspberry Cheesecake [120]

TACO BELL

TACOS/GORDITAS/CHALUPAS 290–760
Crunchy Taco [290] • Fresco Crunchy Taco [290] • Crunchy Taco Supreme [320]
Doritos Locos Tacos [340] • Doritos Locos Tacos Supreme [370]
Volcano Taco [410] • Chicken Soft Taco [460] • Fresco Chicken Soft Taco [460]
Soft Beef Taco [510] • Gordita Supreme Chicken [510]
Crispy Potato Soft Taco [520] • Soft Beef Taco Supreme [530]
Chalupa Supreme Chicken [530] • Grilled Steak Soft Taco [550]
Gordita Supreme Steak [550] • Gordita Supreme Beef [550]

BURRITOS/SPECIALTIES................................... 280–2,020
Cheesy Nachos [280] • Nachos [420] • Cheese Roll-Up [450]
Tostada [530] • Nachos Supreme [690] • MexiMelt [740]
Mexican Pizza [860] • Grilled Chicken Burrito [870] • Chili Cheese Burrito [930]

TACO SALADS.. 1,260–1,340
Chicken Fiesta Taco Salad [1,260] • Express Taco Salad w/chips [1,270]

   DRESSINGS... 50–210
   Avocado Ranch Dressing [50] • Cilantro Dressing [210]

SIDE ITEMS.. 200–770
Mexican Rice [200] • Black Beans [200] • Chips & Corn Salsa [230]

CONDIMENTS/SAUCES................................... 20–170
Reduced Fat Sour Cream [20] • Pico de Gallo [35] • Fire Roasted Salsa [50]
BORDER SAUCE: Mild [35] • Hot [45] • Fire {60]
Creamy Jalapeno Sauce [50] • Salsa Verde [55] • Salsa [80] • Guacamole [105]

DESSERTS... 200–310
Cinnamon Twists [200]

TACO BUENO

BREAKFAST.. 350–2,090
Potato Stix [350] • Potato Egg Burrito [680] • Sausage Egg Burrito [720]

ENTREES... 244–4,150
Party Taco [244] • Chicken Crispy Taco [410] • Beef Crispy Taco [440]
Beef Taco Rollup [462] • Tostada (w/o refried beans) [467]
Flame-Grilled Chicken Fajita Taco [500] • Chicken Taco Rollup [520]
Mini Cheese Quesadilla [533] • SW Empanada [540]
Flame-Grilled Steak Fajita Taco [600] • Chicken Soft Taco [610]
Beef Soft Taco [620] • Beef Potato Burrito (w/o queso) [644]
NOTE: Removing cheese from tacos eliminates about 100mg sodium.

SOUPS/SALADS 691–1,911
Chicken Tortilla Soup, cup w/otortilla strips & cheese [691]

SIDES 10–1,787
Pico de Gallo [10] • Sour Cream [19] • Corn Tortilla Chips [25] • Guacamole [128]

DESSERTS... 160–254
Cheesecake Chimichanga [160]

TACO CABANA

BREAKFAST.. 410–2,560
Potato & Egg Taco [410] • Barbacoa Taco [430] • Chorizo & Egg Taco [510]

ENTREES...180–5,190
Chicken Flauta [180] • Carne Guisada Soft Taco [330]
Bean & Cheese Chalupa [350] • Chicken Crispy Taco [430]
Beef Crispy Taco [430] • Brisket Soft Taco [570] • Bean/Cheese Soft Taco [590]

SIDES/SAUCES..15–1,380
Chips, sm [15] • Pico de Gallo [90] • Pineapple Salsa [95] • Salsa Roja [95]
Salsa Verde [125] • Black Bean & Corn Salsa [150]

DESSERTS..60–580
Dulce de Leche, 1 oz [60] • Tres Leches Parfait [300] • Tres Leches Cake [330]

(TACO DEL MAR)

MONDO BURRITOS 850–2,330
Vegan Burrito [850] • Veggie Mondito Burrito [880]

TACOS..210–680
Kid's Chicken [210] • Kid's Shredded Beef [280] • Kid's Pork [340]
Kid's Ground Beef [340] • Fish Taco [390] • Kid's Carne Asada Steak [410]
Veggie w/Rice [440] • Veggie w/Refried Beans [460] • Chicken Taco [520]
Veggie Taco w/Rice & Refried Beans [550]
NOTE: Substitute corn tortilla for flour and reduce sodium by 190mg per taco.

QUESADILLAS...570–2,000
Kid's Quesadilla [570] • Cheese Quesadilla [1,320]

PLATTERS...1,960–3,020

NACHOS 1,670–2,350

BAJA BOWLS..430–1,520
Mondito Veggie [430] • Mondito Vegan [460] • Mondito Chicken [630]
Mondito Shredded Beef [660] • Mondito Fish [710]

SALADS...1,190–1,520

SIDES/ADD-ONS/SAUCES 5–1,510
Lettuce [5] • Cabbage [10] • Sour Cream [55]
SALSA: Habanero [65] • Roasted Chipotle [95] • Tomatillo [125]
White Sauce [85] • Guacamole [105]
Jalapeno Peppers [170] • Rice [300] • Whole Pinto Beans [310]

DESSERTS..120–230
Choc Chip Cookie [120] • White Choc Macadamia Cookie [120]
Oatmeal Raisin Cookie [130] • Double Choc Chip Cookie [135]

(TACO JOHN'S)

BREAKFAST..135–2,110
French Toast Sticks [135] • Oatmeal, all flavors [150]
Jr Breakfast Burrito w/Bacon [620] • Jr Breakfast Burrito w/Sausage [630]

TACOS..290–1,320
Crispy [290] • Taco Burger [570] • Softshell Taco [580] • Chicken Softshell [680]

BURRITOS 1,090–1,960
Bean Burrito [1,090]

SALADS *(w/o dressing)*............................610–1,070
Cran-Apple Chicken Almond [610] • Chipotle BBQ Chicken [820] • Taco Salad [820]
DRESSING: House Dressing [280] • Creamy Italian [320]

LOCAL FAVORITES 400–2,310
Mexi Rolls, 2 pc w/o cheese [400] • Chili Enchilada [870]

SIDES/SPECIALTIES 800–3,390
Super Nachos, sm [800]

CONDIMENTS **25–520**
   Super Hot Sauce [25] • Sour Cream [40] • Pico de Gallo [85]
   Salsa [110] • Mild Sauce [130] • Hot Sauce [140]

DESSERTS. **55–170**
   Giant Goldfish Grahams [55] • Choco Taco [160] • Churro [170]

TACO MAYO

ENTREES. **243–3,537**
   TACOS: Crispy Beef [243] • Soft Steak [577] • Soft Beef [584] • Soft Chicken [592]

SIDES **371–2,052**
   Guac-N-Chips [371]

DESSERTS. **73–120**
   Cinnamon Crisps [73] • Choco Taco [120]

TACO TICO

ENTREES. **458–4,708**
   Taco [458] • Chicken Soft Taco [467] • Cheese Nachos [571]
   Cheese Quesadilla [595] • Chicken Enchilada [606] • Crispy Flour Taco [635]

TCBY

SOFT SERVE FROZEN YOGURT/SORBET **10–95**
   Sorbets, all flavors [10–15]
   YOGURT: all flavors except those below [60-65] •
     Coffee, Choc, Caramel Supreme, Peanut Butter, or Toffee Crunch [80–95]
   NO SUGAR ADDED: all flavors [65–70]

HAND-SCOOPED FROZEN YOGURT/SORBET **10–105**
   Psychedelic Sorbet [10]
   YOGURT: all flavors except those below [45–65] •
     Choc Chunk Cookie Dough [70] • Butter Pecan Perfection [75] •
     Vanilla Fudge Brownie [75] • Praline & Cream [90] •
     Peanut Butter Delight [100] • Mocha Almond [105]

SMOOTHIES **50–150**
   SMOOTHIES: all flavors except those below [50–55} •
   Peach Palm [85] • Mangolada [90] • Pink Pineapple [120] • Pina Paradise [150]

SPECIALTY ITEMS. **55–760**
   Sorbet Fizz [55–95] • Parfaits [150–330]

CAKES/PIES **120–300**
   PIES: Turtle Ripple [120] • White Choc Mousse Brownie [160] •
   Choc Decadence [160]

TIM HORTONS

BREAKFAST. **210–1,190**
   Hashbrown [210] • Oatmeal, all flavors, sm [220]
   Oatmeal, all flavors, lrg [300–320] • Breakfast Sausage & Biscuit [550]
   Egg & Cheese Breakfast Wrap [690] • English Muffin w/Egg & Cheese [700]

DONUTS **190–350**
   YEAST DONUTS: Honey Dip [190] • Maple Dip [190] • Choc Dip [190] • Dutchie [210]
   FILLED DONUTS: Blueberry [210] • Strawberry [220] • Strawberry Vanilla [220]
   Honey Cruller [220]
   CAKE DONUTS: Old Fashion Plain [230] • Glazed [230] • Sour Cream Plain [230]

TIMBITS **40–75**

SANDWICHES/WRAPS 630–1,450
CHICKEN WRAP SNACKERS: BBQ Chicken [630] • Chicken Ranch [650]
SANDWICHES: Egg Salad [760] • BLT [830] • Chicken Caesar [880]

SOUPS/CHILI 650–1,210
Beef Barley [650] • Minestrone [660]

COOKIES 160–290
Trail Mix w/Fruit & Nuts [160] • Oatmeal Raisin Spice [200] • Triple Choc [220]

SMOOTHIES 30–55

TOGO'S

SANDWICHES/WRAPS 610–5,750
HALF/MINI SANDWICH: Albacore Tuna [610] • Avocado & Cucumber [760]
Farmer's Market Wrap [980]

SALADS *(w/o dressing)* 210–1,420
ASIAN CHICKEN: half [210] • full [400]
FARMER'S MARKET: half [220] • full [550]
Chicken Caesar, half [340] • Santa Fe Chicken, half [48]

  DRESSINGS 530–890

SOUPS *(1 cup)* 600–1,850
Garden Veg [600] • Fresh Mushroom & Brie [700] • Chili [730]

DESSERTS 230–380
Oatmeal Raisin Cookie [230] • Choc Chunk Brownie [260]

UNO CHICAGO GRILL

APPETIZERS 790–5,970

ENTREES *(w/o sides)* 170–3,250
Citrus BBQ Salmon [170] • Baked Haddock [540]
Eggplant, Spinach & Feta Five Grain, sm plate [630]

PIZZA 1,630–4,490

SALADS *(w/o dressing)* 95–1,220
HOUSE SALAD: side [95] • whole [190]
CITRUS AVOCADO: side [95] • whole [250] • w/Salmon [370]
Farro Salad, side [310] • Caesar, side [430] • Walnut Crusted Goat Cheese [430]

  DRESSING 190–530
  Classic Vinaigrette [190] • FF Vinaigrette [200]

SOUPS 930–1,080
Veggie Soup [930]

BURGERS/SANDWICHES 460–1,580
Roasted Veg & Goat Cheese Wrap, half [460] • Chicken Sandwich, half [630]
Turkey Bacon & Swiss Sandwich, half [670] • Grilled Chicken Wrap, half [690]
Uno Burger [820]

SIDES 90–1,290
Steamed Seasonal Veg [90] • Brown Rice [100] • Roasted Seasonal Veg [160]

DESSERTS 140–1,820
Mini Bananas Foster [140] • Mini Choc Peanut Butter Cup [150]

WENDY'S

BURGERS/SANDWICHES/WRAPS 540–1,840
Hamburger, Kids [540] • Jr Hamburger [620] • Grilled Chicken Go Wrap [630]
Jr Cheeseburger [670] • Jr Cheeseburger Deluxe [710]
Crispy Chicken Sandwich [720]

CHICKEN. **370–460**
Kid's 4 Piece Chicken Nuggets [370] • 5 Piece Chicken Nuggets [460]
DIPPING SAUCES **120–240**
Sweet & Sour Sauce [120] • Barbecue Nugget Sauce [120]
SALADS *(w/o dressing and croutons)* **290–1,920**
Garden Side [290] • Caesar Side (w/dressing) [290]
Berry Almond Chicken, half [290] • Apple Pecan Chicken, half [505]
DRESSINGS/TOPPINGS **95–290**
FF French [95] • Ranch or Light Ranch [150] • Pomegranate Vinaigrette [160]
SIDE ITEMS. **0–1,330**
Apple Slices [0] • BAKED POTATO: plain [25] • w/sour cream/chives [50]
Baked Lay's [200] • Value Natural-Cut Fries [250]
CONDIMENTS/TOPPINGS **30–200**
Mayo [30] • Ranch Sauce [50] • Mustard [55] • Honey Mustard [75] • Ketchup [80]
FROSTY TREATS **135–700**
Vanilla Frosty, sm [135] • Choc Frosty, sm [140] • Caramel Apple Parfait [140]
Vanilla Frosty Float w/Coca-Cola [160]
FROSTY SHAKE (SM): Strawberry [180] • Wild Berry [190]

WHATABURGER

BREAKFAST. **280–2,760**
Hash Brown Sticks [280] • Cinnamon Roll [390] • Egg Sandwich [570]
BURGERS/OTHER ENTREES **730–2,410**
Justaburger [730] • Whataburger Jr [730] • Whatachick'n Sandwich [860]
SALADS *(dressing info unavailable)* **6–663**
Side Salad [6] • Garden Salad [220] • Apple & Cranberry Salad [200]
Apple & Cranberry Crispy Chicken Salad [660]
SIDE ITEMS. **170–1,182**
Texas Toast, 1 sl [170] • French Fries, sm [200]
DESSERTS/SHAKES. **0–460**
Apple Slices [0] • Fruit Chew [10] • Choc Chunk Cookie [180]
Strawberry Shake [230] • Vanilla Shake [240] • Strawberry Malt [250]

WHITE CASTLE

BREAKFAST. **200–1,830**
Donuts, all varieties *(select regions)* [150–160]
SLIDERS ON A BUN: Hamburger, Egg [200] • Hamburger, Egg, Cheese [300] •
Egg & Cheese [320] • Bacon, Egg, Cheese [510]
Hash Rounds/Potato Snackers, sm/reg *(depending on region)* [310–460]
Cheese Danish [340] • Apple Danish [350] • French Toast Sticks, 4 pc [410]
SANDWICHES/OTHER ITEMS. . . . . **260 -1,240**
SLIDERS: Traditional Bun w/cheese [260] • Original Slider [340] •
Original BBQ [400] • Fish Slider w/cheese [410]
SIDE ITEMS **50–2,940**
FRENCH FRIES: sm [50] • med [50] • lrg [85] • sack [115]
Onion Rings, sm *(depending on region of the country)* [190–340]
DESSERTS/SHAKES **110–980**
Fudge Dipped Cheesecake on a Stick [110] • Oatmeal Raisin Cookie [115]
White Choc Macadamia Cookie [125] • Choc Chunk Cookie [130]
Shakes, all flavors, sm *(depending on region of the country)* [150-470]

WIENERSCHNITZEL

BREAKFAST **240–1,820**
Hash Browns [240] • French Toast Sticks [460] • Egg/Bacon/Cheese Sandwich [830]

HOT DOGS/BURGERS/SPECIALTIES **490–2,230**
Corn Dog [490] • Mini Corn Dog, 6 Pak [540]
Hamburger [610] • Turkey Plain Dog, standard bun [610]
Sea Dog [640] • Turkey Mustard Dog, standard bun [660]
Turkey Plain Hot Dog, pretzel bun [680] • Double Classic Burger [700]

SIDES **400–1,380**
FRIES: reg [400] • lrg [630]

DESSERTS/SHAKES **115–540**
CONES: 3 oz Kids Plain [115] • 3 oz Kids Choc Dipped [135] • 5 oz Plain [180]
MINI SUNDAES: Strawberry [140] • Pineapple [140] • Hot Fudge [160] •
Choc [170] • Caramel [170]

SHAKES **440–480**

WINCHELL'S

DONUTS **70–980**
Donut Hole, Plain [70] • Glazed [80] • Cinnamon Sugared [85]
Coconut Topping [90] • Choc Sprinkles [90] • Sugared [95]
Powdered Sugar [95] • Cinnamon Crumb [120] • Mini Cake, White [150]
Mini Cake, Plain [150] • Mini Cake, Choc Iced [160]
Choc Iced w/Rainbow Sprinkles [170] • Vanilla Iced w/Rainbow Sprinkle [170]

BAGELS/CROISSANTS **310–940**
Mini Croissant [310] • 9 Grain Bagel [350] • Blueberry Bagel [390]
Cinn Raisin Bagel [390] • Whole Wheat Bagel [390]

MUFFINS **640–990**
Blueberry, Choc Chip, Cranberry Orange, or Pumpkin Nut [640]

BAKERY **20–560**
Creme Horn [20] • Macaroon Cookie [55] • Apple Strudel [210]
Pineapple Strudel [220] • Strawberry Cream Cheese [220]

SANDWICHES **690–2,050**
BREAKFAST (ON WHOLE WHEAT BAGEL) **690–1,840**
Egg & Cheese [690] • Bacon & Cheese [700]
DELI (ON WHOLE WHEAT BAGEL) **740–2,050**
BLTCC [740] • Hot Chicken Breast [940] • Cold Tuna Salad [970]

SPREADS **0–1,170**
Strawberry Jelly [0] • Peanut Butter [150] • Peanut Butter & Jelly [150]
CREAM CHEESE (2 OZ): Reg [200] • Lite [200] • Lite w/Chives [220]

DRINKS **10–580**
Raspado, all flavors & sizes or Chilla, fruit flavors, 16 oz/20 oz [10–70]
COFFEE W/FLAVORING (ALL SIZES): Hazelnut or Vanilla [75–150]
Licuado, all flavors, all sizes [125–170]

ZAXBY'S

APPETIZERS **560–2,780**
Fried White Cheddar Bites (w/o sauce) [560]

ENTREES **160–2,790**
CHICKEN (NO SAUCE): Wings, 5 pc [160] • Finger, 1 pc [250] • Wings, 10 pc [330]

SALADS *(w/o dressing)* **40–2,370**
Side Salad [40]

CAESAR SIDE SALAD (W/DRESSING): w/o Croutons [260] • w/Croutons [440]
THE HOUSE SALAD: w/o Jack Cheese [480] • w/Jack Cheese [710]

DRESSINGS **180–530**
    Thousand Island [180] • Honey French Dressing [230]

SIDES **45–540**
    CELERY STICKS: 4 [45] • 6 [70] • Basket [230]
    Cole Slaw [170] • Texas Toast, 1 pc [270] • Kid's Crinkle Fries [290]

SAUCES. **250–710**
    Sweet & Spicy Glaze [250] • Original Sauce [260]

DESSERTS/SHAKES **120–351**
    COOKIES: Choc Chip [120] • White Choc Macadamia Nut [120] •
    Oatmeal Raisin [130]
    SHAKES: Strawberry [231] • Birthday Cake [251] • Vanilla [256] •
    Strawberry Cheesecake [256]

RESOURCES

DASH DIET

NHLBI Health Information Center (Publication #01-4082)
P.O. Box 30105
Bethesda, MD 20824-0105
301.592.8573 or 240.629.3255 (TTD)
www.nhlbi.nih.gov

LOW-SALT DIET INFORMATION

LowSaltFoods.com

WEBSITES OFFERING LOW-SALT PRODUCTS EXCLUSIVELY

HealthyHeartMarket.com
LowSaltFoods.com

ONLINE GROCERS OFFERING LOW-SALT PRODUCTS

Amazon.com
TheBetterHealthStore.com
GlutenFree.com
GlutenFreeMall.com
Kosher.com
MyKosherMarket.com
ShopNatural.com
ShopOrganic.com
USGrocer.com
Walmart.com
WorldPantry.com

ONLINE PRODUCTS AVAILABLE FROM MANUFACTURERS

4C – **www.4c.com**
Allen Canning Company – **www.AllenCanning.com**
American Spoon – **www.spoon.com**
Arrowhead Mills – **www.ArrowheadMills.com**
Authentic Foods – **www.GlutenFree-Supermarket.com**
Bear Naked – **www.BearNaked.com**
Blazing Blends – **www.BlazingBlends.com**
Bob's Red Mill – **www.BobsRedMill.com**
Bolner's Fiesta Brand – **www.FiestaSpices.com**
Canterbury Naturals – **www.CanterburyNaturals.com**
'Cause You're Special – **www.CauseYoureSpecial.com**
Chatila's Bakery – **www.SugarFreeBakery.net**
Chebe – **www.Chebe.com**
Dixie Diners – **www.DixieDiner.com**
Dr. Praegers – **www.DrPraegers.com**
Eden Foods, Inc. – **www.EdenFoods.com**
Ener-G Foods – **www.Ener-G.com**
French Meadow Bakery – **www.FrenchMeadow.com**
Garden of Eatin' – **www.GardenOfEatin.com**
Gloria's Gourmet Foods – **www.GloriasGourmet.com**
Hodgson Mill – **www.HodgsonMill.com**
HolGrain (Conrad Rice Mill Inc.) – **www.Holgrain.com**

Iveta Gourmet – **www.Iveta.com**
Joseph's Bakery – **www.JosephsBakery.com**
King Arthur Flour – **www.KingArthurFlour.com**
The Lollipop Tree, Inc. – **www.LollipopTree.com**
Med-Diet Labs, Inc. – **www.med-diet.com**
Melissa's – **www.Melissas.com**
Montana Mills Bread Co. – **www.MontanaMills.com**
Mozzarella Company – **www.mozzco.com**
Mr. Spice (Lang Naturals) – **www.MrSpice.com**
Natural Ovens Bakery – **www.NaturalOvens.com**
Nutrifit Spice Blends – **www.NutrifitOnline.com**
Rabbit Creek Gourmet – **www.RabbitCreekGourmet.com**
Robert Rothschild Farm – **www.RobertRothschild.com**
Sami's Bakery – **www.SamisBakery.com**
Schar – **www.Schar.com**
Seitenbacher – **www.Seitenbacher.com**
Seneca Foods – **www.SenecaFoods.com**
Sunshine Food Co – **www.SunshineFoodCo.com**
Tillen Farms – **www.TillenFarms.com**
Tumaro's – **www.Tumaros.com**
Vogue Cuisine, Inc. – **www.VogueCuisine.com**
Wax Orchards Inc. – **www.WaxOrchards.com**
Zadie's Low Sodium Seasonings – **www.Zadies.com**

INDEX

INDATA GROUP, INC.

P.O. Box 256
Allyn, WA 98524
360.432.7844

Visit our website:

www.LowSaltFoods.com

Also available
the perfect companion to the
Pocket Guide to Low Sodium Foods
is our best selling cookbook:

The Hasty Gourmet™
Low-Salt Favorites

*300 Easy-to-Make, Great Tasting Recipes
for a Healthy Lifestyle*